PLANT HEALTH MANAGEMENT

NIPA® GENX ELECTRONIC RESOURCES & SOLUTIONS P. LTD.
New Delhi-110 034

PLANT HEALTH MANAGEMENT

Editor

Gireesh Chand

Chairman
Department of Plant Pathology
Bihar Agricultural University
Sabour-813210, Bhagalpur
(Bihar) India

NIPA® GENX ELECTRONIC RESOURCES & SOLUTIONS P. LTD.
New Delhi-110 034

NIPA® GENX ELECTRONIC
RESOURCES & SOLUTIONS P. LTD.

101,103, Vikas Surya Plaza, CU Block
L.S.C. Market, Pitam Pura, New Delhi-110 034
Ph : +91 11 27341616, 27341717, 27341718
E-mail: newindiapublishingagency@gmail.com
web: www.nipabooks.com

For customer assistance, please contact
Phone: + 91-11-27 34 17 17
Fax: + 91-11- 27 34 16 16
E-Mail: feedbacks@nipabooks.com

ISBN: 978-81-19254-87-3

Composed and Designed by NIPA®.

Preface

Plant diseases in 21st century pose greater challenges for food and nutritional security in the changing climate scenario. Production constraints, especially abiotic stresses, abrupt climatic changes, emergence of new species/ strains of insect-pests and diseases, and increasing deficiency of secondary and micronutrients in the soil. Sustaining food and nutrional security under climate change scenario and increasing the farm income towards zero budget farming is the prime challenges before Indian Agriculture. The extended abstract book intends to address the issues of plant health management in order to move a step closer to achieve the vision of zero budget farming under changing climatic scenario by discussing the problems pertaining to plant health and effective management avenues in their respective areas. Such endeavors will help in upscaling the production technologies by providing better and improved plant health regimes in times to come. In this context, to inculcate recognition and motivation of the young researchers, students and industries to emerging disease threat and to design effective management strategies through various conventional and modern approaches is need of the hour. The chapters in the book provide a current and detailed account of biotic and abiotic constraints that hamper crops. The book has a comprehensive coverage of occurrence distribution, economic importance, symptoms of biotic and abiotic constraints disease cycle, epidemiology and sustainable disease management strategies.

I hope that this edited book would help the students, teachers, researchers, policy makers and stakeholders to foster agricultural development. We sincerely thank all the authors for their valuable contributions for providing us valuable plant disease research material for shaping the book. All the words in the lexicon will be futile and meaningless if fail to express our reference to faculty members and students for their blessing, affection, sacrifice and cheerful cooperation to overcome the hurdle. I thank New India Publishing Agency, Pitampura, New Delhi for accepting such valuable publication.

Gireesh Chand

Contents

1

Standardize The Noble Techniques of Seed Treatments for Wilt Disease of Pigeonpea *in vivo*

Neeraj Kumar Rajvanshi, Subhash Chandra, Ajay Kumar H.K. Singh and Divya Singh

Department of Plant Pathology, Narendra Deva University of Agriculture & Technology, Kumarganj, Faizabad-224229, Uttar Pradesh, India

Abstract

Pigeonpea (Cajanus cajan) is an important pulse crop of India and its production is greatly affected by wilt disease. Pigeonpea wilt is a very destructive soil borne disease caused by Fusarium udum. In the experiments, ten treatments were applied viz.*; Neem leaf extracts (T_1), Garlic extracts (T_2), Tulsi leaf extracts (T_3), bio-agents* Trichoderma viride *(T_4), Pseudomonas fluorescens (T_5), Polymer coating (polycot) @ 4 ml diluted in 5 ml of water per kg of seed (T_6), Polymer coaating + Trichoderma viride @ 6.0 g per kg seed (T_7), Polymer + Pseudomonas fluorescens @ 6.0 g per kg seed (T_8), Polymer coating (polycot) 4 ml diluted in 5 ml of water per kg seed + Vitavax power @ 3g per kg seed (T_9) and T_{10} served as untreated. The observations were recorded six times at 10 days intervals and started from 40 days. These polymer alone @ 4.0ml per kg and in combination with bioagents and fungicides were applied to seed were tested against Fusarium udum. The highest per cent disease control and per cent wilt disease incidence were recorded 96.09 to 64.09 and 2.74 to 33.32, respectively in T_9 (Polymer + Vitavax power @ 3g per kg seed) at 10 days intervals followed by T_8 (Polymer +* P. fluorescens*) gave 94.46 to 53.06 per cent inhibition, T_7 (92.39 to 52.74) and T_6 (90.97 to 49.73) however, the lowest per cent disease control was noticed as 76.19 to 40.13 per cent in T_1 (Neem leaves extract) amongst all treatments except untreated.*

Keywords: Bio-agents, polycot, vitavax power, pigeonpea, *Fusarium udum*

Introduction

Pigeonpea (*Cajanus cajan* L. Millsp.) is one of the major pulse crops grown in the tropics and subtropics belonging to family Leguminaceae. Pigeonpea has multiple uses such as tender green seeds used as vegetables, stem and roots as fuel wood, crushed dry seeds as animal feed and to make huts, baskets etc. besides this, it is mainly used as dal. It has been recognized as a valuable source of protein (17.9 to 24.39/100g) particularly in the developing countries where majority of the population depends on the vegetarian foods for meeting its dietary requirements (Ali and Kumar, 2005). In India, the crop is mainly grown in Andhra Pradesh, Bihar, Uttar Pradesh, Karnataka, Gujarat, Madhya Pradesh, Maharashtra, Orissa and Tamilnadu. In Uttar Pradesh, it is grown 3.0 lakh ha area producing 2.58 lakh tons, with an average yield of 858 kg/ha (Anonymous, 2017). The poor yield of pigeonpea is mainly due to biotic stress like diseases and insect pests but only few of them like wilt, sterility mosaic, *Phytophthora* blight and *Alternaria* blight are major and destructive ones. Among fungal pathogens, wilt disease caused by *Fusarium udum* Butler is an important disease in India, Kenya, Malawi, Nepal, Tanzania and Uganda (Reddy *et al.,* 1990). In India, it is the most serious problem all over the pigeonpea growing states especially in UP, MP, Bihar and Maharashtra. In Bihar and Uttar Pradesh, 5-10 per cent losses in standing crop are common feature every year (Singh, 2006). The fungus is primarily a soil borne facultative parasite and enters the host through fine roots and subsequently colonizes in different plant parts (Khune, 1990). Management of pigeonpea wilt through fungicides applied as soil treatment such as Thiram, Ferbam, Carbendazim and Copper oxychloride have been reported by different workers. Indiscriminate use of these chemicals has led to development of fungicide resistance strain and more importantly, environmental pollution, posing a potential risk to animal and human health. Hence, for minimizing the losses caused by wilt need inexpensive and environmentally safe management practices. It was therefore considered desirable to standardize the Noble Techniques of seed treatments against wilt pathogen of pigeonpea under *in vivo* for effective management.

Material and Methods

The field experiment was conducted at main campus of University is located at Kumarganj, Faizabad. The cultivar Bahar was selected to conduct the experiments in three replications with ten treatments *viz.*; Neem leaf extracts (T_1), Garlic extracts (T_2), Tulsi leaf extracts (T_3), bio-agents *Trichoderma viride* (T_4), *Pseudomonas fluorescens* (T_5), Polymer coating (polycot) @ 4 ml diluted in 5 ml of water per kg of seed (T_6), Polymer coating + *Trichoderma viride* @ 6.0 g per kg seed (T_7), Polymer + *Pseudomonas fluorescens* @ 6.0 g per kg seed (T_8), Polymer coating (polycot) 4 ml diluted in 5 ml of water per kg seed +

Vitavax power @ 3g per kg seed (T_9) and T_{10} served as untreated. The observations were recorded on per cent disease control and per cent wilt incidence at 10 days intervals.

Efficacy of plant extracts against *Fusarium* wilt

The effective concentration of plant extracts found *in vitro* will be further tested *in vivo.* Plant extracts (10 per cent) was thoroughly mixed to determine the effect of plant extract *in vivo*. The treated seeds of pigeonpea variety Bahar were sown in sick plots.

Efficacy of bio-agents against *Fusarium* wilt

Seeds of highly susceptible variety (Bahar) of pigeonpea were treated with *Trichoderma viride* and *P. fluorescence* @ 6.0 g/kg seed before sowing. One treatment was maintained without seed treatment as control. Each treatment was replicate at thrice. The seed of Arhar, variety Bahar, was treated with spore suspension of all these bio-agents. The treated seeds were sown in plots and untreated control was also maintained with three replications. Observation on wilt incidence was recorded at the age of 5 weeks of seedlings.

Efficacy of polymer coating with fungicides

The fresh seed lots were available from Division of Seed Science and Technology, Indian Agricultural Research Institute, New Delhi and four years old seed lots were also collected from pulse laboratories, Indian Agricultural Research Institute, New Delhi. Seeds selected for experiment were bold and free from any damage. T_6- Polymer coating (polycot) 4 ml diluted in 5 ml of water per kg seed. T_7- Polymer coating + *Trichoderma viride* @ 6.0g/kg seed (T_6 + T_4). T8-Polymer + *Pseudomonas fluorescens* @ 6.0g/kg seed (T_6 + T_5). T_9-- Polymer coating (polycot) 4 ml diluted in 5 ml of water per kg seed + vitavax power @ 3g/kg seed. These polymers alone @ 4.0ml per kg and in combination with bioagents and fungicides were applied to seed.

Observations Recorded

First appearance of the disease, disease incidence and disease control were recorded at 40, 50, 60, 70, 80 and 90 days after sowing, respectively. The number of infected plants was counted from the total number of plants in a plot. Per cent disease incidence and per cent diseases control were calculated by using the following formula.

$$\text{Disease incidence (\%)} = \frac{\text{No of infected plants per plot}}{\text{Total plant per plot}} \times 100$$

$$\text{Disesese control (\%)} = \frac{\text{C-T}}{\text{C}} \times 100$$

Where,

C = Per cent disease incidence in untreated

T = Per cent disease plot incidence in treated plot

Result and discussion

The results revealed that all the treatments tested *in vivo*, the disease was controlled significantly in all treatments except untreated plots. The effective control more than 50 per cent was recorded in all treatment at 40 and 50 days after sowing. The highest per cent disease control and per cent wilt disease incidence were recorded 96.09 to 64.09 and 2.74 to 33.32, respectively in T_9 (Polymer + Vitavax power @ 3g per kg seed) at 10 days intervals followed by T_8 (Polymer + *P. fluorescens*) gave 94.46 to 53.06 per cent inhibition, T_7 (92.39 to 52.74) and T_6 (90.97 to 49.73) however, the lowest per cent disease control was noticed as 76.19 to 40.13 per cent in T_1 (Neem leaves extract) amongst all treatments except untreated. Among the bio-agents, seed treatment with *P. fluorescens* had controlled maximum wilt incidence 45.27 to 87.00 per cent followed by *T. viride* (43.11 to 84.14 per cent). It was significantly higher than the check up to 90 days after sowing. Singh (2010) observed that the plant extracts of *A. sativum, A. indica* and *Calotropis procera* significantly reduced the wilt incidence in pigeonpea Singh (2010) also reported the seed treatments with bulb extract of *A. sativum* was the most effective against wilt, which reduced 65.9% disease incidence over the control. These results are also in accordance of Ganie *et al.,* (2013) and Sadana and Didwania (2015)

Table 1: Effect of plant extracts (10% conc.), chemicals and bio-agents on the disease incidence of *Fusarium* wilt of pigeonpea

Treatments	Per cent wilt incidence					
	40 day	50 day	60 day	70 day	80 day	90 day
T_1- Neem leaves Extract	16.67	24.00	33.32	41.67	50.00	55.56
	(24.07)	(29.32)	(35.25)	(40.19)	(45.00)	(48.22)
T_2- Garlic bulb extract	7.75	15.74	23.44	31.66	39.88	47.54
	(16.15)	(23.34)	(28.93)	(34.21)	(39.14)	(43.59)
T_3- Tulsi leaf extract	8.32	16.65	25.00	33.32	41.65	50.00
	(16.74)	(24.07)	(29.97)	(35.23)	(40.18)	(45.00)
T_4- *T. viride*	11.10	19.45	27.78	36.12	44.45	52.79
	(19.45)	(26.16)	(31.78)	(36.92)	(41.80)	(46.61)
T_5- *P. fluorescens*	9.10	17.45	25.78	34.12	42.45	50.79
	(17.55)	(24.66)	(30.48)	(35.72)	(40.64)	(45.45)

(Contd.)

T_6- Polymer coating	6.32 (14.54)	15.00 (22.76)	22.57 (28.34)	30.66 (33.59)	38.44 (38.29)	46.65 (43.07)
T_7-Polymer + *T. viride*	5.33 (13.33)	13.88 (21.85)	21.86 (27.84)	29.67 (32.97)	38.00 (38.04)	43.86 (41.47)
T_8-Polymer + *P.fluorescens*	3.88 (11.35)	11.67 (19.95)	19.74 (26.35)	27.67 (31.72)	36.00 (36.84)	43.56 (41.29)
T_9-- Polymer + VitavaxPower	2.74 (9.52)	5.54 (13.60)	8.34 (16.77)	16.67 (24.07)	24.00 (29.32)	33.32 (35.23)
T_{10}- Untreated	70.00 (56.94)	77.00 (61.75)	80.20 (64.09)	85.20 (67.79)	90.50 (73.36)	92.80 (74.98)
CD at 5%	3.31	4.57	5.25	5.23	6.78	6.09

Figures are given in parenthesis are angular transformed value

Table 2: Effect of plant extracts (10% conc.), chemicals and bio-agents on the per cent disease control of *Fusarium* wilt of pigeonpea

Treatments	Per cent disease control					
	40 day	50 day	60 day	70 day	80 day	90 day
T--$_1$- Neem leaf extract	76.19 (61.09)	68.83 (56.15)	58.45 (49.90)	51.09 (45.63)	44.75 (41.98)	40.13 (39.29)
T_2- Garlic bulb extract	88.93 (71.85)	79.56 (63.59)	70.77 (57.35)	62.84 (52.52)	55.93 (48.43)	48.77 (44.30)
T_3- Tulsi leaf extract	88.11 (71.54)	78.38 (62.46)	68.83 (56.12)	60.89 (51.35)	53.98 (47.30)	46.12 (42.77)
T_4- *T. viride*	84.14 (66.89)	74.74 (59.94)	65.36 (54.06)	57.61 (49.42)	50.88 (45.51)	43.11 (41.03)
T_5- *P. fluorescens*	87.00 (69.43)	77.34 (62.04)	67.86 (55.60)	59.95 (50.79)	53.09 (46.79)	45.27 (42.27)
T_6- Polymer coating	90.97 (72.57)	80.52 (64.42)	71.86 (58.17)	64.01 (53.23)	57.52 (49.36)	49.73 (44.85)
T_7-Polymer + *T. viride*	92.39 (76.00)	81.97 (65.63)	72.74 (58.80)	65.18 (53.92)	58.01 (49.63)	52.74 (46.58)
T_8-Polymer+ *P. fluorescens*	94.46 (78.04)	84.84 (68.59)	75.39 (60.53)	67.52 (55.33)	60.22 (50.95)	53.06 (46.76)
T_9-Polyme- +Vitavax power	96.09 (79.63)	92.81 (76.08)	89.60 (72.89)	80.43 (64.27)	73.48 (59.11)	64.09 (53.22)
T_{10}- Untreated	0.00 (0.00)	0.00 (0.00)	0.00 (0.00)	0.00 (0.00)	0.00 (0.00)	0.00 (0.00)
CD at 5%	12.53	12.50	10.08	8.40	6.79	5.52

Figures are given in parenthesis are angular transformed value

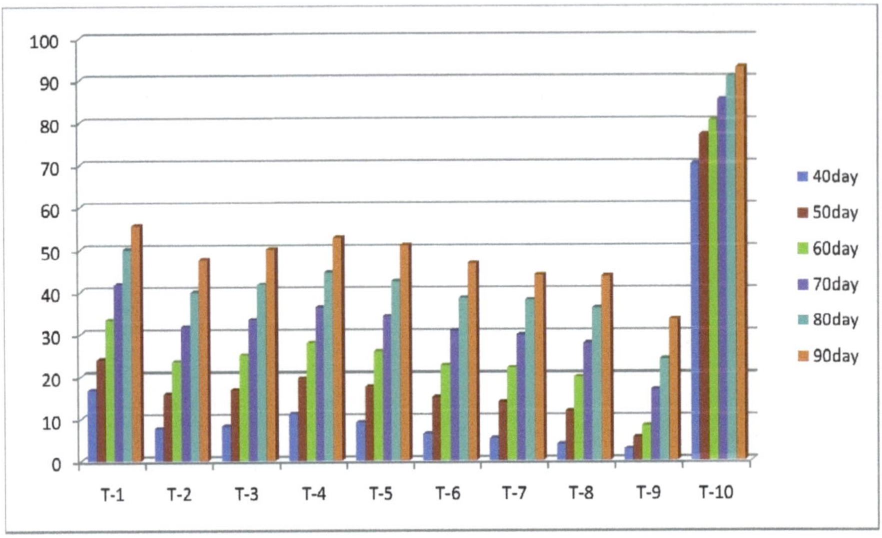

Fig. 1: Effect of plant extracts (10% conc.), chemicals and bio-agents on the disease incidence of *Fusarium* wilt of pigeonpea at 40, 50, 60, 70, 80 and 90 days.

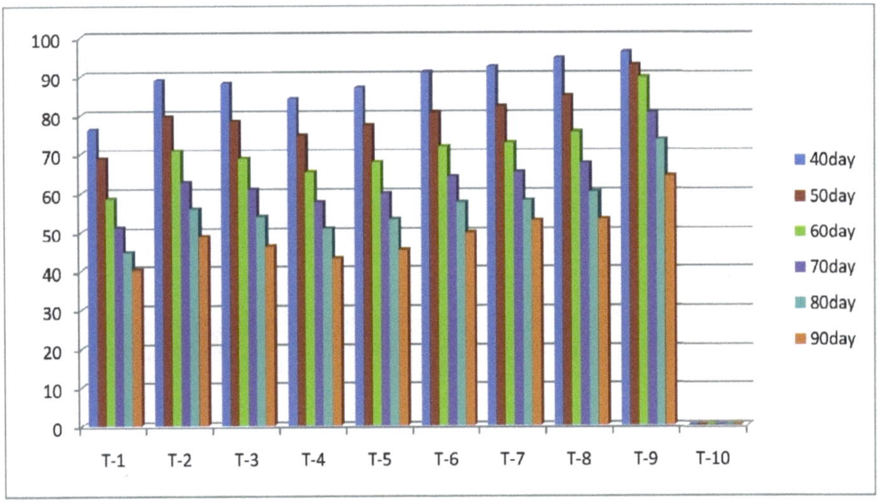

Fig. 2: Effect of plant extracts (10% conc.), chemicals and bio-agents on the disease control of *Fusarium* wilt of pigeonpea at 40, 50, 60, 70, 80 and 90 days.

References

Ali, M. and Kumar, S. (2005). Advances in pigeonpea research. IIPR Kanpur pp-3.

Anonymous (2017). Project Coordinators Report. Annual group meet (*Kharif*) 16-18 May. All India Coordinated Research Project on Mullarp. IIPR, Kanpur.pp.17

Ganie, S.A., Pant, V.R., Ghani, M.Y., Lone, A.H., Anjum, Q. and Razvi, S.M. (2013). *In vitro* evaluation of plant extracts against *Alternaria brassicae* (Berk.) Sacc. causing leaf spot of mustard and *Fusarium oxysporum* f. sp. *lycopersici* causing wilt of tomato. *Scientific Research and Essays,* 8 (37) : 1808-1811.

Khune, R. (1990). Biological control of soil borne plant pathogens. *Indian J. of Mycol. Plant Pathology*.17:1-9.

Reddy, M.V., Sharma, S.B. and Nene, Y.L. (1990). The pigeonpea, In: pigeonpea disease management CAB International, 1990, ICRISAT Patancheru, Andhra Pradesh, 304pp.

Sadana, D. and Didwania, N. (2015). Bioefficacy of fungicides and plant extracts against *Alternaria solani* causing early blight of potato. *International Conference on Plant, Marine and Environmental Sciences*, 38-42.

Singh, P.K., Anis Khan, Robin Gogai and Jaiswal, R.K. (2010). Plant leaf extracts and bio-agents for eco-friendly management leaf wilt of pigeonpea caused by *Fusarium udum*. *Indian Phytopathology*, 63(3): 343-344.

Singh, R.S. (2006). Disease caused by Deuteromycotina, In: Plant Diseases. Oxford and IBH Publishing Co. Pvt. Ltd., New Delhi, pp. 457-463.

2

Efficacy of Plant Extracts, Bio-Agents and Fungicides on Mycelial Growth of *Fusarium udum* Causing Wilt of Pigeon Pea *in vitro*

Neeraj Kumar Rajvanshi, Subhash Chandra, Ajay Kumar H.K. Singh and Divya Singh

Department of Plant Pathology, Narendra Deva University of Agriculture & Technology, Kumarganj, Faizabad-224229, Uttar Pradesh, India

Abstract

Pigeon pea is an important pulse crop of India and its production is greatly affected by wilt disease. Pigeon pea wilt is a very destructive soil borne disease caused by Fusarium udum. In present research work plant extracts (Garlic, Neem, Tulsi), bio-agents (Trichoderma viride and Pseudomonas fluorescens) and fungicides (Vitavax, Bavistin and Thiram + Carbendazim) were tested against Fusarium udum. Among them fungicides were found most effective in inhibiting mycelial growth of Fusarium udum recorded 100% inhibition followed by garlic bulb extract (52.12 to 56.33%). Among bioagents, Pseudomonas fluorescens inhibit the growth up to (46.00 to 51.79%) followed by T. viride (44.32 to 48.79%) amongst all treatments except untreated.

Keywords: Pigeon pea, *Fusarium udum,* bio-agent, fungicide

Pigeon pea (*Cajanus cajan* L. Millsp.) is one of the major pulse crops grown in the tropics and subtropics belonging to family Leguminaceae. It has wide adaptability and low input requirements mostly grown in *kharif* season. In India the crop is mainly grown in Andhra Pradesh, Bihar, Uttar Pradesh, Karnataka

Gujarat, Madhya Pradesh, Maharashtra, Orissa and Tamilnadu. In Uttar Pradesh, it is grown 311.0 thousand ha area producing 325 thousand tons, with an average yield of 1040 kg/ha (Anonymous, 2014). The poor yield of pigeon pea is mainly due to biotic stress like diseases and insect pests but only few of them like wilt, sterility mosaic, *Phytophthora* blight and *Alternaria* blight are major and destructive ones. Among fungal pathogens, wilt disease caused by *Fusarium udum* Butler is an important disease in India, Kenya, Malawi, Nepal, Tanzania and Uganda (Reddy *et al.,* 1990). In India, it is the most serious problem all over the pigeon pea growing states especially in U.P, M.P, Bihar and Maharashtra. In Bihar and Uttar Pradesh, 5-10 per cent losses in standing crop are common feature every year (Singh, 2006). Management of pigeon pea wilt through fungicides applied as soil treatment such as Thiram, Ferbam, Carbendazim and copper oxychloride have been reported by different workers. In discriminate use of these chemicals has led to development of fungicide resistance strain and more importantly, environmental pollution, posing a potential risk to animal and human health. Hence, for minimizing the losses caused by wilt need inexpensive and environmentally safe management practices. It was therefore considered desirable to evaluate botanicals, bio-agents and fungicides against wilt pathogen for effective management.

Material and Methods

Pigeonpea plants showing characteristic symptoms of *Fusarium* wilt were collected from pigeonpea experimental field, Department of Genetics and Plant Breeding, NDUA&T, Kumarganj, Faizabad for isolation and identification. The infected plant parts were cut in to small pieces and surface sterilized with 0.1 per cent mercuric chloride solution and washed thoroughly 3 to 4 times with sterilized water to remove the traces of Mercuric Chloride. The species were transferred in Petri dishes containing potato dextrose agar and incubated at 25 ^{0}C for 6 days.

Efficacy of plant extracts against *Fusarium udum*

In order of find out the efficacy of various plant extracts against the *Fusarium* wilt three plant extracts *viz.*, bulb of Garlic, leaves of Neem and Tulsi were used. Fresh leaves and bulb were collected and washed thoroughly in clean water. Hundred gram of each washed plant material was grinded in Pestle and Mortar by adding equal amount (100 ml) of sterilized water (1: 1 w/v) and heated at 80^0 C for 10 minutes. The materials was filtered through double layered muslin cloth followed by filtering through sterilized Whatman No. 1 filter paper and treated as standard plant extract (100%). The 5.0 and 10.0 per cent concentration were made by adding in requisite amount of sterilized PDA medium. To study the inhibitory effect on mycelial growth of *Fusarium udum*, 5.0 and

10.0 per cent concentration of botanicals were evaluated through poison food techniques under *in vitro* condition by adding five and ten ml plant extract of stock solution to the 95.0 ml and 90.0 ml of sterilized cooled PDA medium. Twenty ml medium was poured into each Petri plate. Three treatments having three replications were maintained. Control treatment was maintained by pouring PDA medium without plant extract. Five mm discs of 7 days old culture of *Fusarium udum* were placed in the centre of plant extract amended Petri plates. The Petri plate having PDA alone were inoculated in the same manner. These Petri plates were incubated at 28 ± 2 ˚C. The observations were recorded on radial growth at 48 hrs, 72 hrs, and 96 hrs of incubation in plant extracts amended Petri plate as well as in control.

Efficacy of bio-agents against *Fusarium udum* using dual culture method

Two bioagents (*Trichoderma viride* and *Pseudomonas fluorescens*) were used against *F. udam* to test the antagonistic effect. Culture of *Trichoderma viride* was obtained from the Department of Plant Pathology, NDUA&T, Kumarganj, Faizabad (UP). For *Pseudomonas fluorescens,* soil sample were collected around the rhizosphere of wilt affected plant from Student Instructional Farm, NDUA&T, Kumarganj Faizabad (UP). Isolates of *Pseudomonas fluorescens* were isolated and identified using Bergey's Manual of Determinative Bacteriology. Bacterial colonies identified as *Pseudomonas fluorescens* were picked and pure culture of isolates was maintained. The potential of cultured *Trichoderma viride* and *Pseudomonas fluorescens* was evaluated *in vitro* using dual culture technique by 5 mm disc cut from the actively growing margins of 72h old culture was placed at the margin of the 90 mm Petri plates containing 20 ml potato dextrose agar (PDA). Disc of 5 mm size of 72h old culture of *Fusarium udum* was placed opposite to the antagonist under aseptic conditions. The plates were incubated at 28 ± 2 °C. Each treatment was replicated thrice. A Petri plate inoculated with pathogen alone served as the control. Mycelial growth of the pathogen was observed regularly from 48 hrs to 96 hrs after the inoculation of pathogen.

Efficacy of fungicides against *Fusarium udum* using poison food technique

Three fungicides (Vitavax Power, Bavistin 25SD, Thiram + Carbendazim) were used in three concentrations of each (0.2, 0.1 and 0.3 per cent). Three concentrations of fungicides were bio-assayed against the test pathogen under laboratory condition to find out their relative efficacy for inhibiting the mycelial growth of the pathogen by poison food technique. The efficacy of fungicides was observed by measuring the radial growth of the fungal colony at 48 hrs, 72 hrs, and 96 hrs after incubation. The percent growth inhibition of mycelia were calculated using the following formula

$$I = \frac{C - T}{C} x100$$

Whereas,

I = Per cent inhibition of fungal growth

C = Radial growth of control

T = Radial growth of treated petridishes

Result and Discussion

During the present investigation of eight treatments namely, Garlic bulb extract, Neem leaves extract, Tulsi leaves extract, *Trichoderma viride, Pseudomonas fluorescens* and Vitavax Power, Bavistin 25SD, Thiram + Carbendazim were evaluated for fungi toxicity against *Fusarium udum*. The results showed that all treatments inhibited the mycelia growth of *Fusarium udum*. It is evident from table 1 and 2 that among plant extracts, maximum per cent inhibition (50.18 to 52.83) was recorded with garlic bulb extract at 5% concentration while, the inhibition percentage increased with the increasing concentration and recorded 52.12 to 56.33 at 10% concentration followed by Tulsi (46.53 to 48.12, 48.00-52.00%) and Neem (38.13 to 40.63%, 40.42 to 43.00%) from 48 hrs to 96 hrs incubation. Devi and Charley (2012) reported the effect of different plant extracts against the mycelial growth of *Fusarium udum*. Among them extract of *A. sativum* showed complete inhibition of radial growth of *Fusarium udum* followed by *A. indica* (74.4%), *Spilanthes acemella* (68.8%) and *Aloe vera* (55.9%). Mehta *et al.,* (2010) found the Garlic bulb extract was significantly superior to inhibit the growth of *Fusarium udum*. Same results were found by Dwivedi and Shukla (2000).

Table 1: Effect of plant extracts (at 5% conc. each) on the per cent mycelial growth inhibition of *F. udum*

Treatment	Per cent inhibition		
	48 hrs.	72 hrs.	96 hrs.
Garlic bulb extract	50.18(45.10)	51.23(45.71)	52.83(46.64)
Neem leaves extract	38.13(38.12)	39.52(38.93)	40.63(39.58)
Tulsi leaves extract	46.53(43.00)	47.86(43.77)	48.12(43.92)
Check	0.00 (0.00)	0.00(0.00)	0.00(0.00)
C.D. at 5%	6.10	6.69	6.98

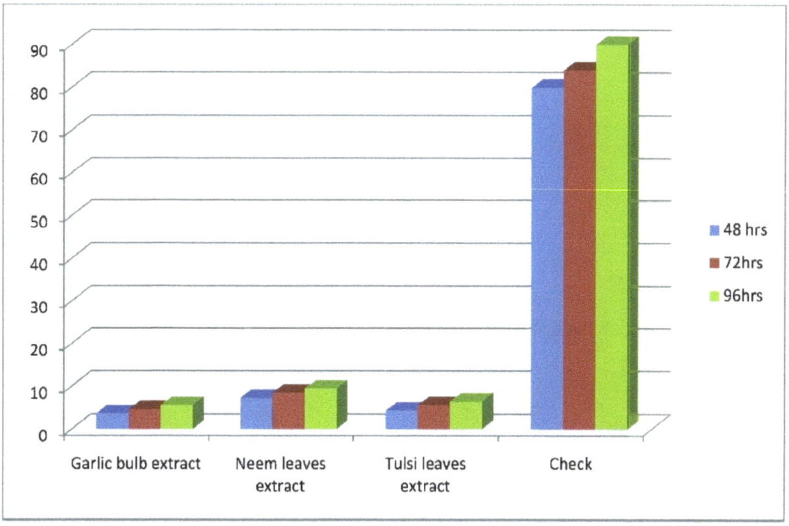

Fig. 1: Effect of plant extracts (5% conc.) on mycelial growth of *F. udum.*

Efficacy of bio-agents against *Fusarium udam* using dual culture method

The results indicated (Table 2) that the antagonist effect on radial growth of *F. udum* was highest in *Pseudomonas fluorescens* which inhibit the growth up to 46.00 to 51.79% followed by *Trichoderma viride* (44.32 to 48.79%). Singh *et al.,* (2015) found that the *Pseudomonas fluorescens* was significantly superior to inhibit the growth of *Fusarium udum*. These findings are in accordance of Khune (1990).

Table 2: Effect of plant extracts (at 10% conc.), bio-agents and chemicals on the per cent mycelial growth inhibition of *F. udum*

Treatment	Per cent inhibition		
	48 hrs	72 hrs	96 hrs
Garlic bulb extract	52.12(46.22)	54.00(47.31)	56.33(48.65)
Neem leaves extract	40.42(39.46)	42.37(40.60)	43.00(40.96)
Tulsi leaves extract	48.00(43.85)	50.13(45.08)	52.00(46.16)
T. viride	44.32(41.73)	46.78(43.15)	48.79(44.30)
P. fluorescens	46.00(42.70)	49.71(44.83)	51.79(46.03)
Vitavax.Power(0.2%)	100.00(90.00)	100.00(90.00)	100.00(90.00)
Bavistin 25 SD (0.1%)	100.00(90.00)	100.00(90.00)	100.00(90.00)
Thiram+Carbendazim (0.3%)	100.00(90.00)	100.00(90.00)	100.00(90.00)
Check	0.00(0.00)	0.00(0.00)	0.00(0.00)
C.D. at 5%	4.23	4.70	4.40

Figure given in parenthesis are angular transformed value

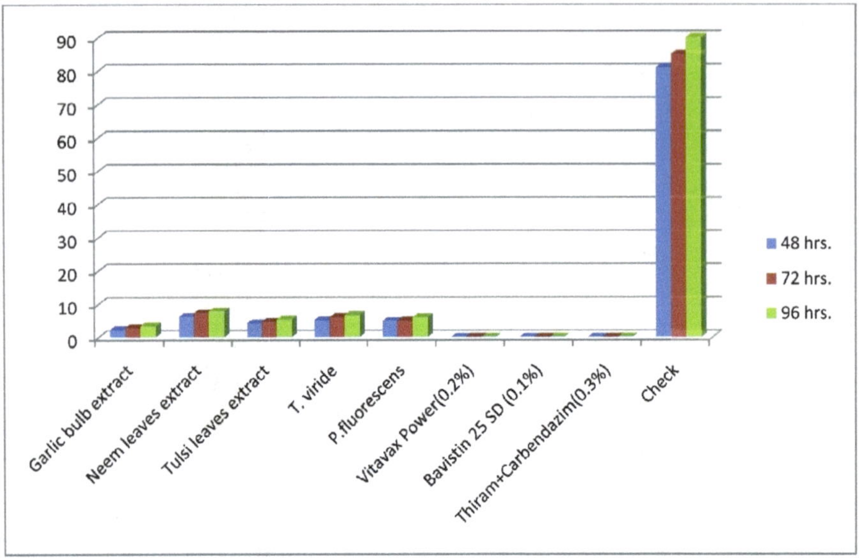

Fig. 2: Effect of plants extracts (10% conc.), chemicals and bio-agents on mycelial growth of *F. udum*.

Efficacy of fungicides against *Fusarium udam* using poison food technique

Three fungicides namely Vitavax Power (0.2%), Bavistin 25SD (0.1%) and Thiram + Carbendazim (0.3%) were tested by poisoned food technique *in vitro*. All of them were found highly effective and resulted cent per cent restriction of radial growth of *Fusarium udum* up to 96 hrs. Karande (2007) reported that Bavistin 25SD (0.1%) and Thiram + Carbendazim (0.3%) at higher concentration gave 100% inhibition of mycelial growth of *Fusarium udum* on PDA medium.

It can be concluded that out of eight treatments tested *in vitro*, Bavistin 25SD (0.1%) and Thiram + Carbendazim (0.3%) were found most effective in inhibiting radial growth of the pathogen followed by Vitavax Power (0.2%), Garlic bulb extract, Tulsi leaves extract, *Pseudomonas fluorescens, Trichoderma viride* and Neem over the check.

References

Anonymous (2014). Project Coordinators Report. Annual group meet (*Kharif*) 16-18 May. All India Coordinated Research Project on Mullarp. IIPR, Kanpur.pp.17

Devi, S. and Chhelry, M. (2012). Effect of extracts of some medicinal plants on the growth of *Fusarium* sp. *J. Mycol. Plant Pathology,* 26:110.

Dwivedi, B.P. and Shukla, D.N. (2000). Effect of leaf extracts of some medicinal plants on spore germination of some *Fusarium* species. *Karnataka Journal of Agricultural Sciences*, 13(1): 153-154.

Karande, M. (2007). Efficacy of fungicides, bio-agents and plant extracts against *F. oxysporum*. *Annals of Plant Protection Science*, 15 (1):267-268.

Khune, R. (1990). Biological control of soil borne plant pathogens. *Indian J. of Mycol. Plant Pathology*.17:1-9.

Mehta, A.N., Chauhan, H.L., Makwara, K.V., Ghel, N.M and Patel, S.L. (2010). Bio efficacy of phytoextrect, antagonist and fungicides against *F. udum* incident of pigeon pea wilt. *Journal of Plant Disease Science,* 5 (1):56-60.

Reddy, M.V., Sharma, S.B. and Nene, Y.L. (1990). The pigeon pea, In: pigeon pea disease management CAB International, 1990, ICRISAT Patancheru, Andhra Pradesh, 304pp.

Singh, P.K., Anis Khan, Robin Gogai and Jaiswal, R.K. (2010). Plant leaf extracts and bio-agents for eco-friendly management leaf wilt of pigeon pea caused by *Fusarium udum*. *Indian Phytopathology*, 63(3): 343-344.

Singh, R.S. (2006). Disease caused by Deuteromycotina, In: Plant Diseases. Oxford and IBH Publishing Co. Pvt. Ltd., New Delhi, pp. 457-463.

3

Efficacy of Botanicals and Bio-Agents Against *Fusarium Oxysporum* f.sp. *Lentils in vitro*

Subhash Chandra, Gireesh Chand*, V.P. Chaudhary, Ajay Kumar and Pankaj Kumar**

***Department of Entomology, N.D. University of Agriculture & Technology Kumarganj, Faizabad-224229, Uttar Pradesh, India*
**Department of Plant Pathology, Bihar Agriculture University, Sabour Bihar, India*

Abstract

Lentil is an important pulse crop and play very important role in the supply of the protein to under nourished vegetarian population of the country. Fusarium wilt of lentil caused by Fusarium oxysporum f. sp. lentis is one of the wide spread and destructive diseases in India under rice-based cropping system. Use of synthetic fungicides has led to the emergence of several problems like environment pollution, residual effect in grains and killing of non-target organism(s). Hence, for minimizing the losses caused by Fusarium wilt, four plant extracts such as Garlic, Neem, Eucalyptus, Tulsi and three antagonistic bio-agents viz. Trichoderma viride, Trichoderma harzianum and Pseudomonas fluorescence were evaluated in vitro. The results clearly showed that all plant extracts were more or less inhibitory to mycelial growth of Fusarium oxysporum f. sp. lentis. The effectiveness of extracts increased with increase of their concentration and maximum growth inhibition was obtained in Eucalyptus followed by Garlic and Tulsi. While minimum per cent inhibition was recorded in Neem. Among bio-agents, T. viride showed maximum growth inhibition of Fusarium oxysporum f. sp. lentis followed by T. harzianum at both 4 and 7 days incubation period.

Keywords: *Fusarium,* bio-agents, plant extracts, *Rhizobium*.

Introduction

Pulses constitute an important ingredient of the vegetarian diet in India sub-continent and play a significant role in Indian farming because of their value in providing quality food to million of peoples and restoring soil fertility through fix atmospheric nitrogen in symbiotic association with root nodule bacterium (*Rhizobium*). Pulses are important source of protein, high in fiber content and provide ample quantity of vitamins and minerals.

Lentil is recognized as one of the most nutritious pulse crop ranking next to chickpea amongst *Rabi* pulses. In India, lentil is mostly grown in northern plains, central and eastern parts of India. The major lentil producing states are Madhya Pradesh, Uttar Pradesh, Bihar, Uttarakhand and Bengal. It can be grown on a wide range of soil from light loam to black cotton soils and can stand even less fertile moderately alkaline soils and rainfed conditions. Lentil is attacked from a numbers of seed and soil borne diseases. *Fusarium* wilt caused by *F. oxysporum* f.sp. *lentis* is the important disease as it caused the significant annual loss in yield, present status of disease problem in the lentil growing areas of the country, non availability of suitable management practices and gaps in our knowledge about this disease. In order to overcome to this disease, a laboratory experiment was conducted to know the efficacy of botanicals and bio-agents against *Fusarium oxysporum* f. sp. *lentis*.

Materials and Methods

The study was carried out in the Department of Plant Pathology, Narendra Deva University of Agriculture and Technology, Kumarganj, Faizabad (U.P.). In order to find out the efficacy of four plants extract *viz*., leaves of Neem, Tulsi and Eucalyptus, Garlic bulb and three bio-agent *viz*., *Trichoderma viride*, *Trichoderma harzianum* and *Pseudomonas fluorescence* against the *Fusarium* wilt were used.

Fresh leaves and bulb were collected and wash thoroughly in clean water and heated with 100 ml of sterilized water at 80^0C for 10 minutes. The material was filtered through double layered muslin cloth. All the plant extract were tested at 5 and 10 per cent concentration under *in vitro* condition by using food poison technique to study the inhibitory effect of these botanicals on radial growth of *Fusarium oxysporum*. ten ml. plant extracts of stock solution were added to the 90.0 ml of sterilized cooled PDA medium. The flasks were thoroughly taken to get uniform mixture of the extracts under aseptic condition before pouring it into the Petri dishes. Twenty ml. medium was poured into each Petri dish in three replications of each extracts. Control treatment was maintained by pouring PDA medium without plant extracts. Five mm discs of 7 days old pure culture of *Fusarium oxysporum* f. sp. *lentis* were cut with sterilized cork borer and placed in the center of plant extracts amended Petri plates. These Petri plates were incubated at 25 ± 2^{0}C. The observation was recorded on radial growth and per cent inhibition at 4 days and 7 days of incubation in plant extracts amended Petri plates as well as in control.

Per cent growth inhibition was calculated using formula;

$$I = \frac{C\text{-}T}{C} \times 100$$

I = Per cent inhibition of fungal growth

C = Radial growth of control

T = Radial growth of treated Petri plates

The antagonistic potential of *Trichoderma viride, Trichoderma harzianum* and *Pseudomonas fluorescence* against *F. oxysporum* f. sp. *lentis* was assessed in dual culture technique. Measuring radial growth of the *F. oxysprum* f. sp. *lentis* as well as that of bio-agents. The mycelial disc of 3 mm diameter from the margin of 7 day old culture of bio-agents and *F. oxysporum* f.sp. *lentis* were placed on solid PDA in paired combination at distance of 2.5 cm from each other in four replication. Control set was made by inoculating *F. oxysporum* f. sp. *lentis* singly on the medium. Dual Petri dishes were incubated at 28^{0}C in BOD incubator and the extent of interaction was observed by measuring area covered by in dual culture and in the control at 4 and 7 days of incubation. The per cent inhibition of the interacting fungi was calculated by using following formula;

$$I = \frac{A1\text{-}A2}{A1} \times 100$$

Where as,

A_1 = Area covered by *Fusarium oxysporum* f. sp. *lentis* in the control.

A_2 = Area covered by the *Fusarium oxysporum* f. sp. *lentis* in dual culture.

Results and Discussion

After 4 days of inoculation, the data presented in Table 1 shows that minimum radial growth was obtained in Eucalyptus (4.0 mm) followed by Garlic (5.11 mm), Tulsi (3.50 mm) and Neem (9.10 mm). The radial growth in control was (22.0 mm). Similarly there was no significant difference observed in radial growth of Garlic and Tulsi at 5 per cent concentration. Maximum per cent growth inhibition was recorded in Eucalyptus (81.81%) followed by Garlic (76.77%), Tulsi (74.59%) and Neem (58.63%) at 5 per cent concentration. At

10% concentration, minimum radial growth was recorded in Eucalyptus (2.48 mm) followed by Garlic (3.25 mm) and Tulsi (3.50 mm) which was at par with each other. In treatment Neem, the radial growth was 6.08 mm which was significantly differed to other treatments. The maximum radial growth observed in control (22.0 mm). Similarly in case of growth inhibition of *F. oxysporum* f. sp. *lentis,* Eucalyptus (88.72%) was significantly superior than Tulsi (84.09%). Garlic (85.22%). Neem (72.36%) was next best treatments to growth inhibition which was at par with each other (Fig. 1).

It was also observed that after 7 days of inoculation Eucalyptus (5.23 mm & 3.36 mm and 87.54% & 92.00%) and Garlic (5.77mm & 3.75mm and 86.26% & 91.11%) showed minimum radial growth and maximum growth inhibition per cent at 5 per cent and 10 per cent concentration level, respectively. Next best plant extract was Neem followed by Tulsi at both concentration level. There was 42.00 mm radial growth of *F. oxysporum* f. sp. *lentis* in control treatment at both concentration i.e. 5% and 10%, however no growth inhibition was found in control (Table 2, Fig. 2). Present results are in conformity with the reports of Singh and Rabi (2000) who reported that higher concentration of leaf extracts of *Eucalyptus globules* (70%) and bulb extract of *Allium sativum* (71%) completely inhibit the mycelium growth of *F. oxysporum* f. sp. *lentis in vitro* & *in vivo.* Kumar *et al.*, (2002) also found that leaf extract of Neem (*Azadirachta indica*), Eucalyptus (*Eucalyptus globules*), Garlic (*Allium sativum*), Tulsi (*Ocimum sanctum*) was effective against wilt *Fusarium oxysporum* f. sp. *lentis* of lentil. Similar results were also obtained by Sinha and Sinha (2004) who reported that Neem (*Azadirachta indica*), Marigold (*Tagetes erecta*) leaf extract and Garlic bulb extract (*Allium sativum*) at 5 per cent as seed treatment reduce wilt incidence and increase yield compared with the untreated control. Mandhore and Suryawansi (2008) screened 35 botanicals and found that *Ocimum sanctum, Eucalyptus* spp. and *Azadirachtra indica* completely inhibited the growth of *Fusarium oxysporum* on agar as well as potato dextrose. Mehta *et al.* (2010) reported that garlic bulb extract was significantly superior to inhibit the growth of *F. oxysporum* f. sp. *lentis* which was followed by Eucalyptus.

The efficacy of bio-agent *Trichoderma viride*, *Trichoderma harzianum* and *Pseudomonas fluorescence* were also tested for radial growth and per cent inhibition of *F. oxysporum* f.sp. *lentis* by using dual culture technique. Minimum radial growth (7.00 and 9.67mm) and maximum growth inhibition per cent (68.18 and 76.97%) were recorded in *Trichoderma viride* at 4 and 7 days incubation period, respectively. Next best bio-agent was *Pseudomonas fluorescence* in suppressing the growth of *F. oxysporum* f.sp. *lentis* which was significantly superior than *Trichoderma harzianum*. After 4 days of incubation, radial growth of *F. oxysporum* f.sp. *lentis* was 22.0 mm that was increased upto 42.0 mm after 7 days incubation in control treatment (Table 3, Fig. 3). Present results are in conformity with the reports of Upadyayay and Mukhopadyayay (1986) who reported antagonistic properties of *Trichoderma viride* and *Trichoderma hariziamum* against *Fusarium oxysporum, Sclerotium rolfsi* and *Rizoctonia soolnai* among the soil borne pathogens of chickpea. Well (1988) also reported that *Trichoderma* and *Gliocladium* has been exceptionally good for bio-control studies because these are ubiquitous in distribution, easy to isolate, grow rapidly on wide variety of substrates, rarely pathogenic on higher plants, better competitive saprophytic ability, enzyme system and antibiotic producing capacity for antagonizing many pathogenic fungi. Present results also endorse the findings of Dolatabadi *et al.* (2010) who found that four antagonistic fungi, namely *Pieiformospora indica, Sebacina vermifera, Trichoderma viride* and *Trichoderma hariziamum* against *Fusarium* wilt of lentil. Similarly Choudhary *et al.*, (2012) studied the antagonistic potential of three *Trichoderma* spp. *viz., Trichoderma harizanum, Trichoderma viride* and *Trichoderma koningii* against *Fusarium oxysporum* f.sp. *lentis* causing wilt of lentil under *in vitro*. All the three bio-agent were found effective in inhibiting the growth of pathogen.

Table 1: Effect of plant extracts against *F. oxysporum* f. sp. *lentis* on radial growth and growth inhibition at 5 and 10 per cent concentration *in vitro* after 4 days incubation

Plant extracts	Concentration (5%)		Concentration (10%)	
	Radial growth (mm)	Growth inhibition (%)	Radial growth (mm)	Growth inhibition (%)
Neem	9.10	58.63 (49.95)	6.08	72.36 (58.89)
Garlic	5.11	76.77 (61.14)	3.25	85.22 (57.37)
Tulsi	5.60	74.59 (59.67)	3.50	84.09 (66.42)
Eucalyptus	4.00	81.81 (64.75)	2.48	88.72 (70.36)
Control	22.0	00.00	22.0	00.00
SEm±	0.82	1.02	0.50	0.77
CD at 5%	2.60	3.21	1.59	2.42

Figure given in parenthesis are transformed value

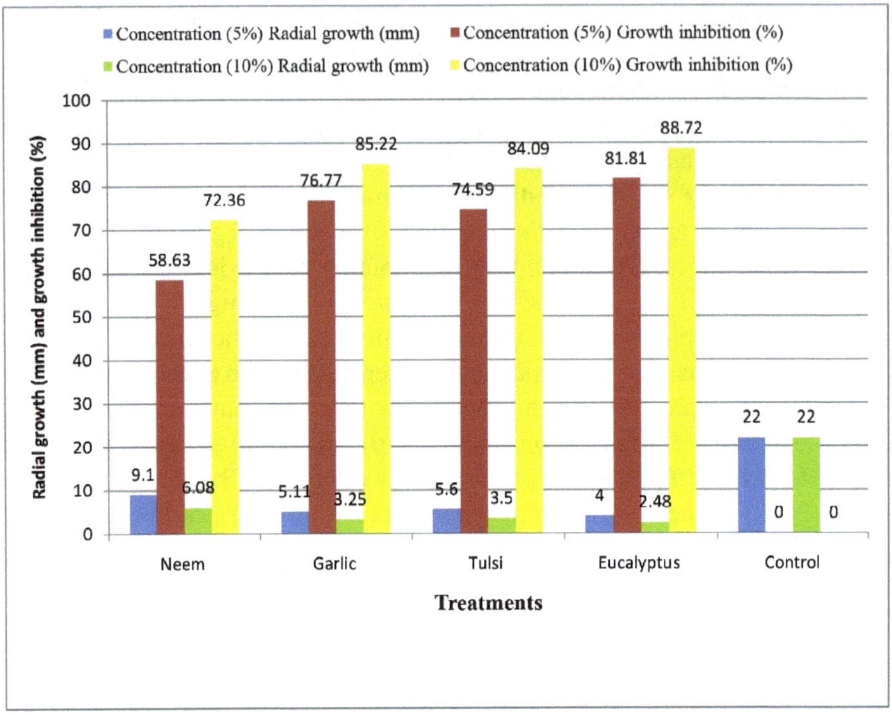

Fig. 1: Effect of plant extracts against *F. oxysporum* f.sp. *lentis* on radial growth and growth inhibition at 5.0 and 10.0 per cent concentration *in vitro* after 4 days incubation

Table 2: Effect of plant extracts against *F. oxysporum* f. sp. *lentis* on radial growth and growth inhibition at 5 and 10 per cent concentration *in vitro* after 7 days incubation

Plant extracts	Concentration (5%)		Concentration (10%)	
	Radial growth (mm)	Growth inhibition(%)	Radial growth (mm)	Growth inhibition(%)
Neem	6.20	85.23 (57.37)	4.87	88.40 (70.09)
Garlic	5.77	86.26 (68.19)	3.75	91.11 (72.64)
Tulsi	12.28	70.76 (57.23)	7.12	83.04 (65.65)
Eucalyptus	5.23	87.54 (69.30)	3.36	92.00 (73.57)
Control	42.0	00.00	42.0	00.00
SEm±	0.58	0.64	0.32	0.38
CD at 5%	1.82	2.04	1.02	1.22

Figure given in parenthesis are transformed value

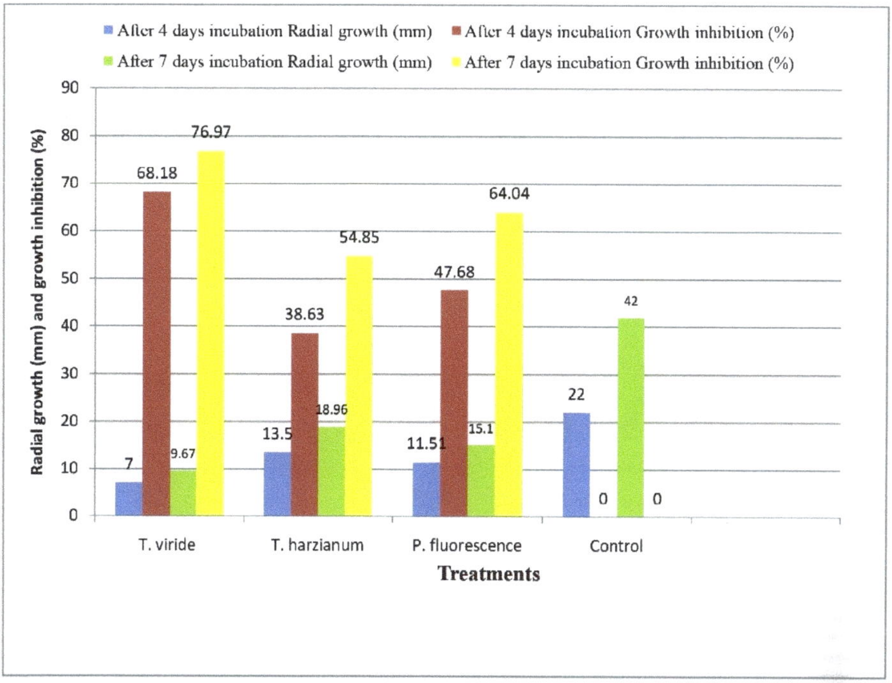

Fig. 2: Effect of Plant extracts against *F. oxysporum* f.sp. *lentis* on radial growth and growth inhibition at 5.0 and 10.0 per cent concentration *in vitro* after 7 days incubation

Table 3: Efficacy of bio-agents against *F. oxysporum* f. sp. *lentis* on radial growth and growth inhibition using dual culture technique after 4 and 7 days incubation

Fungal antagonism	After 4 days incubation		After 7 days incubation	
	Radial growth (mm)	Growth inhibition(%)	Radial growth (mm)	Growth inhibition(%)
T. viride	7.00	68.18 (55.61)	9.67	76.97 (61.27)
T. harzianum	13.50	38.63 (38.41)	18.96	54.85 (47.75)
P. fluorescence	11.51	47.68 (43.62)	15.10	64.04 (53.13)
Control	22.0	00.00	42.0	00.00
SEm±	0.88	0.80	0.64	0.32
CD at 5%	2.89	2.62	2.09	1.05

Figure given in parenthesis are transformed value

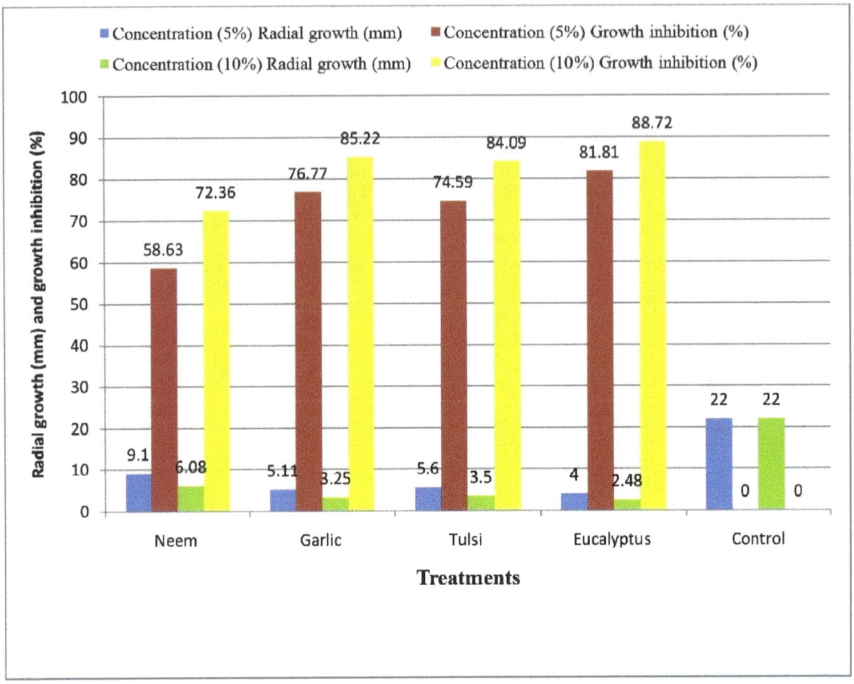

Fig. 3: Effect of bio-agents against *F. oxysporum* .fsp. *lentis* using dual culture technique after 4 and 7 days

References

Chaudhary, M.A.; Iliyar, M.B., Intizor-nl-Horsans and Ghoznafar, M.U. (2008). Source of resistance lentil international *Fusarium* wilt nursery (2006-07). *Pak. J. Phytopathology*, 20 (1): 122-124.

Dolatabadi, H.K., Goltapeh, E.M., Mohammadi, N., Rabiey, M., Rohani, N. and Verma, A. (2012). Bio-control potential of root indophytic fungi and *Trichoderma* species against *Fusarium* wilt of lentil under *in vitro* and greenhouse conditions. *J. Arigc. Sci. and Tech.*, 14 (2): 407-420.

Kumar, D., Sharma, M. and Singh, T. (2002). Bio-prospecting of plant extract against seed born *F. oxysporum* f. sp. *udum* in pigeonpea. *Indian J. Pl. Pathol.*, 20 (1&2): 55-57.

Mandhare, V.K. and Suryawanshi, A.V. (2008). Efficacy of some botanicals against. *Fusarium oxysporum* f.sp. *lentis*. causing wilt disease in lentil. *Journal of Food Legumes*, 23 (7): 172-174.

Mehta, A.N., Chauhan, H.L., Makwara, K.V., Ghel, N.M. and Patel, S.L. (2010). Bio-efficacy of phyto-extract, antagonist and fungicides against *Fusarium udum* incident of pigeonpea wilt. *Arigc. Sci. and Tech.*, 5 (1): 56-60.

Singh, R. and Rai, B. (2000). Antifungal potential of some higher plants against *F. udum* causing wilt disease of *Cajanus Cajan*. *Microbes*,102:165-173.

Sinha, R.K.P. and Sinha, B.B.P. (2004). Effect of potash, botanicals and fungicides against wilt disease complex in lentil. *Ann. Pl. Protec. Sc.,* 12 (2): 454-455.

Upadhyay, J. P. and Mukhopadhyay A. N. (1986). Biological control of *Sclerotium rolfsii* by *Trichoderma harzianum* in chickpea. *Tropical Pest Management,* 32: 215-220.

Well, H.D. (1988). *Trichoderma* as a biological agent. In: Biocontrol of Plant disease, vol. 1, (Eds., K. G. Mukherji and K. L. Garg), CRC Press Inc., Boca Raton, Florida, USA. p 71-82.

4

Screening of Lentil (*Lens Culinaris Medikus* sub sp. *Culinaris*) Genotypes Against Fusarium wilt (*Fusarium Oxysporum* f.sp. *lentis*)

Subhash Chandra, Gireesh Chand*, V.P. Chaudhary Ajay Kumar and Pankaj Kumar**

***Department of Entomology, N.D. University of Agriculture & Technology Kumarganj, Faizabad-224229, Uttar Pradesh, India*
**Department of Plant Pathology, Bihar Agriculture University, Sabour, Bihar India*

Abstract

Fusarium wilt is major disease in Central India, the major lentil growing region of country. The disease is soil borne causing heavy loss, development of wilt resistant varieties is most effective means of controlling this disease. Highly resistant sources of wilt in lentil have not been reported from the Indian lentil breeding programme. One hundred thirty lentil genotypes including one susceptible check were evaluated in control conditions of green house against wilt, based on controlled condition screening- LL 1370, IPL 333, PL4, RLG 195, RVL 14-4, L 4737, RKL 607-1, WBL 77, LL 1320, LL 1397, VL 525, LL1379, VL526, RVL14-5, L4717, VL126, L4076, RLG191 and VL150 have been identified as highly resistant genotypes. These can be used in hybridization programme for wilt resistance breeding and studying the inheritance of wilt resistance in lentil.

Keywords: *Fusarium oxysporum* f.sp. *lentis*, screening, resistant, susceptible

Introduction

Lentil (*Lens culinaris* Medic.) is one of the most important and oldest crop that originated in near east and Mediterranean region. It was known to ancient in Egypt and Greece. Lentil remains stable in Middle Eastern and Indian diets, and popular throughout the world. Pulses are restoring soil fertility through fix atmospheric nitrogen in symbiotic association with root nodule bacterium (*Rhizobium*). It is important source of protein, high in fiber content and provides ample quantity of vitamins and minerals. Lentil is recognized as one of the most nutritious pulse crop ranking next to chickpea amongst *rabi* pulses. Dehuled lentil seed contain 24-26 % protein, 3.2 % fiber and 57-60 % carbohydrate, 1.3 % total fat etc. It is a rich source of minerals containing 69 mg calcium, 300 mg phosphorus and 7 mg Iron per 100 g of seed. It is also rich in 10-15 mg vitamin C, (450 IU) vitamin A, and 9 % riboflavin (Ali and Mishra, 2000).

The total area under lentil in India was 1.49 mha with a total production of 1.61 mt and 1006 Kg/ha productivity (Anonymous, 2017-18). In Utter Pradesh, it is grown on 4.78 lakh hacter area with 4.8 million tonnes production and productivity 936 kg/ha (Anonymous, 2017-18). In India, lentil is mostly grown in northern plains zone, central zone and eastern zone. The major lentil producing states are Madhya Pradesh, Uttar Pradesh, Bihar, Uttarakhand and Bengal. It is grown as a *Rabi* crop or winter crop in India and sown from October to November. However, yield of lentil remains low due to biotic and abiotic stresses. Biotic stresses such as *Fusarium* wilt (*Fusarium oxysporum* f.sp. *lentis*), (Kumar *et al.*, 2013) affect lentil and cause severe yield loss. In India, the incidence of this disease has been reported at seedling, flowering and podding stages at temperature 25°C $\pm$ 2°C .Disease management is required to ensure the stable lentil production. The most sustainable and effective solution to this problem is the development of resistant cultivars (Bayaa *et al.*, 1995; Kraft *et al.*, 1994). Lentil germplasms can be screened in fields but field screening has limitations such as, confounding effect of drought and other root rot pathogens. Hence screening under controlled conditions in glasshouse is required. Stable sources are required for breeding wilt resistant varieties. Hence this study was carried out with specific objective of identifying lentil genotypes resistant to *Fusarium oxysporum* f.sp. *lentis* through pot screening.

Materials and Methods

One hundred thirty genotypes of lentil including one susceptible check (L 9-12) were obtained from the Department of Genetics and Plant Breeding, N. D. University of Agriculture and Technology, Kumarganj, Faizabad and IIPR, Kalyanpur, Kanpur (U.P.). The genotypes were screened against fusarium wilt in wilt sick pot during 2015/16 crop season. Screening under controlled condition was carried out at N. D. University of Agriculture and Technology, Kumarganj, Faizabad. Screening for resistance to lentil wilt. The genotypes will be screened through pot screening techniques in green house using the method by (Nene *et al.*, 1982). The seeds were superficially sterilized in 3% sodium hypochlorite for 3 min, then washed in sterile water and then germinated in towel paper for 10 days. Inoculum of pure culture of *Fusarium oxysporum*, isolated from naturally wilt infected lentil plants was used for multiplication. Single spore culture of *F. oxysporum* was multiplied on 100 g of 9:1 sand lentil meal medium for 15 days at 28$\pm$2 f C. Two hundred gram of these inoculums was mixed well with 2 kg autoclaved soil and placed in one 20 cm plastic pots. The 10-day-old uprooted seedlings were washed under tap water to remove soil particles. Root tips approximately 0.5 cm long were cut to facilitate the entry of pathogen in roots. The roots of the seedlings were then immersed in the spore suspension (5 × 106 conidia ml-1) for 5 min to enable conidia to stick to the roots. Inoculated seedlings were transplanted into a mixture of equal parts of sterile soil, sand, peat and per liter which had been potted and pre-irrigated 2 days previously. Seedlings were irrigated after their planting in pots, and incubated at 25 ± 2°C. The appearance of disease symptoms, the percentage of dead plants was recorded following the method proposed by Bayaa and Erskine (1990). In this study lentil genotypes were screened for resistance to fusarium wilt under controlled conditions. Several accessions with high level of resistance under controlled conditions were identified. The genotypes used in this study along with their origin are listed in Table 1.

Table 1: List of lentil genotypes used for screening:

Name of genotypes
LL 1370, IPL 333, PL4, RLG 195, RVL 14-4, L4737, RKL 607-1, WBL 77, JL3, KLS218. LL1320, LL1397, VL525, LL1379, VL526, RVL14-5, L4717, VL126, L4076, RLG191, VL150, RKL1003-24C, L4726, PL220, L4764, L4735, IPL534, DPL15, BPL15, RL3-5,KLS 09-5, IPL 321, L 4711, IPL 219, IPL 215, L 4076, IPL 315, IPL 324, IPL 513, IPL 316, IPL 526, IPL 220, IPL 225, PL-129, LL-1231, RLS 113, L-4707, L-4588, VL-142, VL- 143, RLG 147, RVL13-7, IPL227, NDL14-22, LL1318, JL3, KLS218, VL 148, LL 151, LL 1375, PL 213, L 4769, L 4147, L 4751, LL 1374, PL 194, DL 14-2, L 4771, K 75, NDL 12-1, K-75, IPL 529, RLG-109, VL-138, PL024, TRCL-1, KLS 14-23, PL 406, LH 84-8, L 4755, PL 210, IPL 406, L 4727, NDL 12-1, KLB 343, IPL-533, NDL 11-2. NDL-7-401, NDL 6-1-10, RLG- 73, IPL-314, VL-133, LL-1020, L-4589, LH 07-27, L-4595, IPL-325, PLO-98, LL 1404, L 4710 , IPL 326, IPL 222, LL 1161, RLG 156, IPL 533, IPL 406, DPL 15, IPL-219, IPL-406, IPL-81, LL1210, PL-101, PL-104, VL- 521, LH-484-8, LH 08-10, NDL-11-1, L-4591, DPL-62, KLB102, LL 1255, NDL 12-2, SKUL 9, RKL 604-5, IPL 529, LL 1203, L 9-12. IPL 220, IPL 325, IPL 221, KLS 113, RLG 147.

After germination, observations, were recorded regularly fort night interval from first disease symptoms Appear of wilt symptoms and severity. The disease was recorded using 1- 9 disease rating scale.

Results and Discussion

The studied genotypes were rated on rating scale (1-9). Rating Scale Reaction [Wilt incidence per cent] 1- 1% or less plants wilted Resistant 3- 2-10% plants wilted Moderately Resistant 5- 11-20% plants wilted Moderately Susceptible 7- 21-50% plants wilted Susceptible and 9 Above 50% plants wilted Highly Susceptible. The uniform distributions of inoculum in sick pots were evident from 90% mortality of L 9-12 (infector row). Out of 130 genotypes screened, nineteen genotypes LL 1370, IPL 333, PL 4, RLG 195, RVL 14-4, L 4737, RKL 607-1, WBL 77, LL 1320, LL 1397, VL 525, LL 1379, VL 526, RVL 14-5, L 4717, VL 126, L 4076, RLG 191 and VL 150 were showed the resistance expression while twenty four genotypes RKL 1003-24C, L 4726, PL 220, L 4764, L 4735, IPL 534, DPL 15, BPL 15, RL 3-5,KLS 09-5, IPL 321, L 4711, IPL 219, IPL 215, L 4076, IPL 315, IPL 324, IPL 513, IPL 316, IPL 526, IPL 220, IPL 225, PL 129 and LL 1231 exhibited moderate resistant reaction against *Fusarium* wilt of lentil. Whereas twenty six genotypes RLS 113, L-4707, L-4588, VL-142, VL- 143, RLG 147, RVL13-7, IPL227, NDL14-22, LL1318, JL3, KLS218. VL 148, LL 151, LL 1375, PL 213, L 4769, L 4147, L 4751, LL 1374, PL 194, DL 14-2, L 4771, K 75, NDL 12-1 and IPL 529. expressed the moderate susceptible reaction, while twenty eight genotypes K-75, RLG-109, VL-138, PL 024, TRCL 1, KLS 14-23, PL 406, LH 84-8, L 4755, PL 210, IPL 406, L 4727, NDL 12-1, KLB 343, IPL 533, NDL 11-2. NDL 401, NDL 6-1-10, RLG 73, IPL 314, VL 133, LL 1020, L 4589, LH 07-27, L 4595, IPL 325, PLO 98 and LL 1404. were revealed susceptibility to Fusarium wilt and rest genotypes L 4710, IPL 326, IPL 222, LL 1161, RLG 156, IPL 533, IPL 406, DPL 15, IPL-219, IPL-406, IPL-81, LL1210, PL-101, PL-104, VL- 521, LH-484-8, LH 08-10, NDL-11-1, L-4591, DPL-62, KLB102, LL 1255, NDL 12-2, SKUL 9, RKL 604-5, IPL 529, LL 1203, L 9-12. IPL 220, IPL 325, IPL 221, KLS 113, RLG 147 were expressed highly susceptible reaction against the Fusarium wilt of lentil. The present results also endorse the findings of Agrawal, *et al.* 1993. Kambj *et al.* (1990) reported 3 genotypes viz. pant L-234, JK- 446 and LP-286, resistant to *Fusarium oxysporum* f. sp. *lentis* screened one hundred fifty varieties of lentil in pots at Kota, Rajasthan, for 3 years for resistance to *Fusarium* wilt none of the variety was found completely free from infection. Kaur and sharma (1995) and Pouralibaba *et al.,* (2008) evaluated 32 lentil promising line in glasshouse. He found two resistant cultivar like ILL6037 and ILL7531. Development of wilt resistant lentil lines was attempted by mutation with gamma rays. Rafique, (2016) tested 23 germplasm and cultivars for *In vitro* for host resistance by root dip method revealed five cultivars viz. Markaz-09, Masoor-86, Masoor-2006, Punjab Masoor-00518 and Punjab Masoor-09 found resistant.

The significant information about host-pathogen biology and interaction is necessary for successful screening. The use of green house screening help in identification and selection of donors for wilt resistance. The screened resistance genotypes would have immense potential for use as resistance sources for breeding wilt resistant lentil varieties and cloning of the resistant genes through differential display expression analysis in future research programs.

Table 2: Performance of Lentil genotypes against *Fusarium oxysporum* f.sp. *lentis* under wilt sick pot during *rabi* crop season 2015-16:

Rating scale	Reaction	No. of genotypes	Name of genotypes
1.	Resistance (≤1%)	19	LL 1370, IPL 333, PL4, RLG 195, RVL 14-4, L4737, RKL 607-1, WBL 77, LL1320, LL1397, VL525, LL1379, VL526, RVL14-5, L4717, VL126, L4076, RLG191, VL150.
3	Moderately Resistance (2-10%)	24	RKL1003-24C, L4726, PL220, L4764, L4735, IPL534, DPL15, BPL15, RL3-5,KLS 09-5, IPL 321, L 4711, IPL 219, IPL 215, L 4076, IPL 315, IPL 324, IPL 513, IPL 316, IPL 526, IPL 220, IPL 225, PL-129, LL-1231,
5	Moderately Susceptible (11-50 %)	26	RLS 113, L-4707, L-4588, VL-142, VL- 143, RLG 147, RVL13-7, IPL227, NDL14-22, LL1318, JL3, KLS218. VL 148, LL 151, LL 1375, PL 213, L 4769, L 4147, L 4751, LL 1374, PL 194, DL 14-2, L 4771, K 75, NDL 12-1, IPL 529.
7	Susceptible (11-50 %)	28	K-75, RLG-109, VL-138, PL024, TRCL-1, KLS 14-23, PL 406, LH 84-8, L 4755, PL 210, IPL 406, L 4727, NDL 12-1, KLB 343, IPL-533, NDL 11-2. NDL-7-401, NDL 6-1-10, RLG- 73, IPL-314, VL-133, LL-1020, L-4589, LH 07-27, L-4595, IPL-325, PLO-98, LL 1404.
9	Highly susceptible (>50 %)	33	L 4710, IPL 326, IPL 222, LL 1161, RLG 156, IPL 533, IPL 406, DPL 15, IPL-219, IPL-406, IPL-81, LL1210, PL-101, PL-104, VL- 521, LH-484-8, LH 08-10, NDL-11-1, L-4591, DPL-62, KLB102, LL 1255, NDL 12-2, SKUL 9, RKL 604-5, IPL 529, LL 1203, L 9-12. IPL 220, IPL 325, IPL 221, KLS 113, RLG 147.

References

Agrawal, S.C., Singh, K. and Lal, S.S. (1993). Plant protection of lentil in India. In: Lentil in South Asia (eds. W. Erskine and M.C. Saxena). ICARDA, Aleppo, Syria. Pp. 147-165.

Ali M., Mishra J.P. (2000). Towards the more efficient use of water and nutrients in food legume cropping *J. of Plant Nutrition* 18: 1391–1402.

Anonymous (2013). Project Coordinators Report, Annual Group Meet, *Rabi* 14-15 septembar. All India Coordinator Report on Mullarp, IIPR, Kanpur. pp. 21.

Anonymous (2018). Project Coordinators Report, Annual Group Meet, *Rabi* 14-15 September. All India Coordinator Report on Mullarp, IIPR, Kanpur. pp. 23.

Bayaa, B. and Erskine, W. (1990). Screening technique for resistance to vascular wilt in lentil. *Arab J. Plant Prot.*, 8: 30-33.

Bayaa, B., Erskine,W. and Hamdi, A. (1995). Evaluation of a wild lentil collection for resistance to vascular wilt. Genet. Resour. *Crop Evol.*, 42 : 231-235.

Kamboj, R.K., Pandey, M.P. and Chaube, H.S. (1990). Inheritances of resistance of Fusarium wilt in Indian Lentil germplasm (*Lens culinaris* Medik.). *Euphytica*, 50 (2): 113-117.

Kaur, A. and Sharma, L. C. (1995). Screening of Lentil varieties against Fusarium wilt. *Indian j. of Mycol. Pl. Pathol.*, 23 (2):172-173.

Kraft, J.M., Haware, M.P., Jim´enez-Diaz, R.M., Bayaa, B. and Harrabi, M. (1994). Screening techniques and sources of resistance to root rots and wilts in cool season food legumes. *Euphytica*.73: 27– 39. .

Kumar, V., Garkoti, A. and Tripathi, H. S. (2013). Management of vascular wilt of lentil through bio control agents and organic amendments in tarai area of Uttarakhand state. *Pak. J. Bot.*, 24 (3): 429-444.

Nene,Y.L., Kannaiyan, J. and Reddy, M.V. (1982). Chickpea resistance screening techniques. Information Bulletin No. 9 ICRISAT, Patancheru, P.O. Andhra Pradesh, India. Pp.3-4.

Rafique, Khola.,Rauf, C. A., Farahulam and Shabbir,ghulam (2016). Management of vascular wilt of lentil through host plant resistance, biological control agents and chemicals. *Pak. J. Bot.* 48 (5) : 2085-2092.

5

Management Approaches for Major Diseases of Chickpea (*Cicer arietinum* L.) and Pigeon pea (*Cajanus Cajan* L. Millsp)

Anil Kumar,[1] Fariha Adan[2] and Thota Gopi Krishna[2] and Gireesh Chand[3]

[1]*Department of Plant Breeding and Genetics, Bihar Agricultural University Sabour-813210, Bihar, India*
[2]*Research Scholars, Department of Plant Breeding and Genetics Bihar Agricultural University, Sabour-813210, Bihar, India*
[3]*Department of Plant Pathology, Bihar Agricultural University Sabour-813210, Bihar, India*

Abstract

Chickpea is one of the major grain legume crops of the tropics and sub-tropics. It is the second most important pulse crop after pigeon pea in India and is commonly known as gram or Bengal gram is a versatile crop among the grain legumes with a total production of 11.6 (Mt) from 13.2m ha. However, it ranks fifth in the productivity after Fababean, pea, lupin, and lentil and ranks first among the pulses both in acreage and production. Whereas, area under pigeon pea 3.90 mha with a total production and productivity of 2.89 mt and 741 kg/ha, respectively and is commonly known as red gram or Arhar is a very old crop of India. The chromosome number of pigeon pea is 2n = 22 chromosomes. They are the rich source of protein and supplies a major share of the protein requirement of the vegetarian population of the country. Chickpea accounts for 70.7% of the world Chickpea production n India followed by Australia, Pakistan, Turkey, Myanmar, Ethiopia, Iran USA, Canada and Mexico. Both crops are used as an important source of protein in human nutrition and cattle feed.

Chickpea is considered to have medicinal effects and it is used for blood purification. Chickpea contains 21% protein, 61.5% carbohydrate, 4.5% fat. Its seed is also rich in protein, starch, fiber, calcium, iron and niacin, malic and oxalic acid, which makes it one of the best nutritionally balanced pulses for human consumption. However, like any other pulses, the chickpea seed also contains antinutrional factors, which can be reduced or eliminated by cooking. Both crops enrich the soil fertility by fixing atmospheric nitrogen in the root nodules and improve the soil structure. It is also to improve soil fertility by biological nitrogen fixation which helps reduce the input cost for the existing crop. These crops usually receive few inputs other than labor, insecticides and seed. Chickpea is a crop of both tropical and temperate regions. Low yield of chickpea attributed to its susceptibility to several fungal, bacterial and viral diseases. In general, estimates of yield losses by individual insects and diseases range from 5 to 10% in temperate regions and 50 to 100% in tropical regions. Whereas, Pigeon pea can be attacked by more than 100 pathogens. These include fungi, bacteria, viruses, nematodes, and mycoplasma like organisms. Fortunately, only a few of them cause economic losses and the distribution of the most important diseases is geographically restricted. The diseases of considerable economic importance at present are Fusarium wilt, sterility mosaic, phytopthera blight and alternaria blight.

Keywords: *Fusarium wilt, sterility mosaic, blight, bacterial and viral diseases*

Introduction

Chickpea (*Cicer arietinum* L.) is the second most important crop after beans, commonly known as gram or Bengal gram is a versatile crop among the grain legumes with a total production of 11.6 (Mt) from 13.2m ha. However, it ranks fifth in the productivity after Fababean, pea, lupin, and lentil and ranks first among the pulses both in acreage and production. India accounts for 70.7% of the world Chickpea production followed by Australia (4.4%), Pakistan (4.3%), Turkey (4.2%), Myanmar (4.0%), Ethiopia (2.8%), Iran (2.5%), USA (0.84%), Canada (0.78%), and Maxico (0.62%) (FAO, 2011). It is used as an important source of protein in human nutrition and cattle feed. Chickpea is considered to have medicinal effects and it is used for blood purification. It contains 21% protein, 61.5% carbohydrate, 4.5% fat. Its seed is also rich in protein, starch, fiber, calcium, iron and niacin, malic and oxalic acid, which makes it one of the best nutritionally balanced pulses for human consumption (Jukanti *et al.*, 2012). However, like any other pulses, the it's seed also contains antinutrional factors, which can be reduced or elimi-nated by cooking. It's enriches the soil fertility by fixing atmospheric nitrogen 141 kg/ha (Rupela, 1987) in the root nodules and improves the soil structure (Asthana and Chaturvedi, 1999). It also improve soil fertility by biological nitrogen fixation which helps reduce the input cost for the existing crop and. Chickpea usually receives few inputs other than labor, insecticides and seed. Chickpea is a crop of both tropical and temperate regions. The two distinct forms of cultivated chickpeas are Desi (small seeds, angular ram's head shape, and colored with high percentage of fiber) and Kabuli (large-seeds, irregular rounded, owl's- head shape, and beige colored seeds with low percentage of fiber) types. Kabuli type is grown in temperate regions while the Desi type chickpea grown in the semi-arid tropics. Low yield of chickpea attributed to its susceptibility to several fungal, bacterial and viral diseases. In general, estimates of yield losses by individual insects and diseases range from 5 to 10% in temperate regions and 50 to 100% in tropical regions (Van Emden *et al.*, 1988). While in case of pigeon pea [*Cajanus cajan* (L.) Millspaugh], it is one of the major food legume crops of the tropics and sub-tropics. In India, after chickpea, pigeon pea is the second most important pulse crop. India has largest area under pigeon pea 3.90mha with a total production and productivity of 2.89 mt and 741 kg/ha, respectively (DAC, 2011). Pigeon pea commonly known as red gram or arhar is a very old crop of this country. The chromosome number of pigeon pea is 2n = 22 chromosomes. It is a rich source of protein and supplies a major share of the protein requirement of the vegetarian population of the country. Pigeon pea can be attacked by more than 100 pathogens. These include fungi, bacteria, viruses, nematodes, and mycoplasma-like organisms. Fortunately, only a few of them cause economic losses and the distribution of the most important diseases is geographically restricted. At present farmers mainly grow pigeon pea landraces and it is possible that they have some degree of tolerance to most of the pathogens. This situation could change once the diverse landraces are replaced by a few improved cultivars. The diseases of considerable economic importance at present are Fusarium wilt, sterility mosaic, phytopthera blight and alternaria blight.

I. Fusarium Wilt

Chickpea production is severely affected by Fusarium wilt caused by Fusarium oxysporum (Schlechtend.:Fr.) f. sp. ciceris (Padwick) Matuo & K. Sato, in most chickpea growing areas of the world which cause annual chickpea yield losses vary from 10 to 15% (Jalali and Chand, 1992). In India, wilt alone causes on an average 10% loss annually and is prevalent in all chickpea growing states (Singh and Dahiya, 1973). In Bihar, it ranges from 2 to 20%. However, it was observed that early wilting causes 77–94% losses while late wilting causes 24–65% loss (Haware and Nene, 1980). It causes complete loss in grain yield if the disease occurs in the vegetative and reproductive stages of the crop (Haware and Nene, 1980; Haware *et al.*, 1990; Halila and Strange, 1996; Navas *et al.*, 2000).

Symptomatology

The disease manifests as mortality of young seedlings (within 25–30 days after sowing) to wilting or death of adult plants. Seedlings that die due to wilt disease can be confused with other diseases of wilt complex, if not examined carefully. Fusarium wilt infected seedlings collapse and lie flaton the ground retaining their dull green color. Adult plants show typical wilt symptoms of drooping of petioles, rachis and leaflets. All the leaves turn yellow and then light brown. The roots of the wilting plants do not show any external rotting but when split open vertically, dark brown discoloration of internal xylem is seen. Vascular discoloration is observed on longitudinal splitting of stem. Seeds harvested from wilted plants were lighter and duller than those from healthy plants (Haware and Nene, 1980).

Causal Organism

The fungus produces white to light orange aerial mycelium and sporodochia on incubated seed. The mycelium is profusely branched, covers the entire seed and is white to light pink in color. Sporodochia are rarely produced, but if present, the aerial mycelium completely covers it. Microconidia are abundant, and are produced on short, unbranched (microconidiophores) in small, dry, false heads. Microconidia are hyaline, single celled, over to cylindrical straight to slightly curved, and measuring 2.5 to 3.5 × 5 to 11 μ in size. Macroconidia are fewer then microconidia and produced on branched macroconidiophores. They are fusoid with pointed ends, hyaline, have 3 to 5 septa and measure 3.5 to 4.5 × 25 to 65μ. Chlamydospores are usually intercalary and are produced singly in pairs or in chains. They are globose to sub-globose, thick walled and smooth surfaced. Chlamydospores like swellings are often seen also on the hyphae.

Disease Cycle and Epidemiology

The Fusarium wilt is soil and internally seed borne disease, facultative saprophyte and can survive in soil more than 6 years in the absence of susceptible host (Haware *et al.*, 1986). Haware *et al.* (1982) showed the fungus to be in the helium of the seed in the form of chlamydospore like structures. The primary infection is through chlamydospores or mycelia. The conidia of the fungus are short lived; however, the chlamydospores can remain viable upto next crop season. Plant species other than chickpea may serve as symptomless carriers of the disease. Gupta (1991) reported *Vigna radiata, V. mungo, Cajanus cajan, Pisum sativum* and *Lens culinaris* as symptomless carriers of the disease. The pathogen may also parasitize several weeds such as *Cyperus rotendus, Tribulus terrestris, Convolvulus arvensis* and *Cardiospermum halicacabum* (Nene *et al.*, 1980). The soil type, reaction, moisture and temperature are known to influence disease development. Rachana *et al.* (2002)

reported that black soil support highest wilt incidence (75.5%). Wilt incidence in sandy-loam, red and clay soil was found to be 64.4, 59.9 and 46.6%, respectively. According to Sugha *et al.* (1994b) soil temperature in the range of 24.8–28.5°C and soil moisture above 25% within the water holding capacity of soil were most conducive for chickpea wilt. Below 17°C, infection remains restricted in the root without any wilt symptoms. The importance of the soil temperature has also been substantiated by the observation that late sowing of the crop reduces the incidence of the disease.

Management of Disease

Deep ploughing during summer and removal of host debris from the field reduces inoculum levels. The soil inoculum can be reduced by addition of 15–20 tons of farmyard manure with Trichoderma sp. @ 4–5 kg/ha before sowing (Singh and Dubey, 2007). Seed dressing with benlate T (Benomyl + thiram) eradicated seed borne inoculum (Haware *et al.*, 1978). The disease can be managed by seed treatment with various seed dressing fungicides. Two years field data clearly indicates that seed treatment with Bavistin + thiram (1:1) @ 2.5 g/kg seed before sowing decreased seedling mortality 7% and increased seed germination 11.2% and grain yield 2.8 Q/ha (Pal and Singh, 1993). The filamentous fungi, Trichoderma have attracted the attention because of their multiprong action against various plant pathogens (Harman *et al.*, 2004). The species of Trichoderma have been evaluated against the wilt pathogen and have exhibited greater potential in managing chickpea wilt under glasshouse and field conditions (Kaur and Mukhopadhayay, 1992). Earlier, Padwick (1941) also observed that a species of Trichoderma was highly antagonistic to wilt pathogen of chickpea. Mane (1995) isolated and evaluated 88 different fungal and bacterial agents against F. oxysporum f. sp. ciceris and four isolates of Trichoderma spp., three isolates of fluorescent Pseudomonas, one isolate of Acrophilophora sp. and three isolates of *Gliocladium* spp. showed antagonistic activity *in vitro*. Under field conditions, maximum wilt reduction (28.3%) in cultivar Pusa 256 was observed when T. viride was applied as seed coating with talc as carrier with gum.(Nikam *et al.*, 2007) tested four oilseed cakes and observed that groundnut cake followed by neem seed and castor cake were found to be most effective in checking percent wilt incidence by 61.91, 52.39 and 47.62%, respectively as against control. Haware *et al.*, 1978 reported seed-borne inoculum can be eradicated by seed dressing with Benlate (benomyl 30% + thiram 30%) at 0.25% rate. Nikam *et al.*, 2007 revealed that foliar sprays of thiram followed by carbendazim and captan proved to be effective in checking the wilt incidence by 42.46, 38.10 and 33.34%, respectively as against control (100% wilting). Kolte *et al.* (1998) effectively controlled chickpea wilt with seed treatment by Rhizobium, *T. viride*, *T. harzianum* and Azotobactor sp.The identification and use of host plant resistance has the great potential in the long-term management of wilt. The genotypes H99–9, Pusa 212, JG 315, JG 322, PCS 1(Sel.ICCV-11), PCS 2 (Sel.KPG 142–1), PCS 5 (Sel.BGD-112), and PCS 6 (Sel. Pusa- 1073) showed resistant (<10% wilt incidence) reaction during 3 years (2001–2004) were deposited to Gene Bank, NBPGR, New Delhi with ACC No. 405202–405209 (Dubey and Singh, 2004). In addition to these a large number of wilt resistant cultivars namely Avrodhi, Haryana Channa 1, BGD 72, BGM 547, GNG 469 (Samrat), GNG 663 (Vardan), RSG 693 (Aadhar), KPG-59 (Uday), K 3256 (Pragati), Phule G-87207 (Vishal), Phule G 9425–9, JG 322, GPF 2, PBG 1, Pusa 372 and Pusa 1053 (Chamtkar) were identified. The resistance to wilt for race 2 in WR 315 is controlled by a single recessive gene (Sharma *et al.*, 2005). Tullu *et al.* (1998) reported single recessive gene for resistance to race 4 and identified a RAPD marker linked with resistance.

II. Dry Root Rot

Dry root rot of chickpea has been reported from India, Iran, Australia, Ethiopia, Pakistan, Spain and USA. Wilt and dry root rot diseases alone affecting the productivity of chickpea, 5–20% loss in yields (Singh, 2010). Rhizoctonia bataticola is a polyphagous soil borne pathogen infecting over 500 plant species worldwide causing huge losses. Dry root rot disease of chickpea is caused by Rhizoctonia bataticola (Taub) Butler = Macrophomina phaseolina (Maubl.) Ashby. It has been reported from Australia, Ethopia, California, India, Iran, Lebaonan, Maxico Pakistan, Syria and Turkey (Allen, 1983 and Nene, 1979).The fungus lacks fruiting bodies and spores. The mycelium is light-brown, thick in which black sclerotia are formed. Sclerotia are variable in form, small and loosely connected by mycelial threads

Symptomatology

The first symptom of the disease is yellowing of the leaves within a day or two; such leaves drop and in the course of the next two or three days, and plant showed completely dried symptoms within a week after the appearance of the first symptom. The tissues were weakened and break off easily. The affected roots are dark brown to black and usually dry, unless the soil is wet. The tap root is quite brittle, show shredding of the bark and can be broken easily. If the plant were pulled out from the soil and examined the basal stem and main root system of diseased plant showed extensive rooting with most of the lateral roots destroyed. In advance cases minute dark black sclerotial bodies can be seen on the surface of the root, as well as in the pith. If the plants are pulled from the soil and examined, the basal stem and the main roots may show dry rot symptoms.

Disease Cycle And Epidemiology

The fungus is seed and soil-borne, facultative parasite and may survive in the soil in the form of sclerotia for long time (Dingra and Sinclair, 1994). Soil borne inoculum is more important in causing infection and disease development. It produces pycnidia when the atmospheric temperature is above 30°C and the pycniospores remain viable for over a year. The fungus is mainly a soil-dweller and spreads from plant to plant through irriga-tion water, tools and implements and cultural operations. The sclerotia and pycniospores may also become air borne and cause further spread of the pathogen. The disease appears suddenly when ambient temperatures are between 25 and 30°C.

Management of Disease

Drenching affected plants and the infested soil with Bordeaux mixture or other effective fungicide may help in reducing the inoculums potential. Field sanitation measures, including cutting down the diseased plants and burning them and deep ploughing in summer help to reduce the diseases intensity during the following season. Drought should be avoided. Sowing should always be done on the recommended time. Seed treatment with a mixture of carbendazim 1.5 g and thiram 1.5 g per kg of seed and with Trichoderma viride formulation + 3 g thiram per kg seed can reduce the disease incidence. Nagamani *et al.* (2011) observed that seed treatment with carbendazim @ 2 g/kg of seed+ seed treatment with T. viride @ 4 g/kg of seed +soil application of FYM fortified with T. viride (T7) was found to control root rot. Hence integrated management of the disease using biocontrol agents and chemicals is the best alternative (Ramarethinum *et al.*, 2001).

I. Fusarium Wilt

In India, the infestation occurs in almost every state in which pigeon pea is cultivated, especially in Rajasthan, Maharashtra, Madhya Pradesh, Uttar Pradesh and Bihar. The wilt is also found in many other countries like Kenya, Malawi and Tanzania. The continuous cultivation of pigeon pea in the same area in each year results up to 50% plant mortality due to the disease. In Bihar and U.P., it loss 5–10% of standing crop is common feature every year (Kannaiyan *et al.*, 1984). The disease incidence is high during flowering and pod formation stages.

Symptoms

Symptoms are more pronounced and the damage is greater when the plants have grown up after the rainy season. The susceptible plants are attacked when young (about 5–6 weeks old). The symptoms are variable. Typically the first symptom is the premature yellowing of the leaves. The next symptom is the wilting or withering of the leaves of the diseased plants. Wilting is characterized by gradual, sometimes sudden, yellowing, withering and drying of leaves followed by drying of the entire plant or some of its branches. Patches of diseased plants are scattered throughout the field indicating locations where pathogen is present and infection started. Examination of main root and the base of stem and infected plant after pulling it out from the soil, the blackened longitudinal streaks are seen on the roots. These black streaks represent the vascular bundles of the infected plants plugged with mycelium and fructifications of the fungus. Partial wilting is also common as only one side gets withered.

Causal Organism

The wilt of pigeon pea is caused by *Fusarium udum* Butler. It is facultative parasite and can survive in the soil in the absence of the host through chlamydospores. The mycelium is restricted to the vascular tissues. It is inter and intracellular, hyaline, branched, geniculate and septate. The profuse growth of mycelium within the xylem vessels completely plugged with the lumen of the vessels and thus, the free flow of water is checked resulting in the disease. Mycelium produces spores of three types within host tissues-macroconidia, micro conidia and chlamydospores. The micro conidia are small, elliptical or curved, thin walled, one or two septate and 5–15 × 2–4 µm. The macro conidia are linear, sickle shaped, pointed at both ends, thin walled, 3–4 septate and measures 15–50 × 3–5 µm. The chlamydospores are usually formed in chains within the tissues of the host plant. They are rounded or oval and thick walled and can remain viable for long time.The perfect stage, *Gibberella* indica, described by Rai and Upadhyay (1982), is usually found on exposed roots and collar region of the stem up to the height of 35 cm above the ground level. The mature perithecia are superficial, aggregate, subglobose to globose, sessile, and smooth walled, dark violet, and 350–550 µm in diameter. Asci are 8-spored, mostely sub-cylindrical, 60–80 × 6–10 µm, broader in the middle and, with short stalk, a narrow apex, and a center apical pore. The ascospores are elliptical to ovate, 10–17 × 5–7 µm, hyline, commonly 2-celled, rarely 3–4 celled and constricted at the septa.

Disease Cycle

Fusarium udum is facultative parasite and lives saprophytically in the soil without host for a long time. The fungal pathogen attacks host roots by germ tubes arising from asexual spores and reached in vascular tissues to establish infection. The fungus can be grow and multiply in the vascu-lar tissues, causing partial or complete wilting of the host plant. The host plant is killing within few days or weeks. When the crop is harvested, the plants are cut at the soil level leaving the infected root system and stubble to infest the soil. Being the saprophytic, the fungus continues to grow and multiply in the soil and remain until the next crop season. The fungus can survive at 4.0–9.0 pH and soil temperature of as high as 35 °C. If the crop is growing continuously on the same field, the disease incidence increases each year.

Management of Disease

The Fusarium wilt disease is soil borne in nature; it is difficult to control wilt of pigeon pea like other soil borne fungal diseases. There are several methods to check the severity of the fungal disease. The crop rotation for long duration of 3–5 years help in reducing the virulence of the pathogen even it can live saprophytically in the soil. Mixed cultivation of sorghum or tobacco in the same field followed by pigeon pea reduces the disease severity. Seed treatment with carbendazim may provide protection in the early stage of plant growth. The most effective aspect of disease control is cultivation of disease resistant varieties of pigeon pea like NP 15, ICPL 96058, ICP 4769, ICP 7118, ICP 7035, ICP 7182, ICP 8863, ICP 9168, ICP 10958 and ICP 11299.Amendment of soil with roots of certain leguminous crops (sweet clover), molasses and oil cakes (groundnut cake) markedly increased the antibiotic (bulbiformin) production by *B. subtilis* and a reduction of 88% in the incidence of wilt. Seedlings gained resistance to Fusarium infection when the seeds were inoculated with B. subtilis before sowing. Trichoderma harzianum effectively suppressed fusarium wilt of pigeonpea. At ICRISAT, three genotypes, ICPL 96047, ICPL 96061 and ICPL 96046 were found resistant to fusarium wilt, powdery mildew and phyllody.

II. Sterility Mosaic of Pigeonpea

Sterility mosaic was first reported from Pusa (Bihar) by Mitra (1931). It is also called Green plague of pigeon pea as it is one of the most damaging disease in most of the arhar growing states in the country. The disease is restricted to Asia and has been reported from Bangladesh, Nepal, Thailand, Myanmar and Sri Lanka. In India, this is a serious problem in Uttar Pradesh, Bihar, Gujarat, Karnataka, Tamil Nadu and Andhra Pradesh. In India, alone annual loss of 205,000 tons of grains (worth Rs. 75 crores) is reported by several workers.

Symptoms

The affected crop plants do not die but remain green even after the crop maturity. The disease affected arhar crop looks from distance as a green forage crop standing in the field. Infected plants appear bushy with yellowish green foliage of reduced size and suppression of flowers, and pods. Severe stunting, reduction in leaf size, increased number of secondary and tertiary branches arising from the leaf axils and complete or partial cessation of development of the reproductive structures are also observed. Mainly three types of symptoms are reported:

a. Severe mosaic of leaflets: Plants do not produce flowers and pods.

b. Ring spot, where there is no sterility; this is characterized by green islands surrounded by a chlorotic halo on leaflets. The rings disap-pear as the plants mature.

c. Mild mosaic with partial sterility.

Disease Cycle

Perennial and ratoon pigeon pea plants infected with the disease appear to be the only source of Pigeon pea Sterility Mosaic Virus (PSMV) and its vectors. *A. cajani* is the only vector of PSMV. Besides pigeon pea, these mites have been observed onto common weeds such as *Oxalis circulate* and *Cannabis sativa*. However the role of these two weeds in the survival of the vectors or virus is obscure.

Management of Disease

a. Seed treatment with 10% aldicarb protected the crop till maturity.

b. Uses of insecticides (Phorate, carbofuran and metasystox) as foliar spray were effective for limited period but failed to provide protection as later stage of crop growth.

c. Resistant varieties: Host resistance is the best solution of the problem. Some pigeon pea varieties show the resistance to the sterility mosaic like Bahar, DA-11, DA-33, ICPL-306, Hy-3C, Pusa-9, Pusa-885, Asha, Sharad (DA-11), Narendra-Arhar-1, etc.

References

Agrios, G. N. (2005). Plant Pathology. 5th ed. Elsevier Academic Press, London

Allen, D. J. (1983). The pathology of tropical food legumes. John Wiley and Sons, New York, p413.

Bakr, M. A., Rahman, M. M., Ahmed, F., Kumar, J. (1993). Progress in the manage-ment of Botrytis gray mold of chickpea in Bangladesh. Haware, M. P.; Gowda, C. L.L.; McDonald, D. (eds.). International Crops Research Institute for the Semi-Arid Tropics (ICRISAT). Recent advances in research on Botrytis gray mold of chickpea: summary proceedings of the second Working Group Meeting to discuss collaborative research on Botrytis Gray Mold of Chickpea. Patancheru, A. P. (India). ICRISAT. pp.17–18.

Common Names of Diseases, The American Phytopathological Society Retrieved from "http://en.wikipedia.org/w/index.php?title=List_of_pigeonpea_diseases & oldid=581610763".

DAC. (2011). Fourth advance estimates of production of Food grains for 2010–11. Agricultural statistics division, Directorate of economics and statistics, Department of agriculture and cooperation, Government of India, New Delhi [http://eands.dacnet. nic.in/advance_estimate/3rdadvance_estimates_2010–11 (English)].

FAO. (2011). FAOSTATS. Food and Agriculture Organization of the United Nations, Rome, Italy. http://faostat.fao.org/site/567/default.aspx#ancor (accessed on 4 Apr. 2013).

Haware, M. P. (1998). Diseases of chickpea. In 'The pathology of food and pasture legumes' (eds. D. J. Allen, J. M. Lenne) pp. 473–516. (ICARDA, CAB International: Wallingford, UK).

Haware, M. P., Nene, Y. L. (1980). Influence of wilt at different stages on the yield loss in chickpea. *Trop. Grain Legume Bull.* 19, 38–40.

Haware, M. P., Nene, Y. L. (1982). Plant Dis. 66, 250–251. 22. Jalali, B. L., Chand, H. (1992). Chickpea wilt. Pages 429–444 in: Plant Diseases of International Importance. Vol. 1. Diseases of Cereals and Pulses. U. S. Singh,N. Mukhopadhayay, J. Kumar, and, H. S. Chaube, eds. Prentice Hall, Englewood Cliffs, NJ

Kannaiyan, J., Nene, Y. L., Reddy, M. V., Ryan, J. G., Raju, T. N. (1984). Prevalence of pigeonpea diseases and associated crop losses in Asia, Africa and the Americas. *Trop. Pest Management* 30:62

Kolte, S. O., Thakre, K. G., Gupta, M., Lokhande, V. V. (1998). Biocontrol of *Fusarium* wilt of chickpea (Cicer arietinum) under wilt sick field condition. Paper submitted, ISOPP at National Symposium on management of soil and soil borne diseases. 9–10th Feb., (1998). p22.

Navas-Cortes, J. A., Hau, B., Jimenez-Diaz, R. M. (2000). Yield loss in chickpea in relation to development to Fusarium wilt epidemics. *Phytopathology*, 90:1269–1278.

Nikam, P. S., Jagtap, G. P., Sontakke, P. L. (2007). Management of chickpea wilt caused by Fusarium oxysporium f. sp. Ciceri. *African Journal of Agricultural Research*, 2(12): 692–697

Singh, N. P. (2010). Annual Group Meet, August 29–31, 2010, Project Coordinator's Report, All India Coordinated Research Projects on Chickpea, IIPR, Kanpur, 20–21.

Singh, R. P. (2008). Plant Pathology. 8th ed. Kalyani Publisher, New Delhi

Singh, R. S. (2005). Plant Diseases. 8th ed. Oxford & IBH Publishing Co., New Delhi

6

Efficacy of Micronutrients on Mycelium Growth of *Fusarium oxysporum* sp. cubense Causing Panama Wilt Disease

Ram Niwas, Gireesh Chand and Chandra Shekhar Azad

Department of Plant Pathology, Bihar Agricultural University, Sabour-813210 Bhagalpur, Bihar, India

Abstract

The major losses of banana at present by Panama wilt disease pathogen of banana and its management is very typical because it is caused by a soil-borne pathogen (Fusarium oxysporum f.sp. cubense). *The micronutrients are used to manage the disease as well as it provides the healthiness of plant and increases the fertility of the soil that's why the plant is free from the disease or less infected. An experiment of micronutrients was conducted in the laboratory of plant pathology BAU, Sabour for* In-vitro *evaluation of the micronutrients* viz. *Zinc Sulfate, Ferrous Sulfate, Ammonium Sulfate, Copper Sulfate, Calcium Nitrate, Borax and Potassium Chloride against Fusarium oxysporum* f.sp. cubense *causing Panama wilt of banana. The results of the experiment revealed that among the micronutrients used, Borax @ 500 and 750 ppm completely inhibited the mycelial growth of FOC followed by Zinc Sulfate (45.7, 42.6, 39.2 and 18.5 mm at 100, 250, 500 and 750 ppm respectively). The incorporation of borax in the solid medium at higher concentrations* viz., *500 and 750 ppm is very effective for the management of Panama wilt disease of banana. This approach leads to maintain our ecosystem sustainability for a longer time and manage the disease.*

***Keywords*:** Banana, *Fusarium*, Micronutrients, Sustainable management

Introduction

Banana is one of the most important food crops after wheat, rice, and maize in the world. To meet the growing food needs of the increasing population in the country and there is a need to raise Banana productivity. In order to the needs of the escalating population, banana production needs to be doubled and estimated pro-duction requirement by 2020 is around 25 million tons (Annon, 1996). Efforts for enhancing productivity are limited by a number of biotic and abiotic stresses. The crop suffers from a number of devastating diseases caused by fungi, bacteria, viruses, nematodes, and a number of environmental factors. Among all these diseases, Panama disease is also known as *Fusarium* wilt or vascular wilt incited by *Fusarium oxysporum* f.sp. *cubense* (E.F. Smith) Snyd. And Hans. In this context, the present study has been undertaken with the aim of managing *Fusarium oxysporum* f. sp *cubense* with micronutrients.

Material and Methods

Potato Dextrose Agar (PDA) medium was mixed with different micronutrients viz., zinc sulfate, ferrous sulfate, ammonium sulfate, copper sulfate, calcium nitrate, borax and potassium chloride at four different concentrations viz., 100, 250, 500 and 750 ppm (weight /volume) and they were tested on the mycelial growth of *Fusarium oxysporum* f. sp. *cubense* using by poisoned food technique following the procedure of Schmitz, (1930) the suitable control was also maintained without mixing any nutrients.

The PDA medium was mixed with borax at four different concentrations *viz.,* 100, 250, 500 and 750 ppm. The amended medium was poured into sterilized Petri plate @ 20 ml/plate. The fungicides are mixed in PDA media before pouring in the 90 mm Petri-plates. The 5 mm bits of pathogen are cut with a cork borer and put in the center of the plates after solidifying the medium. The percent inhibition growth was calculated using below-mentioned formula.

I= C-T/Cx100

Where,

I = Inhibition percentage;

C = Colony diameter in control (mm)

T = Colony diameter in treatment

Table 1: Effect of certain micro nutrients on the mycelial growth of *Fusarium oxysporum* f. sp. *cubense*

Sl.No	Micronutrients	Mycelial growth (mm)				Percent inhibition			
		100 ppm	250 ppm	500 ppm	750 ppm	100 ppm	250 ppm	500 ppm	750 ppm
1.	Calcium Nitrate	85.02	82.18	77.84	74.50	5.53	8.69	13.51	17.22
2.	Ammonium Sulphate	84.30	82.18	77.70	71.74	6.33	8.69	13.67	20.29
3.	Calcium Sulphate	80.08	79.20	71.52	66.90	11.02	12.00	20.53	25.67
4.	Potassium Chloride	73.36	75.04	69.36	67.38	18.49	16.62	22.93	25.13
5.	Borax	73.56	14.66	2.90	0.00	18.27	83.71	96.78	100.00
6.	Ferrous Sulphate	46.00	45.76	40.82	35.86	48.89	49.16	54.64	60.16
7.	Zinc Sulphate	45.70	42.60	39.20	18.50	49.22	52.67	56.44	79.44
8.	Control	90.00	-	-	-	-	-	-	-
	CD(p=0.05)	2.98	2.29	2.23	1.50	-	-	-	-

Results and Discussion

The experiment was conducted to find out the effect of different concentration of micronutrients on the mycelial growth of *Fusarium oxysporum* f. sp. *cubense* causing panama wilt of banana (Table 1). Among the seven micronutrients tested, (calcium nitrate, ammonium sulphate, copper sulphate, potassium chloride, borax, ferrous sulphate and zinc sulphate), borax @ 500 ppm and 750 ppm completely inhibited (Plate-1) the growth of *Fusarium oxysporum* f. sp. *cubense* followed by zinc sulphate (45.7, 42.6, 39.2 and 18.5 mm in 100, 250, 500 and 750 ppm, respectively). (Fig-1) The maximum mycelial growth was recorded in ammonium sulphate. Lakpale *et al.* (1997) reported that micronutrients at 750 ppm concentration retarded the mycelial growth of *Rhizoctonia solani* causing sheath blight of paddy.

The micronutrients are used to manage the disease as well as it provides the healthiness of plant and increases the fertility of the soil that's why the plant is free from the disease or less infected. The mechanism of healthiness of plant will be done at micronutrients are applied in the soil and the plant uptake nutrients at their required amount that's why the plant will be very strong resulting the Panama wilt pathogen does not enter into the plant, remain the plants become healthy.

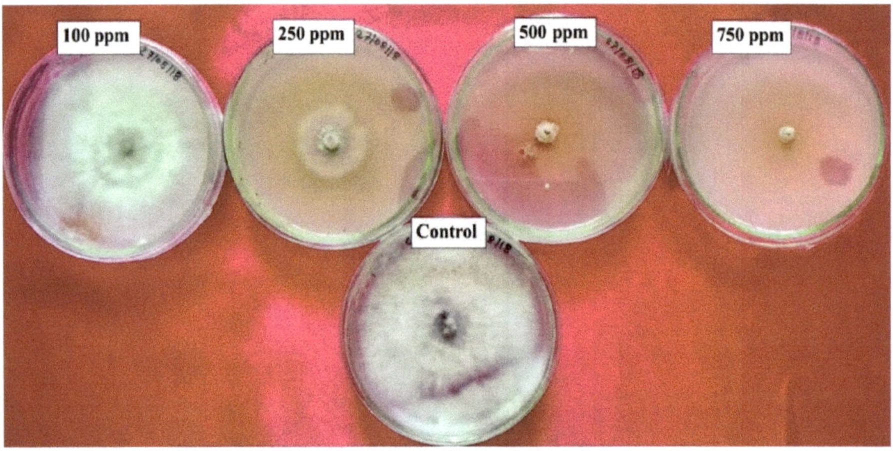

Plate 1: *in-vitro* evalution of Borax against Foc

The mycelial growth of *Fusarium oxysporum* f.sp. *cubense* was find against different microntrientss and finally, we concluded the borax have completely inhibited the growth of *Fusarium oxysporum* f.sp. *cubense in-vitro* that's why the borax will be used for the management of the Panama wilt disease of Banana (Figure 2).

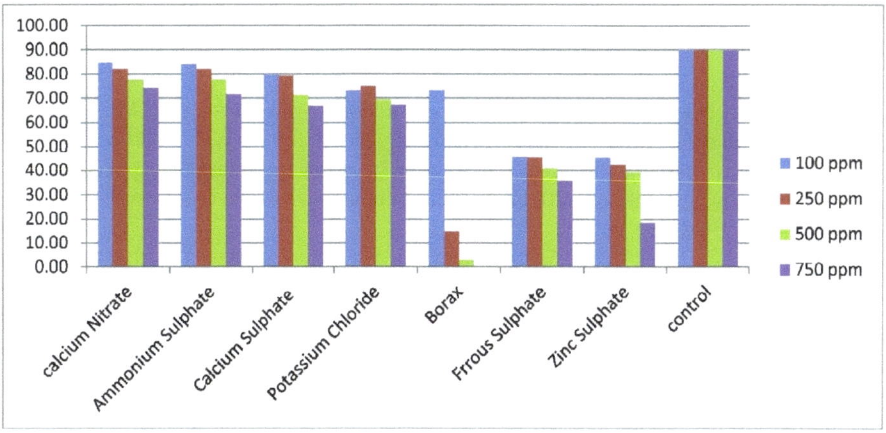

Fig. 1: *Mycelial growth (mm) of Fusarium oxysporum f. sp. cubense against different micronutrients*

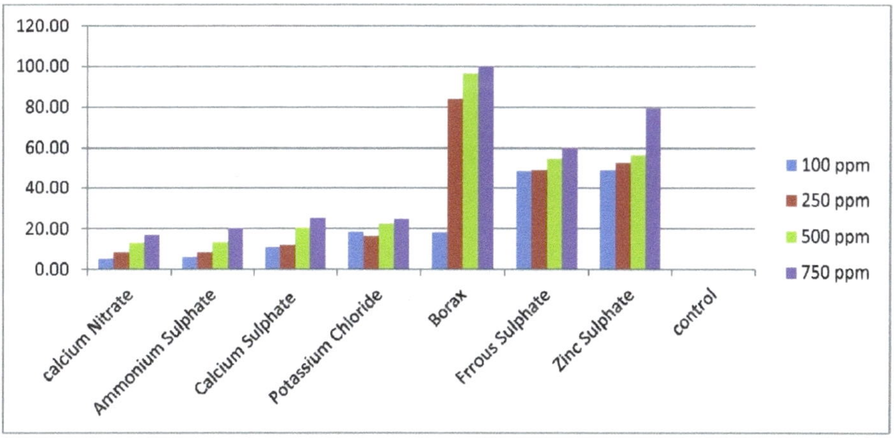

Fig. 2: Percent inhibition of fungal growth of the *Fusarium oxysporum* f.sp.*cubense*

Sundaravadana and Alice, (2006) reported that the micronutrient amended medium generally improved the bio control potential of *T. viride* against *M. phaseolina*. The above findings lend support to the present investiga-tion and the addition of micronutrients particularly borax increased the biocontrol activity of *T. viride.* Hence, this investigation suggests that the borax could be effectively used a viable control strategy for agriculturally important soil-borne diseases.

The above findings lend support to the present investigation and the addition of micronutrients particularly borax suppressed the *Fusarium oxysporum* f.sp. *cubense*. Hence, this investigation suggests that the borax could be effectively used a viable control strategy for agriculturally important soil-borne diseases. This approach leads to maintain our ecosystem sustainability for a longer time and manage the disease.

References

Anonimus (1996) Why NRCB? A beginning, NRCB Newslet, National Research Centre on Banana, Trichy 1:1-4.

Chand G, Jaiswal US, Maru AK (2016) Effect of Micronutrients on Panama Wilt of Banana (*Fusarium oxysporum* f. sp. *cubense*) and its Synergistic action with *Trichoderma viride*. In: Proceedings of International Conference on Innovative Approaches in applied Sciences and Technologies (ICIAsT-2016), from 1-5 February, 2016 held at Kasetsart University, Thailand, Bangkok

Lakpale N, Khare N, Trimurthy K, Agarwal KC (1997) *In-vitro* studies on growth and sclerotial for mation of *Rhizoctonia solani* (Kohn.) causing sheath blight of paddy. *Journal of Soil and Crops* 7: 43-45.

Molina A B, Valmayor RV (1999) Banana production systems in South East Asia. Bananas and Food Security, Pica C., E. Foure, E.A. Frison (eds.), INIBAP, Montpellier, France, 423-436.

Roja V (2006) Studies on the role of abiotic factors on the biocontrol poten tial of *Trichoderma viride* against *Macrophomina phaseolina* (Tassi) Goid, an incitant of dry root of groundnut. M. Sc (Agri.) Thesis, Annamalai University, Tamilnadu, India.

Sanjeev K K, Eswaran A. (2008) Efficacy of Micro Nutrients on Banana Fusarium wilt (*Fusarium oxysporum* f. sp. *cubense*) and its Synergistic action with *Trichoderma viride. Not. Bot. Hort. Agrobot. Cluj.* 36 (1): 52-54.

Schmitz H. (1930). Poisoned food technique. *Industrial and Engineering Chemistry Analyst* Ed. 2:361.

Sundravadana S. and Alice D. (2006) Antifungal activity of zinc sulphate on *Macrophomina phaseolina* (*Tassi*) Goid and its synergistic action with *T. viride*. *J. Biol. Control* 20: 213-218.

7

Biotic and Abiotic Stresses of Mungbean: Breeding Aspects, Diseases and Their Management

Thota Gopi Krishna[1], Anil Kumar[2] and Fariha Adan[1]

[1]*Research Scholar, Department of Plant Breeding and Genetics Bihar Agricultural University, Sabour, 813210, Bihar, India*
[2]*Department of Plant Breeding and Genetics, Bihar Agricultural University Sabour, 813210, Bihar, India*

Abstract

Mungbean [*Vigna radiata* (L.) Wilczek] *is an important pulse crop grown in India. It is a short duration annual with yellow flowers and fuzzy brown pods. Majority of the mungbean grown in India is under rainfed conditions and the productivity of mungbean is not upto the mark to meet the daily dietary requirement of a populous country like India. The biotic and abiotic stresses in mungbean, majorly MYMV, powdery mildew, drought, salinity, water logging etc leaves a severe yield loss in mungbean crop. Among them, MYMV and powdery mildew diseases show yield losses accounting upto 85% and 40%, respectively in severe conditions. The present review paper is based on the study of both biotic and abiotic stresses and the recent advances in breeding for resistance to stresses. A detail explanation of major diseases and insect pests affecting mungbean are discussed along with the information of genomic resources and research done in mungbean in recent years. Recently SSR's have been using widely for all molecular level research work like genetic diversity, constructing linkage maps for identifying QTL's, marker assisted breeding etc. in mungbean. The resistant varieties developed against these biotic and abiotic stresses are listed which are very important for attaining a prominent yield in mungbean.*

***Keywords*:** Green gram, biotic and abiotic stresses

Introduction

Mungbean [*Vigna radiata* (L.) Wilczek] which is also known as green gram or moong is a short duration pulse crop mainly grown in India, Pakistan, Bangladesh, Sri Lanka and other south east asian countries. It belongs to fabaceae family have yellow flowers and fuzzy brown pods with upright or annual vine growing habit. Based on scientific discoveries now it was confirmed that its origin lies in India and Indo-Burma region (Vavilov, 1951). India is the largest global producer & consumer accounting for about 65% of global acreage and 54% of world's production (Singh 2011). In India, mungbean is used as food legumes and is a major proteinary diet for many vegetarians. Orissa, Andhra Pradesh, Madhya Pradesh, Maharashtra, and Rajasthan are the states with majority of area under mungbean cultivation in India .

In India, mungbean is grown in all the 3 seasons namely- kharif, rabi and zaid where former (kharif) crop is grown in rainfed conditions and the latter (rabi and zaid) crops are grown in irrigated conditions. Due to its short duration nature, it fits well in all cropping systems and also enrich the soil fertility by symbiotic nitriogen fixation with rhizobium bacteria. *Vigna radiata* var *sublobata,* occur wild in India, is discovered to be the putative progenitor of mungbean. The total area covered under mungbean in India was 30.41 lakh hectares with a total production of 14.24 lakh tonnes and productivity of 468 kg/ha (Tiwari and Shivhare, 2016). The area covered under mungbean in Bihar was 1.57 lakh hectares with a production of 1.04 lakh tonnes and productivity of 664 kg/ha (Tiwari and Shivhare, 2016).

Among the biotic stresses, the MYMV disease is the most devastating disease accounting for about 85% yield losses in severe infections (Karthikeyan *et al.,* 2014). For the acclimatization of a crop to new environments, tolerance to abiotic stresses is more important than the biotic stresses. Abiotic stresses affect plant metabolism, disturbs cellular homeostasis and imbalance major physiological and biochemical processes (Arora *et al.*, 2002). As compared to cereals, less attention was given for mungbean but in recent times, some progress have been done in mungbean improvement by developing resistance to biotic and abiotic stresses. Keeping all these things in view, the present review attempt has been made to cover the various aspects of genetic improvement of mungbean for resistance to biotic and abiotic stresses and also the detailed explanation of major diseases, pests of mungbean and their management.

Major Biotic and Abiotic Stresses Affecting Mungbean Production

Mungbean is a cheap and rich source of vegetable protein and is a good supplement to regular intake of diet. It is a minor pulse grown all over India. The following are the nutritional components of mungbean which areprotein of

24-26%, carbohydrates of 51%, minerals of 4% and vitamins of 3% (Karthikeyan *et al.*, 2014). The major Abiotic stresses affecting the mungbean production are as follows:

Terminal heat stress, drought stress, water logging stress and salinity stress.Terminal heat and drought stresses may cause considerable dropping of flowers and reduced pod set. Excess moisture and water logging conditions causes crop lodging and turning it vulnerable to a number of diseases and insect-pests which results in reduction of yield and quality of the grains.

The major biotic stresses affecting the mungbean production are as follows: Economically important diseases considered are mungbean yellow mosaic virus (MYMV), cercospora leaf spot, powdery mildew and bacterial leaf spot and insect pests including bruchids, pod borer, bean fly and other pests. Among them, MYMV and powdery mildew diseases show yield losses accounting upto 85% and 40% respectively in severe conditions.

Breeding for Resistance to Biotic Stresses in Mungbean

Mungbean is affected by different biotic agents like fungi, bacteria, virus and insect pests etc. And these biotic stresses cause severe yield losses in mungbean.

MYMV disease

MYMV disease caused by begomoviruses, popularly known as gemini viruses which are the most important genus within the family, geminiviridae. They are single stranded DNA viruses and mainly occurs in monopartite (a single DNA) or a bipartite (DNA-A and DNA-B) condition. It was first observed in mungbean field in India, 1955at the experimental farm of the IARI, New Delhi, India. It was mainly transmitted by white fly *(Bemesia tabaci)*in persistent manner and also by grafting technique but not possible by wind, sap, seed and soil. Severe infected plants possess few flowers and yellow colured pods with immature seeds. Disease infection lowers the photosynthetic efficiency and as a result the crop yield is reduced or affected (Malathi and John 2008). In Mungbean, resistant lines for MYMV are identified by screening the mungbean germplasm based on the visual symptoms seen in the field. And here a highly susceptible line like example CO-9 is used as susceptible check for spreading the disease. Based on the visual symptoms observed, the mungbean genotypes are categorised into different types like immune, resistant, moderately resistant, moderately susceptible and highly susceptible according to the (0-9) scale given by (Mayee and Datar 1986). For breeding resistant cultivars, the details of inheritance and sources of resistant genes are important. The inheritance of resistance to MYMV has been reported in mungbean and is conferred by a single recessive gene (Reddy & Singh 1995), a dominant gene (Sandhu *et al.*

1985), two recessive genes (Verma and Singh 1988) and complementary recessive genes (Shukla and Pandya 1985). *Vigna radiata* var *sublobata*, wild sp., which is a good source of MYMV resistance. The first MYMV resistant variety released was Pant M 2 in 1983. Other resistant varieties are as follows: Samrat, Pant moong 4, Narendra Mung 1, Ganga 8 and GM 3 which lead to the increase in mungbean cropping areas in recent years. Breeding methods for MYMV resistance includes, selection from landraces, intraspecific hybridization (most common), interspecific hybridization and mutation breeding.

Powdery Mildew Disease (PM)

Besides MYMV, powdery mildew is a serious disease for the mungbean grown in both kharif and rabi seasons. Powdery mildew is caused by *Sphaerotheca phaseoli* and it shows high yield losses in severe conditions. Powdery mildew disease accounts for yield loss up to 20-40%. Resistance to powdery mildew is governed by single dominant gene (AVRDC, 1979) and also several reports which showed it is governed by additive gene action, recessive polygenes. The identification of resistant donars such as Raipur Utera Mung (RUM) in 1987 created a major breakthrough for further development of resistant varieties in mungbean. The first high yielding variety resistant to PM disease was TARM 2, released in 1992 for rabi cultivation. Some other important resistant sources identified are RUM 5, ATF 3640 and VC 6468-11-1A which lead to development of PM resistant cultivars like TARM 1, TARM 2, TARM 18, JM 721 and Pusa 9072 that are notable for rabi cultivation in south India.

Other diseases and pests

Cercospora leaf spot causes severe yield losses in mungbean accounting upto 23% (Quebral and Cagampang, 1970). Resistant sources identified for cercospora leaf spot includes M-98, 98cmg-003, C2/94-4-42, NM-1, NM-2, 98 cmg-018, BRM188, CO-3, Basanti, PDM-11, BARI Mung-2 and VC3960-88 (Iqbal *et al.*, 2004). Less importance has been given for insect resistance breeding in mungbean in past years but recently attention for bruchid resistance in mungbean is given. Bruchid beetles are the most devastating storage insect pest of grain legumes and cause significant loss to mungbean. Some resistant sources are identified and used for breeding purposes. Resistance to bruchid is governed by single dominant gene in *Vigna radiata* var. *Sublobata* (Kitamura *et al.* 1988). Mungbean variety TC1966, completely resistant to two species of bruchid beetles, *Callosobruchus chinensis* (adzuki bean weevil) and *C. maculates* (cowpea weevil), which cause major damage to mungbean during storage.

Breeding For Resistance To Abiotic Stresses In Mungbean

Majority of the mungbean cultivation in india is under rainfed conditions. In these conditions the crop is subjected to different types of Environmental stresses or Abiotic stresses like Drought, Water logging, salinity and higher temperature (Terminal heat) etc. To increase the area under mungbean cultivation and its productivity in India, there is need of acclimatization of the mungbean cultivars for these abiotic stresses. For attaining this objective, there is need to develop the abiotic stresses tolerant mungbean varieties.

Drought stress

Water deficit stress disturbs various physiological processes linked with growth, development and yield of a crop (Hsiao and Acevedo 1974). Water deficit results in increase of root shoot ratio, thickness of cell walls, amount of cutinization and lignifications & decrease of leaf area index of plants. Mungbean is highly susceptible to water deficits than many legumes (Pandey *et al.* 1984). Due to its short duration nature, it is reported that mungbean is tolerate to drought stress. But the drought stress condition during flowering stages highly reduces the flowering & proper pod growth and development and further reduces the productivity of mungbean. Severe drought decreases vegetative growth, flower initiation and setting of pods (Morton *et al.* 1982). Genotypes developed with better water use efficiency helps to improve grain yield in dry areas. Drought resistance is of two types: (i) dehydration avoidance involving morphological and physiological adaptations to manage the cellular water status and (ii) dehydration tolerance facilitating remobilization of reserves of stem and accumulation of some protectants that provide functioning under water deûcit conditions. Drought escape is facilitated when phenological development is perfectly matched with periods of soil moisture availability, where the growing season is shorter and terminal drought stress predominates (Farooq *et al.* 2009). Screening of genotypes to drought tolerance and inserting the trait into high-yielding lines has been greatly practised at The World Vegetable Centre (AVRDC). The genotypes, 'V 1281', 'V 2013' and 'V 3372' were noted as drought tolerant at AVRDC. For spring/summer season, short duration varieties with more harvest index, determinate habit and decreased photoperiod sensitivity are well suited.

Water logging stress

Water logging is the serious problem in mungbean by which productivity also decreases. So there is need to develop water logging tolerant mungbean varieties. Mungbean cannot tolerate water logging mainly during the initial stages of growth (Singh and Singh 2011). Flooding or water logging decreases the oxygen concentrations in soil to least amounts and also disturbs the nodule activity of nitrogen fixation and thereby affecting the crop yield. Hence mungbean cultivation is not good for tropical wet lands where the annual rainfall is greater than 1000 mm (Fernandez and Shanmugasundaram 1988). The heavy rain damages the crop causing severe yield losses. Water logging affects many physiological processes like reduction in photosynthesis (Ahmed *et al.* 2002). Kumar *et al.*, (2013), in his studies reported that after 9 days of exposure to flooding, the photosynthesis rate and yield losses in sensitive genotypes (Pusa Baisakhi & MH–1K–24) were 83 and 85 %, respectively. On an average, photosynthetic loss at 3, 6 and 9 days of water logging was 43, 51, and 63 %, respectively, while grain yield loss was 20, 34 and 52 % respectively. Islam *et al.*, (2008), reported that the flooding tolerant genotypes like GK48 and VC3945A has less extent of seed yield reduction compared to other genotype.

Temperature stress

Mungbean is grown all over India at different photoperiods and temperatures. In general, mungbean is sensitive to photoperiod and temperature which shows affect on flowering and finally yield loss. Hence there is need to develop photoperiod and temperature insensitive mungbean varieties for having that factor with nill effect on yield. As the photoperiod is lengthened from 12 to 16 h, flowering in some short-season early strains may be delayed only a few days; but in photoperiod sensitive strains, it may be delayed to as many as 30 to 40 days and some strains may even fail to flower. High temperature stress shows direct negative impact on flower retention and finally on pod formation (Kumari and Verma 1983). The terminal heat stress is a serious problem in India for spring and summer mungbean. However, in kharif crop, more than 40° C temperature is seen during the initial stages which causes great reduction in seed yield due to pollen inviability, lack of fertilization and high or complete flower shedding. Khattak *et al.*, (2006), evaluated 14 commercial mungbean varieties, 77 mutants and 24 advanced genotypes for maximum flowers' retention capability under high temperature (above 40°C) and agronomic traits during summer. NFM-6-5 and NFM-12-14 showed high seed yield when compared to NM 92. NM 92 showed susceptibility to the flowers shedding under high temperature (above 40°C). Kaur *et al.* (2015), conducted experiment on two mungbean varieties (SML 832 and 668) grown in pots at different sowing dates. At flowering and podding stages stomatal conductance, photosynthetic efficiency and chlorophyll concentration were inhibited in two genotypes under heat stress. CE studies showed that temperatures mainly 43/30 degree celsius, 45/32 deg.celsius (day/night) were too bad for pod set, reproductive function and yield traits for mungbean.

Salinity stress

Salinity stress cause prominent amount of yield loss in mungbean. Salt stress affect seed germination, shoot growth, root growth, root length, biomass and seedling vigour. Mungbean production of 455 kg/ha in Pakistan is comparatively low to other countries of the world due to the fact that mungbean cultivating areas are salt affected. Ahmed, (2009) conducted experiment with 5 mungbean genotypes to see the effect of salt stress on the yield and its components. Salt stress was more effective at vegetative, flowering and seed filling stages rather than seed development stage in all the five accessions/genotypes. NM-92 showed adaptability under saline conditions. Kumar *et al.* (2012), conducted the experiment in Annamalai university to see the response of eight parents and 5 hybrids under different salt stress. All the hybrids show higher levels of salinity tolerance compared to their respective parents. VRMGG1/VBN1 was observed as relatively salt tolerant from the research.

Genomic resources and research

Mungbean is an autogamous or self pollinated diploid plant with 2n =2x =22 somatic chromosomes and having a genome size of 515 Mb (Tangphatsornruang *et al.* 2009). Small genome size, short life-cycle, self-pollinating, and close genetic relationship to other legumes are the characters of mungbean that facilitates itself to be used as a model organism among legume crops. The reference genome of the cultivated mungbean (V. *radiata* var. *radiata* VC1973A) is recently released and the genome sequencing of the wild progenitor (*Vigna radiata* var. *Sublobata*) paves the way for further mungbean genome research and identifying the genes related to particular desirable traits. The wild mungbean genome has many beneficial genes that helps in widening the genetic base or genetic diversity of the cultivated mungbean varieties. The genetic linkage maps which were constructed from a commercial mungbean cultivar and a wild mungbean accession giving precious information about important traits like seed quality, weathering tolerance, and pest/disease resistance (Lambrides *et al.* 2000). Molecular techniques like RAPD, RFLP, SSR and SNP's have been using in the modern research programmes for the clear cut understanding of the mungbean at a molecular (DNA) level. Recently SSR's have been using widely for all molecular level research work like genetic diversity, constructing linkage maps for identifying QTL's etc. in mungbean. More recently, AVRDC-The World Vegetable Center made a core collection consisting of 1,481 accessions and a mini-core consisting of 296 accessions (Schaieitner *et al.* 2015) for efficient use of genetic resources and easy access by breeders. Many studies have focused on molecular mapping and locating QTLs for traits in mungbean based on RFLPs (Humphry *et al.* 2005). It will be difficult to resolve the 11 linkage groups and to saturate the linkage map without the use of highly accurate SSR and SNP markers. The success of generating a genome map of black gram based on adzuki bean markers has paved the way for the use of adzuki bean SSR markers in mungbean. SSR's have been broadly used to identify disease resistance QTLs in legume species that assists in marker-assisted selection in crops.

Number of QTLS identiûed in mungbean by comparative analysis with soybean QTLS. (Chen *et al.*, 2007).

Trait	Soyabean QTLs	Mungbean QTLs
First flower	104	54
Leaflet length	66	53
Leaûet width	61	55
Plant height	268	171
Pod maturity	196	142
Pod number	59	40
Seed oil	236	178
Seed oil to protein ratios	16	0
Seed protein	356	140
Seed weight	272	245
Seed weight per plant	16	11

Major Mungbean Diseases And Their Management

1. Mungbean Yellow Mosaic Disease

Causal organism

The causal agent of the Yellow mosaic disease is mungbean yellow mosaic virus belonging to the Geminiviridae family and is transmitted by white fly (*Bemisia tabaci*). Nariani (1960) reported this disease first in the fields of IARI, New Delhi. The name mungbean yellow mosaic virus was given by (Nene, 1968). The transmission is also done by grafting but not by seed, soil or sap. Whitefly transmits the virus to hosts within 10-15 min after aquisition.10 viruliferous whitefly agents are needed for 100% transmission (Nene, 1973). It has several alternate and collateral hosts that act as sources of inoculums. Rathi and Nene (1974) reported that host range of MYMV is limited to Leguminosae, Compositae and Gramineae families.

Symptoms

The presence of yellow spots scattered on the young leaves is the first diagnosable visible symptom.The trifoliate leaf with alternate yellow and green patches irregularly which later turns yellow.The field affected with this disease can be diagnosed from a distance. The leaves appear as slightly puckered and with reduced size.The late maturity, presence of few flowers and pods are the characteristics of infected plants. The pods also turn yellow and contain deformed or malformed or under developed seeds.The major factors for reduction in yield are decrease in number of pods/plant, seeds/pod and seed weight (Nene, 1973). Yield losses varying from 5-100% based on susceptibility of cultivars, disease severityand whiteflypopulation (Rathi, 2002).

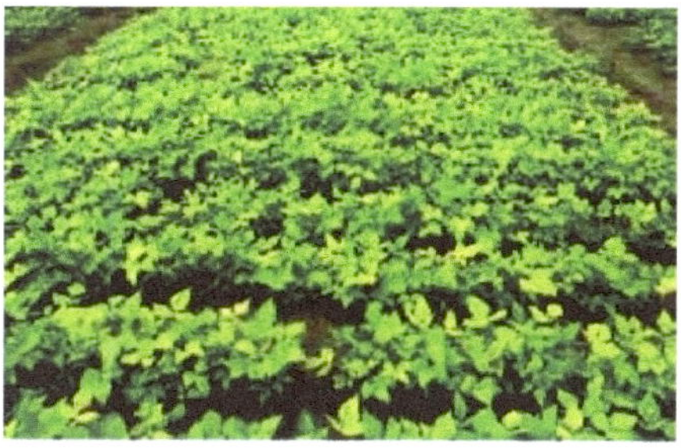

Field view showing severity of MYMV

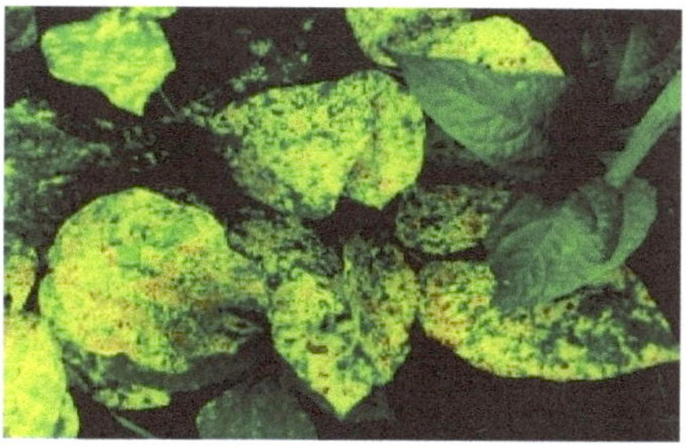

MYMV infected plant

Management

- Growing of resistant varieties:Narendra Mung1, Pant Mung 3, PDM 139 (Samrat), PDM-11 (Spring Season),ML 131, ML 267, ML 337, Pusa 105 and MUM 2.
- Intercropping with non host crops- sorghum, pearl millet and maize.
- Roguing of diseased plants to prevent furthur disease spread.
- Application of metasystox or triazophos 40 EC @ 2.0 ml/L or malathion 50 EC @ 2.0 ml/L or oxydemeton methyl 25 EC @ 2.0 ml/L at 10–15 days intervals in foliar manner.

1. Powdery Mildew

Causal organism

The causative agent of Powdery mildew is *Erysiphe polygoni*, which is one of the most devastating diseases of mungbean in india. It is the major problem of rice based cropping systems (Abbaiah 1993). The fungus is ectophytic and obligate in nature. It spreads on the host surface and directs haustoria into the epidermal cells to uptake nutrients. The hoste range of this organism is limited to leguminosae family. Conidial or cleistothecial form existence of fungus on the host tissues act as source of primary infection. The secondary infection is done by air borne conidia. Yield losses in cool, dry months by high infection of the powdery mildew have been estimated to be 20 to 40% (Reddy *et al.* 1994). The yield losses by powdery mildew for winter mungbean are greater than rainy season mungbean.

Symptoms

The disease starts as faint dark spots, turns to small white powdery spots which furthur turns to white powdery coating on all parts of the plant above the surface of soil. The dirty white powdery mass appears in advanced infection stages. Defoliation too takes place in severe infection stages. It induces forceful maturity of diseased plants pertaining to drastic yield losses.

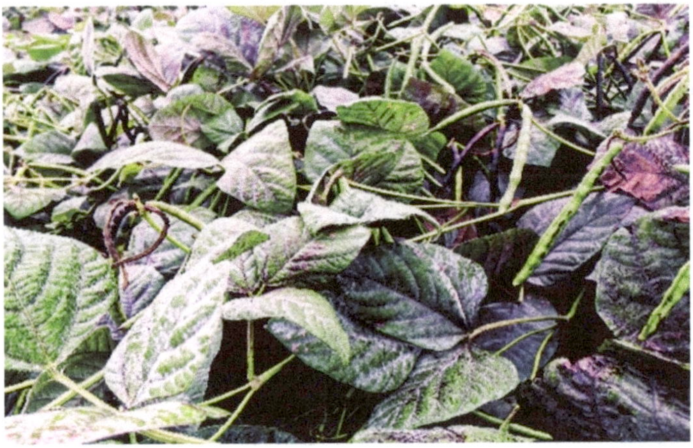

Mungbean Plants affected with powdery mildew

Management

- Roguing and destroying of diseased plants.
- Delayed sowing with wider spacings reduces disease severity.
- Growing of resistant varieties: LM 223, LM 24, P115, ML 131, MI 322, ML 337, ML 395 SS1, JRUM 1, TARM 1 and AVRDC 1381
- Spraying of NSKE @ 50 g/L or neem oil of 3000 ppm @ 20 ml/L twice at 10 days interval from initial disease seen or Spraying of eucalyptus leaf extract 10% at initiation of the disease or Spraying of water soluble sulfur 80 wp @ 4 k g/L or carbendazin 50 WP @ 1 g/L (0.05%), benlate (0.05%) and topsin-M (0.15%).

3. Cercospora Leaf Spot

Causal organism

The causative agent of the Cercospora leaf spot (CLS) is *Cercospora canesens* or *Cercospora cruenta* which cause drastic yield losses under warm and humid weather conditions. Mungbean is highly susceptible to CLS than urdbean. The infected seeds and crop debris are used for fungul survival (Grewal 1978). Rath and Grewal (1973) reported that high sporulation is at 96% relative humidity and 27°C temperature.

Symptoms

The disease starts with Leaf spots of circular to irregular shape. The central portion turns gray with reddish brown to dark brown margin. Varied lesion size is depending on the isolate and the host (Ilag 1978). The pathogen also affects the petioles, stems and pods. The spots grow in size during flowering and pod filling stage finally leading to defoliation under favourable conditions. Singh *et al.* (2000) reported that yield losses of 50% in highly affected field.

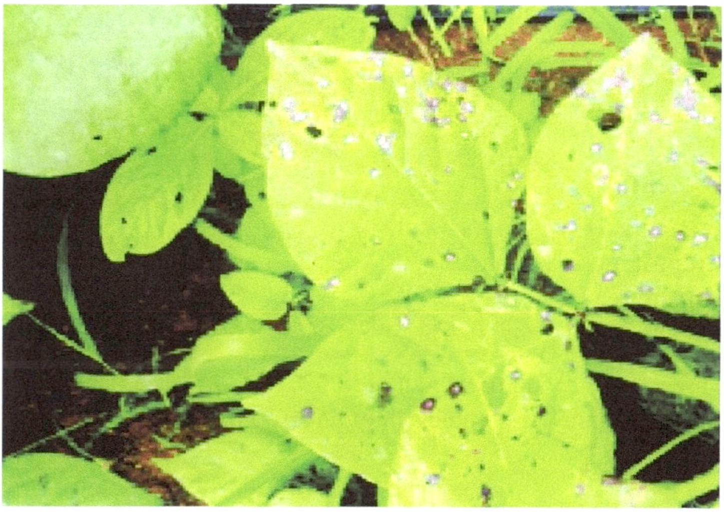

Mungbean plant affected with cercospora leaf spot

Management

- Removal and destroying of infected crop debris and collateral hosts.
- Rotation of crop with non legume crops.
- Treating of seeds with thiram or captan @ 2.5g/kg of seed.
- Growing of resistant varieties: LM 113, LM 168, LM 170 and JM 171
- Spraying of carbendazim 50 WP @1.0 g/L or mancozeb 45 WP @ 2.0 g/L or copper oxychloride @ 3 to 4 g/L.

4. Bacterial Leaf Spot

Causal organism

The causative agent of bacterial leaf spot is *Xanthomonas phaseoli,* which is a gram negative and rod shape bacteria. During off-season, the bacteria survives in seeds, plant debris and other host plants. The disease development is favoured by warm, humid weather and a optimum temperature range of 30–33°C.

Symptoms

The small, brown and dry raised spots on leaves and stem are the characteristic symptoms of this disease. Leaf spots starts initially as superficial eruption and later turns into corky or rough by invading tissues. Yellowing of leaves and premature defoliation of leaves occurs. The infection also spreads to stem and pods.

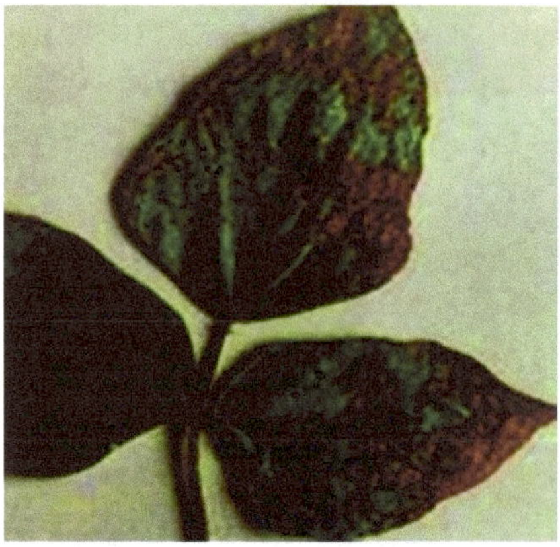

Mungbean leaf affected with bacterial leaf spot

Management

- Treating the seeds with streptomycin sulfate @ 500 ppm or captan @ 0.3% or bleaching power @0.025%.
- Three spray of streptomycin @ 0.025% + 0.1% carbendazim or three protective spray of streptocycline @ 100 ppm or zineb @ 0.3% or benomyl @ 0.2%.

5. Mosaic Mottle

Causal organism

The causative agent of the mosaic mottle is Bean common mosaic virus belonging to poty virus group. Transmission is done by sap, mechanical manner, and by seed (Nene, 1972). Singh and Nene (1978) reported that mosaic mottle is also transmitted by aphids, *Aphis craccivora* and *A. gossypii*. The virus host range is restricted to leguminosae family (Srivastava *et al.* 1969).

Symptoms

The mosaic pattern of irregular broad patches of light and dark green areas, blistering and puckering of leaf blade are the characteristic symptoms of the disease. The leaves appear rough and brittle. The decrease in overall growth and excessive branching is shown by infected plants. At times of severe infection, the whole inflorescence turns into leaf like structures and thus causing 100% seed yield loss (Nene 1972).

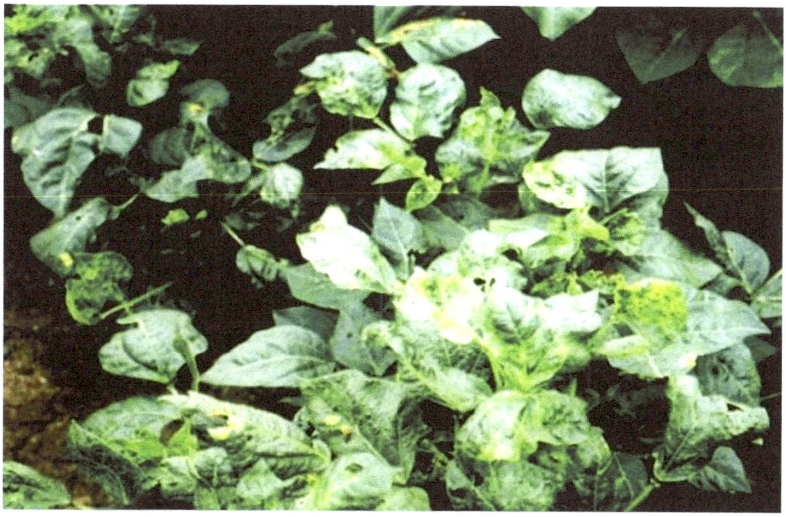

BCMV affected plant with stunted growth, yellowing and mottling symptoms on leaves

Management

- Usage of diseased free seeds.
- Roguing of infected plants.
- Spray with insecticide (dimethoate 30 EC @ 1.7 mL/ha) on 30 days after sowing in foliar manner.

6. Leaf Curl

Causal organism

The causative agent of leaf curl is Tomato Spotted Wilt Virus, which is an significant potential killer of mungbean and urdbean plants (Nene, 1972). The virus is transmitted through sap, grafting and the thrip, *Frankliniella schultzei* (Amin *et al.* 1985).

Symptoms

The symptoms initiates with Chlorosis around some lateral veins and their branches close to the margin of the youngest trifoliate leaf. The characteristic symptoms are the downward curling of margin of leaves and also rolling and twisting of young leaves. During early infection after sowing, plants remain stunted and die due to top necrosis. While it shows only veinal chlorosis during late infections. Few Pods production with small seeds are seen.

Management

- Spray with rogor (0.05%) on first appearance of the disease and later at 10 days interval in foliar manner.
- Cultivation of resistant/tolerant varieties : Pant mung 3.

7. Anthracnose

Causal organism

The causative agents of anthracnose in mungbean are *Colletotrichum capsici* and C. *lindemuthianum* mainly. The infected seeds and crop residue serves as survival for pathogen from one crop season to next one (Singh *et al*., 1981). Primary leaves and the hypocotyls act as secondary infections. Rains at frequent manner is favourable for epidemic development of disease. And the favourable conditions are temperature of 17–24°C and relative humidity of 100%.

Symptoms

The symptoms of the disease are characterised by presence of circular brown sunken spots with dark centers and bright red orange margins on leaves and pods. The disease occurs on foliage, stems and pods. Diseased part will be withered off during severe conditions. Seedling blight occurs when infection is occured after immediate germination.

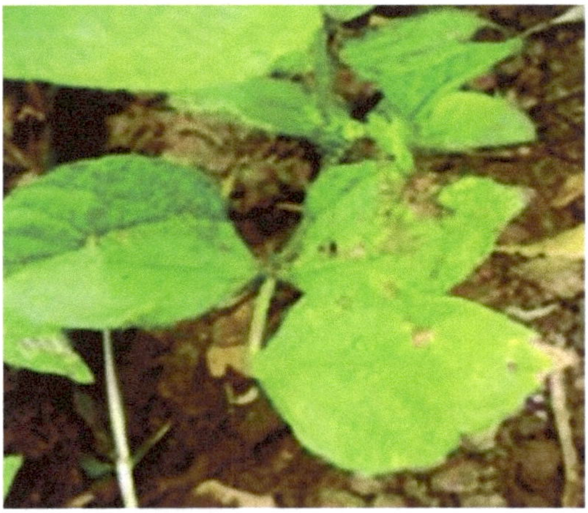

Green gram anthracnose symptoms on leaves

Management

- Treating of seeds with hot water at 58°C for 15 minutes for seed borne infection.
- Treating of seeds with thiram 80% WP @ 2 g/L or captan 75 WP @ 2.5 g/L helps in removing the seed borne infection.

- Spraying of 0.2% zineb 80% WP @ 2 g/L or ziram 80% WP @ 2 g/L with initial appearance of symptoms on the crop and repeat after 15 days if needed.

8. Macrophomina Blight

Causal organism

The causative agents of the macrophomina blight is *Macrophomina phaseolina*, a fungus which causes root rot, collar rot, seedling blight, stem rot, leaf blight, pod and seed infection. It causes seed rot and germinating seedlings mortality during pre-emergence stage. Seedling blight disease is seen in post-emergence stage. The jet black coloured sclerotia survived in soil and host residues act as primary infection. Also spreads through infected seeds. It has a wide host range. The aerial spread of the disease is done by pycniospores. The pathogen is favoured by 30°C temperature moisture of 15%.

Symptoms

As the identification of disease in early stages is difficult but dark lesions on main stem near soil level turns into localized dark green patches. The affected parts will be weak and shredded easily. The decaying of secondary roots and shredding of tap root cortex region are major symptoms. By pulling of plants shows the dry rot symptoms of basal stem and root. Black coloured sclerotia is seen on rotten stem and root. High temperature and water stress conditions are favourable for occurence of this disease.

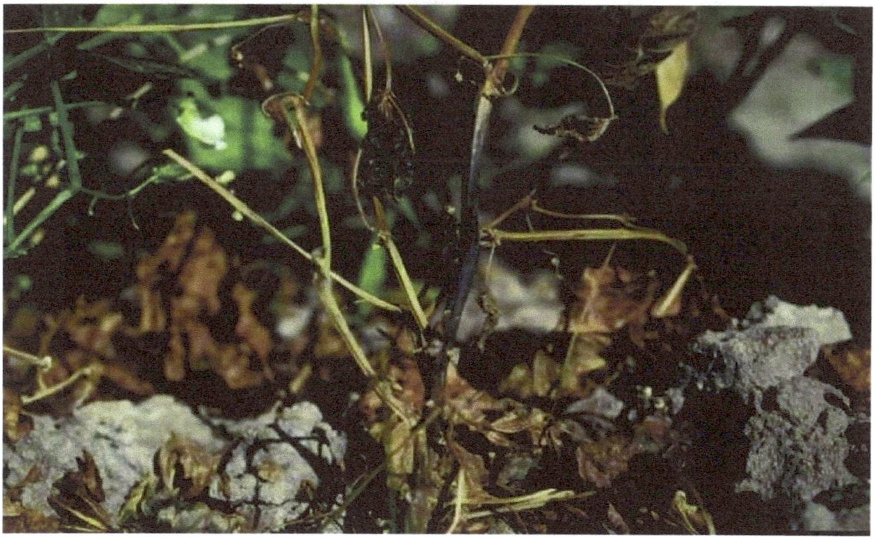

Mungbean plant affected with Macrophomina blight

Management

- Application of zinc sulfate @ 25 kg/ha or neem cake @ 150 kg/ha or soil application of Pseudomonas fluorescens (1 x 101°Cfu/g) or Trichoderma viride (1 x 10–8 cfu/g) @ 2.5 kg/ha + 50 kg of well decomposed FYM during sowing in basal manner.
- Seeds treated with Trichoderma (1 x 108 cfu/g) 5–10 g/kg of seed or captan 75 WP @ 2.5 g/L and thiram 80% WP @ 2 g/L before sowing.
- Roguing of diseased plants.
- Spraying of carbendazim 50 WP @ 1.0 g/L at an interval of 15 days after the appearance of the symptoms.

Major insect pests of green gram and their management

1. Gram Pod Borer

The gram pod borer, *Helicoverpa armigera* is a polyphagous pest and likely to cause severe damage in mungbean too. The larva has variation of colour from greenish to brown. The adults are light pale brownish yellow stout moth. The fore wings appear grey in colour to pale brown with a v shaped speck.

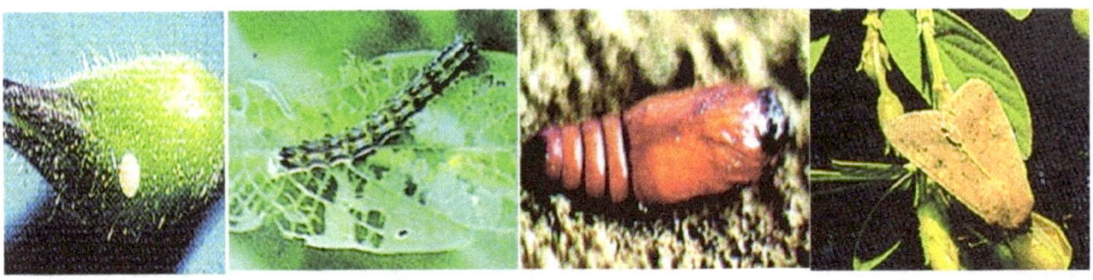

Egg Larva Pupa Adult

Symptoms

Defoliation is seen in early stages. Larva's head is seen inside the pods feeding and rest of the body hanging outside. Pods with prominent round holes is also seen.

Management

- ETL 10% of affected pods.
- Arranging pheromone traps at 12/ha.
- Application of Azadirachtin 0.03 % WSP 2500-5000 g/ha.
- Collection of grown up larva and blister beetle mechanically.

1. Spotted Pod Borer

As similar to gram pod borer, the spotted pod borer-*Maruca testulalis* also cause severe damage to mungbean pods and thus yield of the crop. Larva is having green white to brownish head. The forewings are light brown colour with white markings.

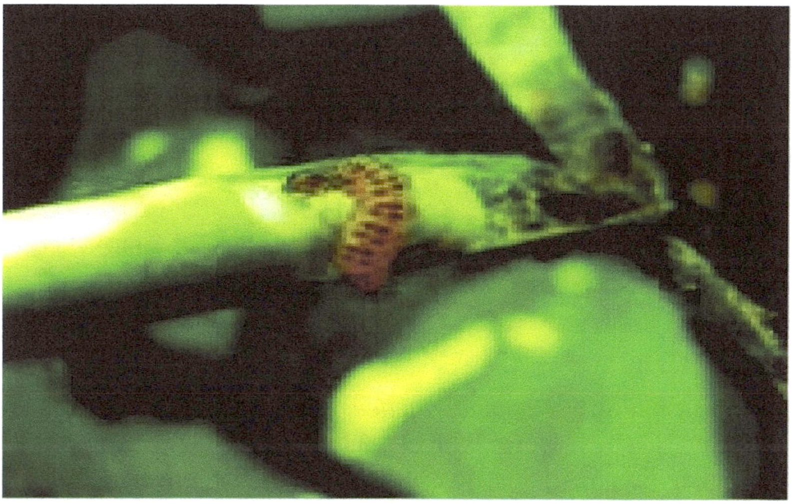

Larva feeding on pods with head inside and body out

Symptoms

Defoliation with larva's head inside the pod feeding and the pods with prominent round holes.

Management

- ETL 3/plant.
- Phosalone of 0.07% (Spray fluid 625 ml/ha).

1. Spiny Pod Borer

The spiny pod borer, *Etiella zinckenellacauses* dropping of flowers and young pods. The older pods are with brown spot indicating the larval entry. Larvae are green in colour at early stages but later turns to pink before pupation. There is the presence of 5 black spots on prothorax for larva. Adults are brownish grey moths with orange coloured prothorax and forewing with a white stripe.

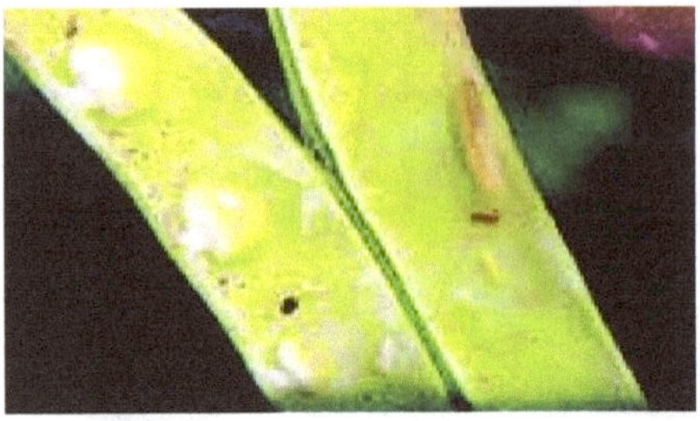

Larva

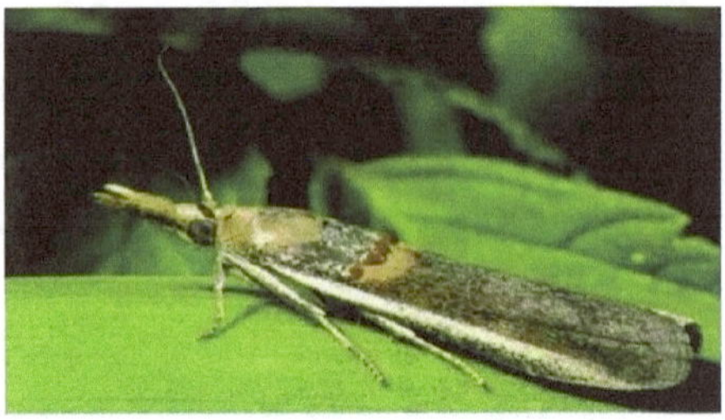

Adult

Management

- ETL 10% affected parts.
- Conservation of natural enemies like Tetrastichus sp., Bracon hebetor etc.
- Spray NSKE 5% twice followed by triazophos 0.05%.

4. Blue Butterfly

The pest, blue butterfly-*Lampides boeticus* cause damage to the buds flowers and young pods, which appear with bore holes. Honey dew secretion and slug like caterpillar is seen. Adult moth is greyish blue with prominent black spots in the hind wings.

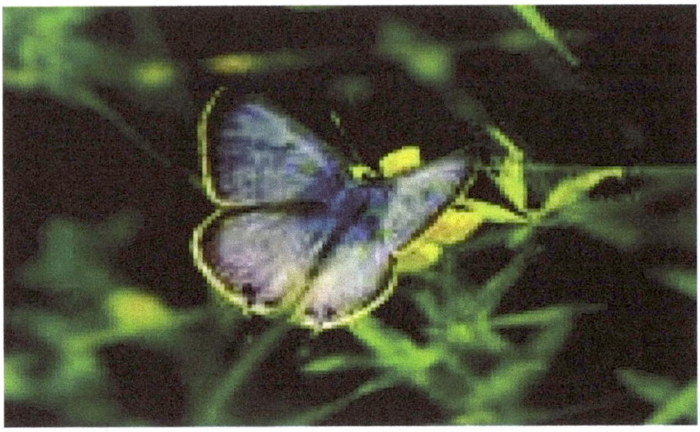

Adult feeding on flowers

Management

- Spraying of indoxacarb 15.8% SC 333 ml/ha.
- Spraying of neem oil 2%.

5. Grass Blue Butterfly

The grass blue butterfly, Euchrysops cnejus shows the symptoms like buds, flowers and young pods with bore holes indicating the presence of slug like caterpillar. The holes on pods are filled with excreta. Larve are pale green to yellow in colour. Adult is blue coloured and characterized with 5 black spots in the hind wings and two black spots in the inner margin.

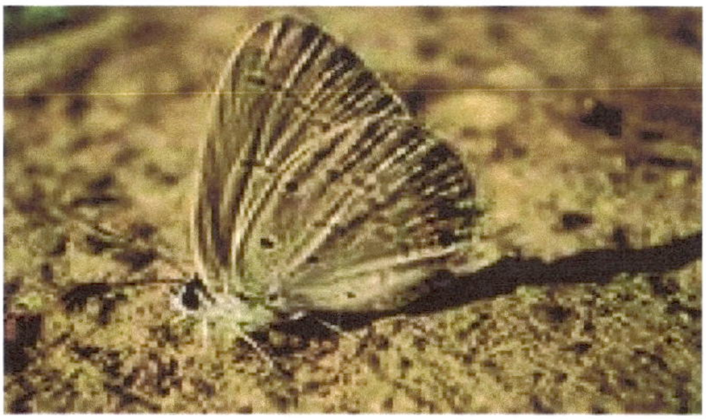

Adult blue butterfly

Management

- Try to avoid closer spacing of plants.
- Recommendation of deep summer ploughing for removing quiescent pupa.
- The ETL of 10% affected parts.
- Control by releasing of *Trichogramma chilonis* at 1.5 lakh/ha/ week for four times.
- Spraying of Quinalphos 25 EC @ 1000 ml/ha.

6. Bean Aphids

The bean aphids *Aphis craccivora* is a prominent pest of mungbean. The symptoms involve damaged leaves, inflorescence stalk and young pods covered with dark coloured aphids. Also accompained with honey dew secretion and black ant movements. Adults are dark coloured with cornicles in the abdomen.

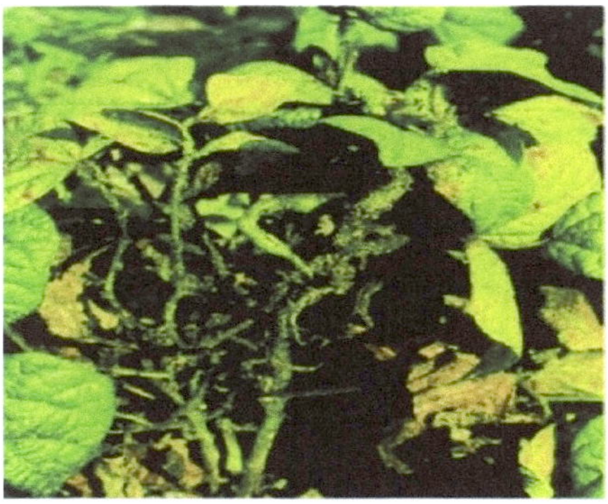

Symptoms on plant

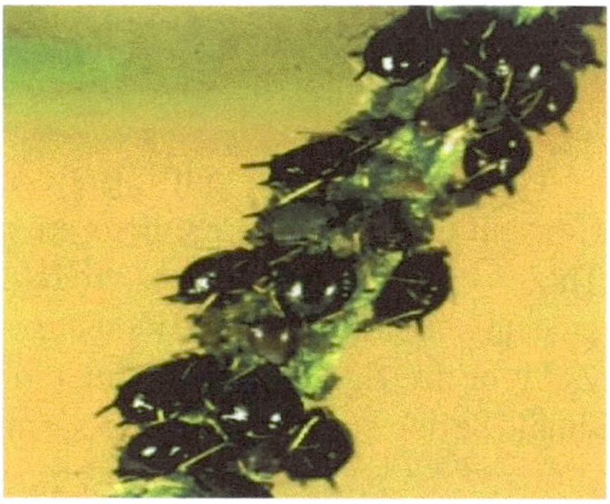

Nymphs & Adults

Management

- Spraying of Emamectin benzoate 5% SG 220 g/ha.

7. Bruchids

Bruchid beetles are the most devastating storge insect pest of grain legumes and cause significant loss to mungbean. Thecowpea bruchid, *Callosobruchus maculatus* (Fabricus) is mainly responsible for most infestations in mungbean. The adults are tear shaped, small brown beetles. They are orange brown coloured with dark markings on their body. The eggs are small, 0.6 mm long, visible on the surface of seeds. The larvae are short cream coloured maggots that feed within grains.

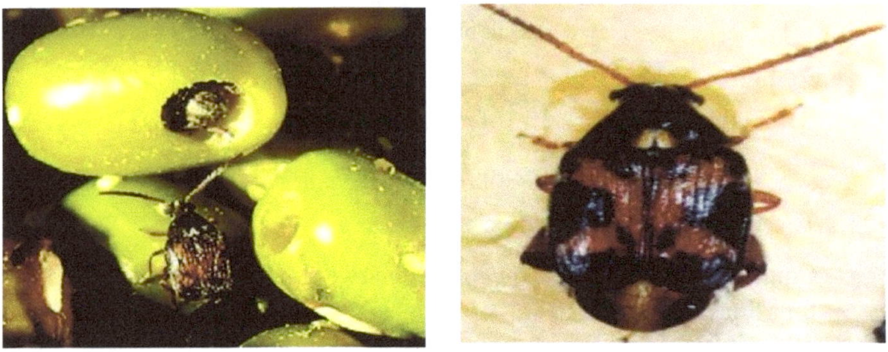

Mungbean seeds with adult and eggs on seeds

Management

- Sun drying is the most common management practice.
- Field disinfestation (0.05% malathion spray at mature green pod and yellow pod stage).

Future prospects in mungbean breeding

It is known that importance of mungbean as proteinary diet and a regular food legume for many people. The objective of optimum and sufficient yield will not be achieved without putting stop check to biotic and abiotic stresses. Conventional breeding methods are not adequate for achieving this objective. There is need to incorporate modern breeding methods like Marker assisted breeding, tissue culture and biotechnological principles for better and prominent yield for the vigorously growing global population. Hence, the deep research should be done in the fields of biotic and abiotic stresses resistance of mungbean.

A brief view of biotic and abiotic stresses

Type of stress (biotic/abiotic)	Causal organism/ Scientific name	Symptoms/ affects	Resistant sources	Resistant/Tolearant varieties	Management
1. Mungbean Yellow mosaic disease	Mungbean yellow mosaic virus (MYMV)	Yellow spots scattered on the young leaves	*Vigna radiata* var *sublobata*, wild sp.,	Pant M 2, Samrat, Pant moong 4, Narendra Mung 1, Ganga 8 and GM 3	Application of metasystox or triazophos 40 EC @ 2.0 ml/L
2. Powdery mildew (PM)	*Erysiphe polygoni*	White powdery coating on all parts of the plant above the soil surface	RUM5, ATF 3640 and VC 6468-11-1A	TARM 1, TARM 2, TARM 18, JM 721 and Pusa 9072	Spraying of NSKE @ 50 g/ L or neem oil of 3000 ppm @ 20 ml/L
3. Cercospora leaf spot	*Cercospora canesens*	Circular to irregular leaf spots with greyish centre and reddish brown margin	M-98,98cmg-003, C2/94-4-42, NM-1, NM-2, 98 cmg-018, BRM188	LM 113, LM 168, LM 170 and JM 171	Spraying of carbendazim 50 WP @1.0 g/L or mancozeb 45 WP @ 2.0 g/L
4. Bruchid beetles	*Callosobruchus maculatus*	Presence of circular holes and small whitish eggs on seeds	*Vigna radiata* var. *Sublobata*	TC1966 (completely resistant to both cowpea weevil and adzuki bean weevil)	Sun drying, Field disinfestation with 0.05 % malathion spray on young pods
5. Drought	------------	Increase of root shoot ratio, thickness of cell walls, amount of cutinization and lignifications	V 1281', 'V 2013' and 'V 3372'	K-851, PS-10, Pusa Baisakhi (Dutta P & Bera AK, 2008)	Usage of tolerant varieties
6. Water-logging	------------	Decrease of oxygen conc. In soil and nodule nitrogen fixation activity	GK48 and VC3945A	T 44 & MH–96–1	Usage of tolerant varieties

(Contd.)

7. salinity	------------	Affects seed germination, shoot growth, root growth, root length, biomass and seedling vigour	NM-92	VRMGG1/VBN1	Usage of tolerant varieties
8. Temperature	------------	Causes pollen in viability, lack of fertilization and high or complete flower shedding.	------------	NFM-6-5 and NFM-12-14	Usage of tolerant varieties

References

Abbaiah K (1993). Development of powdery mildew epidemics in urd bean in relation to weather factors. *Indian Journal of Pulses Res* 6: 186–188.

Ahmed S (2009). Effect of soil salinity on the yield and yield components of mungbean. *Pak. J. Bot* 41(1): 263-268.

Ahmed S, Nawata E, Sakuratani T (2002a). Effects of waterlogging at vegetative and reproductive growth stages on photosynthesis, leaf water potential and yield of mungbean. *Plant Prod Sci* 5:117–123.

Amin PW (1985). Apparent resistance of groundnut cultivar Robut 33–1 to bud necrosis disease. *Pant Dis*. 69: 718–719.

Arora A, Sairam RK & Srivastava GC (2002) Oxidative stress and antioxidative system in plants. *Current Science* 1227-1238.

AVRDC (1979). AVRDC Progress Report 1978. Asian Vegetable Research and Development Centre, Shanhua, Tainan 173.

Chen QS, Zhang ZC, Liu CY, Xin DW, Qiu HM, Shan DP and Hu GH (2007). QTL analysis of major agronomic traits in soybean. *Agricultural Sciences in China* 6(4): 399-405.

Dutta P and Bera AK (2008). Screening of mungbean genotypes for drought tolerance. *Legume Research* 31(2): 145-148.

FarooqM, Wahid A, Kobayashi N, FujitaD and Basra SMA (2009). Plant drought stress: effects, mechanisms and management in sustainable agriculture Springer, Dordrecht. 153-188.

Fernandez GCJ and Shanmugasundaram S (1988). The AVRDC mungbean improvement program. The past, present and future. In: J Fernandez and S Shanmugsundaram (Eds), Mungbean. Asian Vegetable Research and Development Centre, Shanhua, Tainan. 58-70.

Grewal JS (1978). Diseases of mungbean in India. First Intl. Mungbean Symp. Proc., Univ. Philippines 165–168.

Hsiao TC and Acevedo F (1974). Plant response to water deficits, water use efficiency and drought resistance. *Agricultural Meteorology* 14: 69-84.

Humphry ME, Lambrides CJ, Chapman SC, AitkenEAB, Imrie BC, Lawn RJ & Liu CJ (2005). Relationships between hard seededness and seed weight in mungbean (Vigna radiata) assessed by QTL analysis. *Plant Breeding* 124(3): 292-298.

Ilag LL (1978). Fungal diseases of mungbean in the Philippines. First Intl. Mungbean Symp. Proc., Univ. Philippines 154–156.

Iqbal SM, Zubair M and Haqqani AM (2004). Resistance in Mungbean to Cercospora leaf spot disease. *Int. J. Agric. Bio*. 6 (5): 792-793.

Islam MR, Hamid A, KarimMA, Haque MM, Khaliq QA and Ahmed JU (2008). Gas exchanges and yield responses of mungbean (*Vigna radiata* L. Wilczek) genotypes differing in flooding tolerance. *Acta Physiologiae Plantarum* 30(5): 697-707.

Karthikeyan A, ShobhanaVG, Sudha M, Raveendran M, Senthil N, Pandiyan M and Nagarajan P (2014). Mungbean yellow mosaic virus (MYMV): a threat to green gram (Vigna radiata) production in Asia. *International Journal of Pest Management* 60(4): 314-324.

KaurR, Bains TS, Bindumadhava H & Nayyar H (2015). Responses of mungbean (Vigna radiata L.) genotypes to heat stress: Effects on reproductive biology, leaf function and yield traits. *Scientia Horticulturae* 197: 527-541.

Khattak GSS, Saeed IQBAL & Muhammad T (2006). Breeding for heat tolerance in mungbean (Vigna radiata (L.) Wilczek). *Pak. J. Bot* 38(5): 1539-1550.

Kitamura K, Ishimoto M and Sawa M (1988). Inheritance of Resistance with Adzukibean weevil in Vigna radiata spp. sublobata and Successful Incorporation to Vigna radiata. *Japan. J. Breeding* 38:459-464.

Kumar BS, Prakash M, Narayanan S & Gokulakrishnan J(2012). Breeding for salinity tolerance in mungbean. *APCBEE Procedia* 4: 30-35.

Kumar P, Pal M, Joshi R & Sairam RK (2013). Yield, growth and physiological responses of mung bean [Vigna radiata (L.) Wilczek] genotypes to waterlogging at vegetative stage. *Physiology and Molecular Biology of Plants* 19(2): 209-220.

Kumari P& Varma SK (1983). Genotypic differences in flower production/shedding and yield in mungbean (Vigna radiata). Indian journal of plant physiology.

Lambrides CJ, Lawn RJ, Godwin ID, Manners J& Imrie BC (2000). Two genetic linkage maps of mungbean using RFLP and RAPD markers. *Australian Journal of Agricultural Research* 51(4): 415-425.

Malathi VG & John P (2008). Geminiviruses infecting legumes. Characterization, diagnosis and management of plant viruses. Studium Press, Houston 97-123.

Mayee CD & Datar VV (1986). Phytopathometry. Phytopathometry.

Morton F, Smith RE and Poehlman JM (1982). The Mungbean. University of Puerto Rico, Mayaguez. 136.

Nariani TK (1960). Yellow mosaic of mung (Phaseolus aureus). *Indian Phytopathology* 13: 24–29.

Nene YL (1968). Annual report (No. 1) project, FG-In-358, U.P. Agric. Univ., India.

Nene YL (1972). A survey of viral diseases of pulse crops in Uttar Pradesh, G.B. Pant Univ. Agric. Tech., Pantnagar, Res. Bull. 4.

Nene YL (1973). Viral diseases of some warm weather pulse crops in India. *Plant Disease Reporter* 57: 463–467.

Pandey RK, Herrera WAT, Villegas AW and Penletion JW (1984). Drought response of grain legumes under irrigation gradient. III. Plant growth, *Agronomy Journal* 76: 557-560.

Quebral FC and Cagampang IC (1970). Influence of Cercospora leaf spot Control on Yield of Mungbean. *Agriculture at Los Banos* 10: 7-12.

Rath GC, Grewal JS (1973). A note on Cercospora leaf spot of Phaseolus aureus. *Indian, J. Mycol. Plant Pathol* 3: 204–207.

Rathi YPS (2002). Epidemiology, yield losses and management of major diseases of Kharif pulses in India. In: Plant Pathology and Asian Congress of Mycology and Plant Pathology, University of Mysore, Mysore, India.

Rathi YPS, Nene YL (1974). The additional hosts of mungbean yellow mosaic virus. *Indian Phytopathol* 27: 429–430.

Reddy KR & Singh DP (1995). Inheritance of resistance to mungbean yellow mosaic virus. Madras Agric J, 88: 199-201.

Reddy KS, Pawar SE, Bhatia CR (1994). Inheritance of powdery mildew (Erysiphe polygoni DC) resistance in mungbean (Vigna radiate, L. Wilczek). *Theoretical & Applied Genetics* 88: 945–948.

Sandhu TS, Brar JS, Sandhu SS, Verma MM (1985). Inheritance of resistance to mungbean yellow mosaic virus in green gram. *J. Res. Punjab Agric. Univ.* 22: 607-611.

Schafleitner R, Nair RM, RathoreA, Wang YW, Lin CY, Chu SH & Ebert AW (2015). The AVRDC–The World Vegetable Center mungbean (Vigna radiata) core and mini core collections. *BMC Genomics* 16(1): 344.

Shukla GP, Pandya BP (1985). Resistance to yellow mosaic in greengram. *SABRAO J.* 17: 165-171.

Singh BB (2011). Project coordinators report. All India coordinated research project on MULLaRP. Annual group meet; 11-13; Kanpur: Indian council of agricultural research, Indian Institute of Pulses Research.

Singh DP & Singh BB (2011). Breeding for tolerance to abiotic stresses in mungbean. *J Food Legumes* 24(2): 83-90.

Singh DP (1981). Breeding for resistance to diseases in greengram and blackgram. *Theor. Appl. Genet.* 59: 1–10.

Singh RA, De, RK, Gurha SN, Ghosh A (2000). Yellow mosaic disease of mungbean and urdbean. In: Advances in Plant Disease Management, (Eds.) U. Narain, K. Kumar, M. Srivastave. Advance Publishing Concept, New Delhi, India 337–348.

Singh RN, Nene YL (1978) Further studies on the mosaic mottle disease of urdbean, *Indian Phytopath.* 31: 159–162.

Srivastava KM, Verma GS, Verma HN (1969). A mosaic disease of blackgram (*Phaseolus mungo*). *Sci. Cult.* 35: 475–476.

Tangphatsornruang S, Somta P, Uthaipaisanwong P, Chanprasert J, Sangsrakru D, Seehalak W, Sommanas W, Tragoonrung S, Srinives P (2009). Characterization of microsatellites and gene contents from genome shotgun sequences of mungbean (Vigna radiata (L.) Wilczek) *BMC Plant Biology* 9(1): 137.

Tiwari AK, Shivhare AK (2016). pulses in India: Retrospect and prospects. Department of agriculture, cooperation and farmers welfare. DPD/Pub.1/Vol. 2/2016.

Vavilov NI (1951) The origin, variation, immunity and breeding of cultivated plants. *LWW* 72 (6): 482.

Verma RPS, Singh DP (1988) Inheritance of resistance to mungbean yellow mosaic virus in greengram. *Ann Agric Res.* 9: 98-100.

8

Lentil Diseases and Its Integrated Management Approach

Fariha Adan[1], Anil Kumar[2] and Thota Gopi Krishna[1]

[1]Research Scholar, Department of Plant Breeding and Genetics Bihar Agricultural University, Sabour, 813210, Bihar, India
[2]Department of Plant Breeding and Genetics, Bihar Agricultural University Sabour, 813210, Bihar, India

Abstract

*Lentil (*Lens culinaris *Medik) is an important rabi leguminous annual herb with rich source of protein and other balanced nutrition. Lentil is susceptible to many insect-pests and diseases which causes significant yield loss which may range from 50 to 100% leading to one of the most important biotic constraints in productivity. The major fungal diseases in lentil are* Fusarium *wilt, Ascochyta blight and rust which causes severe losses in lentil production. Other minor diseases like botrytis grey mould, anthracnose, alternaria, stem rot, collar rot and some viral diseases also infect the lentil field under condusive environment conditions. Coming to major insect pests of lentil viz. helicoverpa, aphids, leaf weevils and lygus bugs with several noteworthy minor field pests such as thrips and cutworm with few storage pests that infest the crop. With an integrated blueprint of disease management, one can minimize risk of yield loss by following modified package and practices with need based use of pesticides, thus maximizing profit in lentil production.*

Keywords: *Lens culinaris*, biotic constraints and *Fusarium* wilt

Introduction

The cultivated species of lentil i.e *Lens culinaris* Medik , commonly known as masoor is a herbaceous rabi pulse crop with highest protein content ranging from 15.9% to 31.4% (Grusak *et al.* 2009). Presently, lentil occupies area of about 43.45 lakh hectares with annual production of 49.52 lakh tones giving productivity of 1140 kg/ha (FAO 2013). Globally, lentil is grown in area of Canada, India, Turkey, Nepal, Australia, USA, Iran. India ranks first in the area and second in the production with 43% and 37% of world area and production respectively. In India, lentil is cultivated in Madhya Pradesh, Uttar Pradesh, Bihar, Rajasthan, West Bengal and Assam. Bihar records highest yield productivity i.e 1209 kg/ha (Source: DAC&FW, DPD/Pub.1/ vol. 2/ 2016). Two sub species of lentil viz, (i) sub species *Macro sperma* (Bold seeded) that weighs more than 25g in test weight and mainly cultivated in Bundelkhand region of UP/MP and Maharashtra state , (ii) sub species *Micro sperma* (small seeded) having test weight less than 25g and grown in Indo-gangtic plains of NEPZ (Uttar Pradesh, Bihar, West Bengal and Assam). The lentil crop gives an average yield of 10-15 q/ha but this yield can be compromised with different biotic stress like incidence of disease and pests. Lentil is susceptible to many diseases caused by fungi, bacteria, virus, nematodes. Some severe fungal diseases are wilt (*Fusarium oxysporum* f. sp. *lens*), rust (*Uromyces fabae lentis*), ascochyta blight (*Ascochyta lentis*), stemphylium blight (*Stemphylium botryosum* Wallr), grey mould *(Botrytis fabae*), dry root rot (*Rhizoctonia bataticola*), collar rot (*Sclerotium rolfsii*), stem rot (*Sclerotinia sclerotiorum*), anthracnose (*Colletotrichum truncatum*). Insects belonging to different species damage various parts of plant like seedling, surface feeders, feed on foliage, pods, stored grains etc. Thus looking into the gap for proper identification, diagnosis and correct management strategies of major diseases and pests in lentil crop which are discussed in detail

1. Fusarium Wilt

Causal agent : *Fusarium oxysporum* f. sp. *lentil*

Padwick (1941), first observed wilt disease in lentil in India in experimental field in Delhi and Karnal. First authenticated record of vascular wilt of lentil with 67% disease incidence was published by Vasudev and Srinivasan in 1952. In 1979, Khare and others reported that F. oxysporum is seed associated fungus and it occurs in field at three stages i.e. pre-emergence, post emergence and at maturity stages (Vasudeva and Srinivasan, 1952 ; Khare *et al.*, 1979). In pre-emergence, seedling die during or immediately after seed germination. At post emergence stage, seedling is infected after 4-5 days of emergence exhibiting stunted, droop brown radicals and collapse later. Isolated patches are seen later in adult stage.

Symptoms

- Infected plant growth is stunted, leaves turn yellow and curl from lower to upper part of the plants, the crown droops and ultimately the plant dies.
- Roots turn yellowish-brown to dark brown partially or wholly and root nodules are poorly developed but no external rotting is seen.
- Stem exhibits reddish discolouration.
- At flowering to late pod filling stage, diseases start by yellowing of leaves from lower parts and extending upwards, epinasty and drying of whole plants.
- Brown discolouration of xylem vessels showing tyloses.

Pathogen diversity

Great variability is exhibited by *F. oxysporum* although being highly host specific. Sharma and Agnihotri (1972) identified, "A", "B" and "C", three isolates on the basis of virulence in lentil. Bhalla and others (1984) screened a more virulent strain 82A of *F. oxysporum* causing complete necrosis of lentil seedling within 7 days.

Epidemiology

The pathogen, *F. oxysporum* f. sp. Lentil has very limited host range as it only infects lentil in nature. Favourable conditions for wilt is moist soil, warm and humid conditions with an optimal temperature of 22-25 C. Lentil wilt is favoured at 25% soil moisture, at soil pH 7.5 to 8.0 and 20-30 C soil temperature.

Disease cycle

The fungus may be seed-borne but survives in infected plant debris in soil. The primary infection is through chlamydospores in soil, which remain viable upto next crop season. The secondary spread is through cultural operations, irrigation water and implements.

Management

- Seed treatment with Carbendazim or Thiram at 2 g/kg or treat with *Tricoderma viridae* at 4 g/kg or Pseudomonas fluorescens @ 10 g/kg of seed.
- Kannaiyan and Nene reported Thiram 37.5% DS + Carbendazim 25% WP (1:1) as effective seed dressing mixture.

- Heavy doses of organic manure is recommended.
- Crop rotation with non host crops for 5 years.
- Selection of early maturing cultivars and proper adjustment of sowing date to escape weather conditions favourable to the disease.
- Growing of resistant or moderately resistant lentil cultivars.

2. Dry Root Rot

Causal agent : *Rhizoctonia bataticola*

The perfect stage of this pathogen is *Macrophomina phaseolina*. It is a soil borne disease. Dry weather and high temperature is the most condusive factors for fungus.

Symptoms

- Occur at both seedling and maturity stages.
- Characteristics symptom is sudden drying of the plant without showing any yellowing.
- Plants are pulled out easily as secondary root rot. Affected roots are ash to black coloured having numerous minute sclerotia on and inside the roots.

Management

- Crop rotation for 3-4 years to reduce soil borne inoculums.
- Seed treatment with *Tricoderma* 1% WP (10 g/kg of seeds) or with carbendazim 50% WP (2 g/kg of seeds)

3. Black Root Rot

Causal agent : *Fusarium solani*

It is the soil borne fungus and survive in soil as chlamydospores. Severe in light soil with high moisture content and favoured by 22-23 C temperature.

Symptoms

- The disease occur at any stage of plant growth.
- Yellowing of leaves from lower to upper leaves.
- The main and secondary roots show rotting which give characteristically black colour to root.

Management

- Crop rotation for 3-4 years to reduce soil borne inoculums.
- Seed treatment with *Tricoderma* 1% WP (10 g/kg of seeds) or with carbendazim 50% WP (2 g/kg of seeds).

4. Collar Rots

Causal agent : *Sclerotium rolfsii*

Disease is prevalent in warm areas with 25-30 C temperature followed by good sunshine after rain particularly in North India where crop is grown after rice which causes early stage death of plant. The primary source of inoculums is sclerotia.

Symptoms

- At seedling stage, damping off occur and plant gradually turn pale, drop and dry.
- Collar region of plant is infected causing yellowish-brown discoloration and rotting of tissue (Beniwal *et al.* 1993).
- Plants are pulled out easily as root system are poorly developed.

Management

- Adjust sowing date to avoid coincidence of seedling stage with high soil temperature and temperature above 25 °C
- Treat the seed with thiram 75% WS or captan 75% FS @ 3 g/kg seed with carboxin 75% WP @ 2.5 g/kg seed
- Combination of thiram 37.5% DS + carbendazim 25% WP @ 2.5 g/kg seed helps controlling seedling stage mortality.
- Mukhopadhyay reported that using *Tricoderma harzianum* or *Bacillus subtilis* to seeds with 2% molasses solution reduce 80% collar rot incidence.

5. Stem Rot/ Blight

Causal agent : Sclerotinia sclerotium

Symptoms

- Characteristic symptoms appear as rotting of stem tissues above the collar region and yellowing and drooping of leaves above infection point.

- Shredding occur and presence of white fluffy mycelia on rotten stem with irregular shaped dark brown sclerotia.
- Disease is favoured by wet weather and dense crop canopy.
- Affected field gives patchy and blight like appearance.

Management

- 3-4 year of crop rotation and crop debris should be cleaned.
- Spraying dithane M-45 75% DG @ 3 g/l or chlorothalonil 75% WP i.e 2-3 ml/l to prevent stem rot.

6. Lentil Rust

Causal agent : *Uromyces viviae fabae*

Rust is the most widespread foliar disease capable of total crop failure. The yield loss is upto 60-69% in India as reported by Singh *et al.* in 1986. It is considered as one of the major biotic production constraints.

Symptoms

- Characteristic rust symptoms starts during flowering / early podding stage is yellowish-white aecial and pycnidial cups on leaflets, pods, singly or in small groups in circular form (Agarwal *et al.* , 1993).
- Later, brown conidial pustules oval to circular shaped about 1 mm in diameter are formed on stem, leafs and pods.
- The telia is formed late in the season, as dark brown to black colour, present on stems.
- In severe infection, plant dries without forming any seeds in pods.

Epidemiology

Lentil rust occurs in January to February with high humidity, drizzly weather with 20-22 C temperature (Khare *et al.* 1981). The fungus survives as teliospores in legume weed *Trigonella polycerata* during summer months which is primary source of infection.

Management

- Destroy weed host
- Dust sulphur at 20 kg/h or spray M-45 75% DG @ 32 g/ha at disease incidence.

7. Ascochyta Blight

Causal agent : *Ascochyta lentis*

Ascochyta blight is one of the biotic constraints in lentil production. All above ground parts of the plants are affected. The disease is prevalent throughout the globe and report of yield loss is upto 70% , 30-50% , and 50% in Canada, USA and Australia respectively (Gossen and Morrall, 1983; Brower *et al.* , 1995)

Symptoms

- The disease appear at flowering and podding time as patches of blighted area in field. It affects all above ground parts of the plant.
- Small water-soaked necrotic lesions appear that enlarge rapidly on leaves enclosing total leaves area.
- The lesions are elongated or round with grey centres surrounded by brownish margin on leaflets, stem and pods.
- Pycnidia is arranged in concentric circles as minute black dots on spots.
- Plant stem breaks at the point of infection due to girdling and if collar region is girdled, whole plant dies.

Epidemiology

The night temperature of 10 C and day temperature of 20 C accompanied by rain is most favourable for the disease to spread. Fungus survives as pycnidia in plant debris. The pathogen is externally and internally seed-borne. The primary source of infection is seed borne pycnidia. The secondary spread is mainly through air-borne conidia.

Management

- Destroy infected plant debris in the field.
- Crop rotation for 2-3 years along with deep ploughing.
- Intercropping with wheat, barley and mustard.
- Seed treatment with systemic fungicides like Benomyl 50% WP (0.2%), chlorothalonil 75% WP.
- Exposure of seed at 40-50 C to reduce survival of pathogen by 40-70%.
- Spraying carbendazim @ 0.1% at early bloom to early pod set stage.

8. Stemphylium Blight

Causal agent : *Stemphylium botryosum* Wallr

Stemphylium blight of lentil is caused by the pathogen is Stemphylium botryosum. The disease has the potential to cause yield losses of upto 62% under favourable conditions (Bakr, 1993).

Symptoms

- Small pin-headed light brown to tan coloured spots on leaflets (Beniwal *et al.*, 1993). Spot covers entire leaf within 2-3 days.
- The twigs dries, bend downward, turn ashy white, shed severely leaving only terminal leaves on the twigs but pods remain green.
- White mycelia growth is observed on infected twigs and stems.

Epidemiology

Air-borne ascospores or resting mycelium over infected crop debris can be primary source of inoculum. The infection commence with ambient night temperature above 8 C and mean day temperature exceeding 22 C. The relative humidity inside crop canopy must be 94% , a mean of 7.7 hour or less of daily sunshine and drizzling weather are all favourable conditions.

Management

- Remove and destroy old crop residues, crop rotation as cultural method of control.
- Delayed sowing to escape condusive conditions for fungus.
- Foliar spray of mancozeb 75% WP, sulphur 85%, roval 50 WP, three times at weekly interval.

9. Alternaria Blight

Causal agent : *Alternaria tenius*

Pathogen survives all round the year as it has wide host range.

Symptoms

- Symptom starts at tips of leaflets as small pale spots on margins and it enlarges giving concentric ring like appearance and dark brown in colour.

Management

- Foliar spray of dithane M-45 @ 3 g/l over severe incidence of disease.

10. Grey Mould

Causal agent : *Botrytis fabae* or *Botrytis cinerea*

In lentil, grey mould is caused by pathogen *Botrytis fabae* or *B. cinerea* (non host specific pathogen). It is sporadic disease. Knights first reported this disease in Australia in wet year of 1983.

Symptoms

- Symptoms first appear on flowers (Beniwal *et al.* 1993)
- Discrete lesions on lower leaves initially as dark green but turn greyish-brown that enlarges and infect whole plant.
- Flowers are covered with white dirty moldy growth of mycelia of pathogen which is visible distinctly.
- Infected portion of stem are light brown or blanched and covered with white moldy mycelium at plant crown.
- Infected pods fail to fill properly, rot and turn brown covered with mould, discoloured and shriveled seeds.

Epidemiology

The condusive environment of disease is moist and cool temperature of about 18-22 C , thick plant canopy, relative humidity > 95%. Sclerotia is the survival structure of *B. cinerea* and *B. fabae* and it is the source of inoculum.

Management

- Avoiding creation of microclimate at canopy by adjusting sowing dates and seed rates, wide row spacing weed control, avoid high nitrogen dose.
- Treat seed with fungicide such as benomyl 50% WP or chlorothalonil 75% WP @ 2-2.5 g/kg seed to reduce seed borne inoculums.

11. Anthracnose

Causal agent : *Colletotrichum truncatum*

Environment in which fungus is favoured is high humidity and temperature of 25-30 C. Pathogen survive as microsclerotia in crop residue and spreads in field through air borne conidia and by splashing water.

Symptoms

- Prior to flowering or shortly after bloom, appearance of tan lesions with darker borders on leaves and dropping of diseased leaves prematurely.
- Presence of tan to brown lesions with dark margin on lower stem, pods and coalesce to cover large area.
- Shriveled and discoloured seeds are formed in infected pods.

Management

- Treat seed with fungicide such as benomyl or thiabendazole which controls seed borne fungus.
- Foliar application of fungicide such as benomyl or chlorothalonil.

Management for virus control

- Planting disease-free seed
- Controlling insect vectors by spraying neem oil 3000 ppm or systemic insecticides like dimethoate 30% EC (400 g a.i/l) @ 0.8 l/ha or metasystox @ 0.04%.
- Growing resistant varieties of lentil.

Sustainable lentil production through Integrated Pest Management

Considering the myth that IPM can eliminate the use of chemical pesticides is just unlikely to happen. The FAO International Code of Conduct, on the distribution and use of Pesticides (Article 2) suggested IPM definition: IPM means the careful consideration of all available pest control techniques and subsequent integration of appropriate measures that discourage the development of pest populations and keep pesticides and other interventions to levels that are economically justified and reduce or minimize risks to human health and the environment. IPM emphasizes the growth of a healthy crop with the least possible disruption to agro-ecosystems and encourages natural pest control mechanisms (FAO, 2002).

Thus, IPM is the combine set of cultural, biological and chemical measures that provides the most cost effective, environmentally sound and socially acceptable method of managing diseases, insects, weeds and other pests. This system maintains pest population below threshold level and is ecologically safe and sound with integrated use of need based pesticides with non chemical methods. IPM works on knowledge of pests and crop interaction to pests utilizing locally available pest management tools. Since pests can co-evolve through natural selection by use of single product through "integrated" approach is most effective for sustainable management strategies. The concept of IPM does not

Table 1: Summary of viral diseases in lentil

In the given table, some important viral diseases of lentil with its causal agent, vectors and characteristic symptoms are summarized below :

Sr.no.	Diseases	Causal agent (virus group)	Vectors	Symptoms
1.	Lentil yellow disease	Bean leaf roll virus (BLRV), Turnip yellow virus (TuYV) (luteo virus group)	• Aphids	• Interveinal chlorosis later whole leaf become yellow • Reduction in leaf size, pod setting • Leaf rolling
2.	Bean yellow mosaic lesions	Bean yellow mosaic virus (BYMV) (poty virus group)	• By aphids in non persistant manner • Through sap	• Mild mosaic followed by leaf narrowing • New leaves from leaf axils are elongated narrow and light green
3.	Pea seed borne mosaic disease	Pea seed borne mosaic virus (PSbMV) (poty virus group)	• Virus is seed borne in lentil • By aphids in non persistent manner	• Mild mosaic • Malformation of leaves • Stunted and twisted stem • Small and deformed seed
4.	Cucumber mosaic disease	Cucumber mosaic virus (CMV) (Cucumo virus group)	• By aphids in non persistent manner • Through sap • By infected seed	• Vein clearing • Mild systemic mottle • Infected plant show stunted growth
5.	Alfalfa mosaic disease	Alfalfa mosaic virus (AMV) (Alfamo virus group)	• By aphids • Seed transmitted	• Heavy loss in large aphid population areas • Leaves become twisted, deformed leading to necrotic tip growth

Table 2 : Summary of lentil pests

Following table explains briefly about the lentil crop pests with identification marks of insects, damage symptoms caused by them with its possible management methods:

Sr.no.	Pests of lentil	Identification marks	Damage symptoms	Management
1.	Pod Borer (*Helicoverpa armigera*)	• Egg- spherical, yellowish eggs, several hundered of eggs on undersides of leaflets • Larva- 40 mm long, vary in colour, usually brown, distinct light and dark bands along sides of body • Pupa- pupates inside soil in an earthen cell • Adult- Moth is stout with brownish forewings with dark cross band near outer margin and dark spots near coastal margin	• Small larvae feed by scrapping the surface of leaflets • Full grown larvae feed on foliage and bore into green pod to eat the seeds	• Spray monocrotophos 36% SL, chlorpyriphos 20% EC at flowering and at early pod filling • Encourage natural enemies of borer like mynah, assassin bugs, trichogramma spp., B. thuringiensis var. kurstaki, yellow traps, entopathogenic nematodes (EPNs)
2.	Lime bean pod borer (*Etiella zinckenella*)	• Egg- lay eggs near calyx of the flowers or on pods • Larva- 10-12 mm long with brown head capsule, greenish body with brown line • Pupa- pupates in soil • Adult- Moths are 10-12 mm long with wingspan of 22-28 mm having brown grey forewing with white anterior margins	• Larva feed on soft green seeds in the pods cause webbing which is secondary infestation in lentil crop	• Spray cypermethrin 10% EC @ 0.02%, methomyl 40% SP @ 0.03%, monocrotophos 36% SL @ 0.04%
3.	Cowpea aphid (*Aphis cracivora*)	• Eggs- laid on growing region • Nymphs- slate grey in colour • Adult- shiny black having white	• Feeds on plant sap leading to reduction in root and nodulation growth	• Spray neem oil 3000 ppm with systemic insecticides like dimethoate 30% EC (400 g a.i/l) @ 0.8 l/ha,

(Contd.)

Table 3: Storage pests of lentil

This table briefly explains about two major storage pests in lentil accounting damage symptoms and its management -

Sr.no.	Pests of lentil	Identification marks	Damage symptoms	Management
1.	Lentil seed beetle *(Bruchus spp.)*	• Egg- yellow transparent in colour • Adult- brown in colour	• Adult infect lentil fields at flowering time by feeding on nector and pollen • Tiny Nymph feed on developing seeds by penetrating inside pod, old nymph exit from seed surfac leaving only thin circular window of epidermal membrane intact. • Adult remain inside the seed for hibernation	• Fumigation with CO_2 of infested seeds before storage, increase shelf life
2.	Callosobruchus beetles (*Callosobruchus cinesis ; C. maculates*)	• Adult- C. cinesis has triangular white spot at the base of the thorax and rust colour elytra with two brown spots • Adult- C. maculates have large round spot on elytra at mid length with black tips	• Occasionally infest fields at end of harvest • Eggs remain attached to the seeds and later adult exit leaving emergence holes on seed	• Remove all residues from warehouse of earlier stored products and spray malathion disinfectant on wall. • Fumigate with phosphine pellets • Seeds before storing should be treated with malathion • Mixing seed with mustard oil and salt (5 ml and 20 g/kg seed) or neem seed oil (3 ml/kg seed) provide adequate pest control

		appendages with black tips, are 1.9-2.5 mm long (winged aphid) and 1.5-2.2 mm (wingless aphid) with whitish fine dusting over body	• Severe infestation cause deformation, stunted growth and lower seed set	metasystox @ 0.04% • Natural enemies are spread like ladybird beetles, syrphid flies, damsel bug, green lacewing and aphid parasitoids like aphidius spp. • Using imidacloprid for seed dressing.
4.	Thrips (*Thrips frankiniella*)	• Eggs- white, kidney bean shaped eggs developing within leaf tissue • Adults- 1-2 mm long body with four extremely slender wings or wingless, light coloured	• Damage during flowering period • Suck sap from leaves, flower, pods by puncturing the plant organs causing silvery blotches	• Insecticides like malathion, dimethoate controls thrips • Encourage pirate bugs and Orius spp. As natural enemies of thrips
5.	Lygus bugs	• Eggs- curved slightly with eye shaped, laid on stems and leaves of plants • Young nymph are light green and wingless old nymph have black dots on top of thorax and abdomen • Adults- bud is 3 mm wide 6 mm long, pale green to reddish brown to black colour, characteristic "V" shaped marking on upper centre of body and wingtips are membranous	• Adult bugs suck the sap from flowers and developing seeds and inject toxic saliva into plant • Characteristic chalk spot on seeds	• Spray monocrotophos @ 31% SL @ 2 ml/ha
6.	Leaf weevils (*Sitona macularius*)	• Larva- white larvae with brown head capsules • Adult- grayish brown coloured body, a pronotum has three longitudinal light line and elytra have three rows of dark and white spots	• Root nodules are affected by grub in soil which affect N_2 fixation capacity of plant • Adult weevil feed on foliage making semicircular notches from leaf edge • It is a vector of broad bean stain comovirus (BBSV)	• Application of carbofuron 75% WP reduces nodule damage • Seed treatment with chlorpyriphos 20% EC @ 720 g a.i/ha or malathion 50% EC @ 1300 a.i/ha

(Contd.)

7.	Cut worm (*Agrotis ipsilon*)	• Larva- dark green or grayish colour larvae with two bright lines • Adult- Moth is grey brown with 40 mm wingspan. The forewings are light brown and hindwings are creamy white with brown edges	• Young larvae damage foliage of plant • Mature larvae cut the plant above root crown and move to another plant without consuming after cutting	• Deep ploughing of the fallow field • Go for spot application of insecticides at affected patches with cypermethrin @ 0.02%

only involves trade-off between pest control but also to minimize the adverse effects on non-target organisms such as natural enemies, pollinators, wildlife and plants, contamination of soil and water.

Tools of IPM

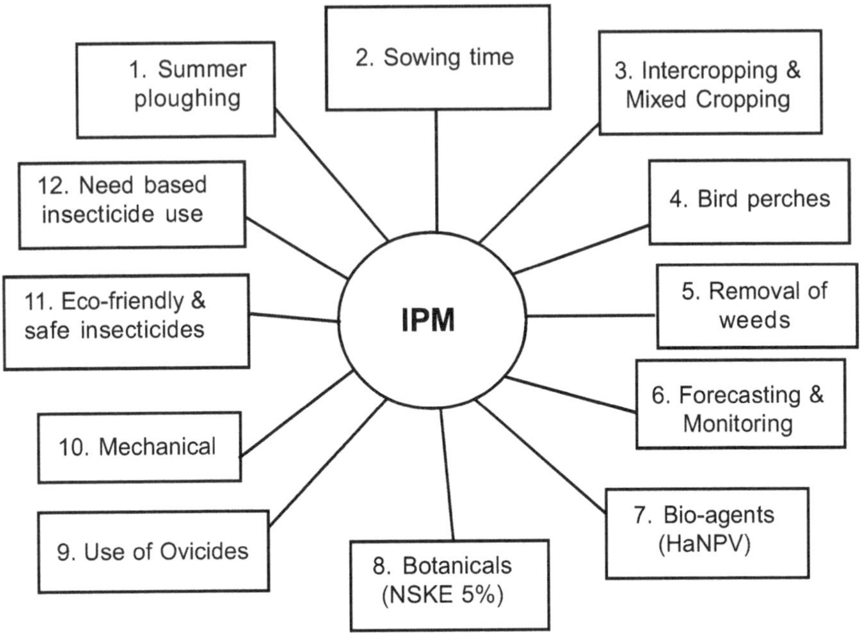

Source: Field guide of lentil pest and their management, ICAR, NCIPM, GOI Technical bulletin : 36

The core of sustainable agricultural i.e IPM includes following management plan e.g., monitoring, cultural, mechanical, biological and chemical control having compatibility among them. In pulses, urgent need was felt to summarize efficient integrated pest management module. Publication by Reed and Lateef (1990), Lal and Katti (1998) and Shanower and Romeis (1999) were reviewed and updated with following salient findings:

Cultural Working Plan

- Adjustment of sowing date to escape the condusive environment for pest development.
- Seed borne diseases can be minimized by field sanitation and summer ploughing.
- 2-3 years of crop rotation is necessary to reduce wilt incidence.

- For endemic area of wilt disease, mixed cropping with sugarcane (3:2) and lentil with toria or barley or safflower (4/6:1) had proved to be effective.
- Application of neem cake @ 50-75 kg/ha is recommended in nematode endemic area and also manages *Fusarium* wilt.
- Managing time and frequency of crop harvesting for storage insect pests. For e.g. timely harvest reduces C. maculates infestation by 50–90%. Also mixing seeds with olive oil (3 ml/kg seed) before storage help in controlling *Callosobruchus* beetles for 3-4 months.

Genetical Working Plant

- Planting resistant varieties of lentil for control of pest and diseases.
- Higher content of total soluble sugar (TSS), crude fiber, reducing sugar and lower content of starch, these factors affect the incidence of the pest.
- Pest avoidance in Northern India is the result of varietal phenology and growth habit as cold winter suppress their activity.
- Delayed planting or selecting a landrace/ varieties of desired maturity duration and resistance offers control over pest population.

The following table given below contain lentil varieties with specific resistance or tolerant to particular disease in suitable zone:

Variety	Resistant/Tolerant to disease	Suitable Area for production
BR 26	-	North Bihar
PL 77-12 (Arun)	Tolerant to wilt	All Bihar
BR 25	-	Bihar and Madhya Pradesh
L4147 (Pusa vaibhav)	Resistant to rust and tolerant to Pod borer	North-Western plain
P-927 & P-202	Resistant to Pod borer	-
Pant L 406	Resistant to rust and wilt	North-Western plain zone
LH-84-8	Resistant to rust	North-Western plain zone
VL-4	Tolerant to wilt	Hilly area of North Western and Eastern states
Pant L 639	Moderately resistant to shattering, resistant to rust and wilt complex	NWPZ, NEPZ and Central zone
VL-3	Tolerant to Ascochyta blight	Uttar Pradesh

Bold Seeded Varieties

Variety	Resistant/Tolerant to disease	Suitable Area for production
Pant L 234	Tolerant to wilt and rust disease	Uttar Pradesh
NFL 92 (Narendra Masoor1)	Resistant to rust and tolerant to wilt	Uttar Pradesh
DPL 15 (Priya), and DPL 62 (Sheri)	Resistant to rust and tolerant to wilt	NWPZ
IPL 81 (Noori)	Tolerant to wilt and rust	CZ
K 75 (Malika)	-	NEPZ and CZ
Pusa 4076 (Shivalik)	Resistant to rust and affected from drought in comparison to desi lentil	NWPZ and CZ
Pusa 1	-	Bihar, Uttar Pradesh, Madhya Pradesh, Haryana and Orissa
Pusa 4	-	Uttar Pradesh, Bihar and West Bengal
JLS 1	Tolerant to wilt	Central plain region

Source: Field guids of lentil pest and their management, ICAR, NCIPM, GoI, Technical Bulletin

Mechanical Working Plan

Effective treatment against *Bruchids* is to apply diatomaceous earth (DE) at 1 to 2% and sand treatment. It works when insect bodies trap DE paeticles which damage the cuticle and insects die due to water desiccation.

Botanical Working Plan

- Plant derived products e.g. Neem in the form of neem seed kernel extract, green neem berries, neem oil (1 to 15 ml/kg of grain) is effective with insecticidal activity, inhibit moult formation, antifeedant, growth retardation, reduced fecundity.
- Beetle infestation is managed by edible and non edible oils reported in pulses. The oil coating cuts the oxygen supply to the embryo and cause suffocation resulting in insect death.
- Plant essential oils viz. turmeric oil, ocimum oil, clove oil, sweet flag oil, and eucalyptus oil have fumigants as well as contact insecticidal properties such as antifeedant, repellant and insect growth regulator.

Biological Working Plan

- IPM supports conservation and introduction of native natural enemy population which restrict pest population without damaging the crops.

- Significant success have been reported with augmentative biocontrol with *Campoletis chloride, Campoletis flayicincta, Hyposter annulipes* etc
- One should maintain balance use of pesticides so that destruction of favourable natural enemy pest does not occur.

Here's a list of predators and parasitoid associated with insect pest of lentil:

Pests	Natural enemy/pathogen/nematode	Stage of pest
Insects		
Aphis craccivora	*Menochilus sexmaculatus*	Nymph/ Adult
	Coccinella septumpuctata	Nymph/ Adult
	Brumus sutularis	Nymph
	Chrysopa carnea	Nymph
Agrotis ipsilon	*Bracon kitcheneri*	Larva
	Fileanta ruficanda	Larva
	Broscus punctatus (Predator)	Larva
	Liogryllus bimacultus (Predator)	Larva
Helicoverpa spp	*Apanteles ruficus*	Larva
	Bracon brevicornis	Larva
	Campolestis chloridae	Larva
	Chrysopa	Egg
	Chelonus heliopae	Egg-larva
	Clubiona	Larva
	Enicospilus spp.	Larva
	Erioborus argenteopilosus	Larva
	Exorista fallax	Larva
	Delta spp. (Predator)	Larva
	Goniophthalamus halli	Larva
	Microplitis	Larva
	Neosconathis (Predator)	Larva
	NVP (pathogen)	Larva
	Ovomermis albicans (Nematode)	Larva
	Polistes olivaceus (Predator)	Larva
	Rogas spp.	Larva
	Thomisus	Larva
Diseases		
Root rot	*Trichoderma viride*	
Wilt	*Trichoderma harzianum*	
Soft rot	*Pseudomonas flurorescens*	
	Bacillus subtilis	

Source: Field giude of Lentil pest and their management, ICAR, NCIPM, GoI Technical Bulletin: 36

Chemical Working Plan

- Chemical control is recommended in epidemic situation and when pest crosses ETL level.

- The synthetic chemical insecticides works for long lasting protection as it degrade slowly. Some synthetic insecticides are monocrotophos 36% SL, dimethoate 30% EC, chlorpyriphos 20% EC, cypermethrin 10% EC etc have been recommended (Lal and Katti 1988).
- Some insecticides used in storage grain protection are Pyrethroid, Deltamethrin, Organophosphates viz ; Pirimiphos-methyl, chlorpyrprifos-methyl, synthetic pyrithroids etc.

Lentil Integrated Disease Management (IDM) Blueprint

Integrated disease management strategies to minimize disease incidence in lentil crop are as follows

1. On-farm hygiene

- Burying or burning stubbles reduces inoculum of many diseases.
- Seed present on-farm should be from "cleanest" paddocks.
- Keeping early control on volunteer lentils, faba beans, chickpea, lathyrus etc.

2. Paddock selection

- Previous season lentil crop stubble should be kept at a distance of at least 250m from next season lentil crop.
- Avoiding lentil sowing near canola or other broad leaf crops in an area with high risk of sclerotinia.
- Paddocks under high soil nitrogen should be avoided as greater vegetative growth predisposes disease.
- Since herbicide residues weaken plants resistance to disease, thus maximum plant-back period is ensured.

3. Seed source

- Seed used should not be from infected paddocks with fungus and viruses. Threshold of less than 1% for fungus and range og 0.1% to 0.5% threshold for virus is accepted.
- Using more than one year old seed which is frosted, diseased, damaged increases disease attack.

4. Seed dressing

- Proper seed treatment should be done especially for disease which affect at early stage like wilt, root rot, collar rot etc with thiram or thiram plus thiabendazole.

5. Canopy management

- Plant population of 100-120 plants per square metre is recommended as higher seeding rates increases grey mould risk due to dense canopy growth.
- Also wide row spacing of 23-42 cm is recommended in grey mould prone areas.
- Generally early sowing is beneficial in low rainfall areas.

6. Virus control

- Sowing seed with less than 0.1% seed infection.
- Remove volunteer weeds regularly which act as alternate host of fungi.
- Spraying insecticides for aphid control which is vectors of many viruses.

7. Fungicide spraying periods

- Three critical period of fungicides spraying – seedling stage, mid flowering/ early pod filling stage, and seed setting stage.
- Grazing withholding periods should be noted before spray.
- Spraying should be done before canopy closure for better fungicide penetration.
- Using high water rates (generally 100 l/ha by ground or 30 l/ha by air) with surfactants to improve spray redistribution.

8. Early harvest

- To minimize botrytis and ascochyta infection on seed, early harvest should be ensured.
- Harvest lentil crop early to prevent poor seed quality and colour.

References

Agrawal SC, Khare MN, Agrawal PS (1976) Control of lentil rust by use of fungicides. *Indian Phytopath.* 29; 90-91.

Agrawal SC, Khare MN, Agrawal PS (1978) Biological control of lentil rust by use of fungicides. *Indian Phytopath.* 30; 176-179.

Agrawal SC, Khare MN, Joshi LK (1975) Effect of pre –sowing treatments of seeds on pre- and post- emergence losses in lentil. Proceeding of the Annual Conference of Madhya Pradesh Academy, Bhopal, India 5,107 (abstr.).

Bakr MA (1993) Plant Protection of Lentil in Bangladesh. In: Lentil in South Asia (pp 177-186). Erskine W and Saxena MC (eds), International Centre for Agricultural Research in the Dry Areas, Aleppo, Syria.

Beniwal SPS, Bayaa B, Weigand. Makkouk K, Saxena MC (1993) Field Guide to Lentil Diseases and Insect Pests. International Centre for Agriculture Research in the Dry Areas, Aleppo, Syria, 106pp.

Bhalla MK, Nozzolillo C, Schneider EF (1984) Pathogenicity of soil fungi associated with a root rot of lentils. *Can. J. Pl. Path.*, 6: 21-28.

Brower JB, Bretag TW, Materne MA (1995) Coordinated improvement program for Australian lentils. Proceeding of 2nd European Conference on Grain Legumes, Copenhagen, Denmark. p. 25.

DAC&FW, DPD/Pub. 1/2/2016.

FAO.2002. Proceedings of the workshop on Rural Radio and food security 5-9, November 2001. FAO, Rome.

Field guide of lentil pest and their management, ICAR, NCIPM, GOI Technical Bulletin: 36

Gossen BD, Morrall RAA (1983) Effect of ascochyta blight on seed yield and quality of lentils. *Canadian Journal of Plant Pathology* 5: 168-173.

Grusak M (2009) In: The lentil: botany, production and uses. W. Erskine *et al.* (Eds.). CAB International. pp. 368-390.

Kannaiyan J, Nene YL (1976) Reaction of lentil germplasm and cultivars against three root pathogens. *Indian journal of Agricultural Sciences* 46;165-167.

Khare MN (1981). Diseases of Lentil (in) Lentils, pp 163-172. Lbs C and dauti G. (Eds.) *Com Commonality* Agricultural Bureau International, England, UK.

Khare MN, Agrawal SC, Jain AC (1979) Lentil diseases and their control. Technical Bulletin. Jawaharlal Nehru Krishi Vishwa Vidyalay. Jabalpur. Madhya Pradesh. India. Pp.1-29.

Knights EJ (1987) Lentil: A potential winter grain legume crop for temperate Australia. *Journal of the Australian Institute of Agricultural Science* 53: 271-280.

Lal SS, Katti G (1998) IPM of pod borer complex infesting pigeonpea (In) IPM system in Agriculture Vol IV Pulses. Aditya books Pvt. Ltd., New Delhi, pp. 79-128.

Mukhopadhyay AN, Kaur N, Saxena HC (1989) Biological control of soil borne diseases of chickpea and lentil. *Indian Phytopathology* 42; 315.

Padwick GW (1941) Report of the Imperial Mycologist. Sci. Rep. Agric. Res. Institute, New Delhi, pp. 94-101.

Paul taylor, Kurt lindbeck, Weidong chen, Rebecca ford. (2007). Lentil diseases. Chapter 18. 291: 313.

Reed W, Lateef, SS (1990) Pigeonpea: pest management In: Nene YL Hall SD, *Shield* Vk (Eds.) The pigeonpea, CAB International *Wallingford*, UK, pp 349-374

Shanower TG and Romeis J. (1999) Insect pests of pigonpea and their management. *Annual Review of Entomology* 44:77-96.

Sharma KB, Agnihotri JP (1972) Pathogenicity and variability of lentil wilt Fusarium. Indian *Journal of Mycology and Plant pathology*, 2: 170.

Sharma OP, Singh SK, Vennila S, Bhagat S, Saini M R, Kumari A, Chattopadhyay C (2014) Field Guide of Lentil Pest and their Management Technical Bulletin No. 36. Pp 36.

Singh K, Jhooty JS, Cheema HS (1986) Assessment of losses in lentil yield due to rust caused by Uromyces fabae. *Lens Newsletter* 13.28.

Vasudeva RS, Srinivasan KV (1952) Studies on the Wilt Disease of Lentil (Lens esculenta Moench). *India Phytopath*. 5: 23-32.

Wayne Hawthorne, Michael Materne, Jenny Davidson, Kurt Lindbeck, Larn McMurray, Jason Brand (2012) Lentil disease management strategy. *Southern Pulse Bulletin*. P- 1 to 8.

9

Bio-efficacy of Different Herbicides on Microbial Population Dynamics of Soil in Maize

Rajeev Kumar Ranjan, Shashank Tyagi, N. Chattopadhyay and M. Haque

Department of Agronomy, Bihar Agricultural University, Sabour Bhagalpur - 813210, Bihar, India

Abstract

A field experiment was carried out during rabi *2012-13 at Bihar Agricultural College farm, Sabour, Bhagalpur to assess the effect of different herbicides on microbial population dynamics of soil in winter maize (Zea mays L.). The experiment comprised of ten weed management treatments involving various herbicides (acetochlor @ 1.125, 2.25 and 4.5 kg a.i. ha^{-1}, atrazine @ 1.0 kg a.i. ha^{-1}, pendimethalin @ 0.5 kg a.i. ha^{-1} + atrazine @ 0.5 kg a.i. ha^{-1}, alachlor @ 0.5 kg a.i. ha^{-1} as pre-emergence and 2,4-Diethyl ester @ 0.6 kg a.i. ha^{-1}and topramezone @ 0.04 kg a.i. ha^{-1}+ atrazine @ 0.25 kg a.i. ha^{-1} as post-emergence including weed free and weedy check laid in randomized block design with three replications. Results indicated that all the herbicides' treatment showed significant adverse effect on microbial population in rhizospheric soil of winter maize up to 45 days after sowing. Further, there was reduction in soil microbial population occurred in all the herbicides treated plots up to said time period as compared with weed free and weedy check. Initially the soil microbial population in weed free plot was much higher than that of weedy check, however, it was found in reverse trends in rest of the time intervals as well as harvest. Thereafter, soil microbial population was gradually increasing at different time intervals and at harvest, their population increased considerably in herbicidal treated plots though the weed free and weedy check showed higher soil microbial population than other herbicide treated plots.*

***Keywords*:** Herbicides, Maize, Microbial counts, Soil actinomycetes, bacteria, fungi

Maize (*Zea mays* L.) is third most important cereal of India after rice and wheat. Maize is versatile cereal over diverse environment for human food, poultry feed and fodder for livestock as well as raw material for industries. In Bihar, maize is cultivated in 0.65 million ha area, 2.10 MT production and 32.25 q ha^{-1} productivity (Anonymous, 2010-11).

Maize is heavily fertilized and wide spaced crop with initial slow growth during winter season favors the emergence of weeds, which leads to severe weed infestation which compete the crop for growth factors which ultimately reduced yield and increased cost of production (Porwal, 2000). *Rabi* season maize suffers from severe weed competition depending upon intensity, nature, stage and duration of weed infestation causes yield losses varying from 28-100% (Patel *et al.*, 2006). Weeds being the major yield limiting factor reduced crop yield by 20-40% depending upon weed species and density (Oerke & Dehne, 2004). Weeds harbor insects and disease organisms by acting as alternate host for these pests and increase cost of production.

Several methods are available to minimize the losses by weeds. Cultural methods are still useful but are costly, laborious and time consuming. Farmers are using alternative methods like chemical weed control. Post emergence herbicides have achieved adequate weed control method due to its broad spectrum activity, convenience and flexibility in maize. Use of herbicides in agriculture system may usually disturb and alter the biological equilibrium in soil (Grossbard, 1976). Shivashankar *et al.* (1981) reported that bacterial, fungal and actinomycetes population were affected considerably up to 45 days after spraying of alachlor and metribuzin, they showed no adverse effects in the subsequent period. Fungal population was inhibited up to 45 days with herbicide doses and recovered at harvest. The higher herbicide doses gave lower populations of bacteria, fungi and actinomycetes.

To manage the complex weed flora in maize, there is need to evaluate different herbicides alone and in combination to have broad spectrum weed control and their impact on microbial population dynamics of soil. Keeping these issues in view, the present investigation was undertaken with the aim to assess the impact of use of herbicides on microbiological status of the soil.

Materials and Methods

A field experiment was conducted during winter (*rabi*) season of 2012-13, at the research farm of Bihar Agricultural University, Sabour, Bhagalpur, Bihar to assess the effect of herbicide molecules on soil microbial population equilibrium in winter maize (*Zea mays* L.). The soil test values indicated that the experimental plot had medium textured soil categorized as silt loam with soil reaction falling in neutral range. Fertility status of the experimental plot as envisaged through organic carbon, N, P_2O_5 and K_2O indicated that available nitrogen (195.6 kg ha^{-1}) was low and available phosphorus (25.0 kg ha^{-1}) and potassium (152.1 kg ha^{-1}) was in medium range during 2012-13.

The experiment comprised of ten weed management treatments involving various herbicides (acetochlor @ 1.125, 2.25 and 4.5 kg a.i. ha^{-1}, atrazine @ 1.0 kg a.i. ha^{-1}, pendimethalin @ 0.5 kg a.i. ha^{-1} + atrazine @ 0.5 kg a.i. ha^{-1}, alachlor @ 0.5 kg a.i. ha^{-1} as pre-emergence and 2,4-Diethyl ester @ 0.6 kg a.i. ha^{-1} and topramezone @ 0.04 kg a.i. ha^{-1} + atrazine @ 0.25 kg a.i. ha^{-1} as post-emergence including weed free and weedy check laid out in randomized block design with three replications.

Soil samples from the experimental plots were collected from the space between the rows at a depth up to 0-15 cm at initial (pre-treatment of herbicide) in maize were air dried, ground and sieved with 20 mesh sized sieve. These samples were subjected to analyze for pH, EC, available N, P_2O_5 and K_2O as per standard methods as described by Bouyoucos (1962), Jackson (1973) and Olson *et al.* (1954) to determine the nutrient status of the soil. The soil samples from different replicates for the same weed control treatment were pooled together and then requisite composite samples of each herbicidal treatment were taken for microbial analysis by dilution plating technique following standard methods. Soil dilutions were prepared in sterile distilled water by constant shaking and plating was done separately in replicates in specific media such as Thornton's agar medium at 10^{-6} dilutions for bacteria, Martin's rose bengal streptomycin agar medium at 10^{-4} dilutions for fungi and Jensen's agar medium at 10^{-5} dilutions for actinomycetes. The plates were incubated at 28±1°C for a maximum duration of 7 days in BOD incubator and observations in terms of counting of number of colonies/plate were made. The experimental data for different characters were subjected to statistical analysis by adopting the methods appropriate to the design (Cochran and Cox, 1963). The results were interpreted on the basis of 'F' test (Fisher, 1935) and critical difference (CD) between treatments mean. Whenever the variance ratio (F value) was found significant, critical differences (CD) values were computed for the comparisons among the treatments means. The data collected from the experiment were analyzed statistically following the standard statistical procedures. The level of significance used in 'F' and 't' tests was P=0.05.

Results and Discussions

Microbial population dynamics of soil

The impact of the herbicides on soil micro-flora *viz*., fungi, total bacteria, and actinomycetes (Table 1, 2 and 3) was recorded at different time of observations i.e. initial, 45, 75 days after sowing and at harvest stage.

Soil fungal counts (CFU x 10^4 g^{-1} soil)

Data on population of fungi in soil at different time intervals of maize is presented in Table 1. All the herbicide treatments showed significant adverse effect on the population of fungi in rhizosphere soil of winter maize up to 45 days after sowing exhibiting soil fungi population in lower range with increasing herbicide doses. Reduction in their population occurred in all herbicide treated plots up to that period over the weed free and weedy check. Thereafter, fungi population was gradually increasing at subsequent time interval i.e. 75 days after sowing and at harvest, their populations increased considerably in herbicide treated plots though weed free (T_2) and weedy check (T_1) exhibited higher fungi population than other herbicide treated plots. Initially fungi population in weed free plot (T_2) was lower than weedy check (T_1), however, it remain continued for rest of the time intervals and harvest. But at harvest, the data showed increase in population and higher than the initial population of the fungi (Table 1).

Table 1: Fungal population in soil as influenced by different weed control treatments

	Weedy check	Fungal population (CFU x 10^4 g^{-1} soil)		
		45 DAS	75 DAS	Harvest
T_1	Weed free check	63.82	77.79	115.33
T_2	Acetochlor @ 1.125 kg a.i. ha^{-1}	55.17	71.76	110.89
T_3	Atrazine @ 1.0 kg a.i. ha^{-1}	47.57	59.89	94.83
T_4	Pendimethalin @ 0.5 kg a.i.ha^{-1} + atrazine @ 0.5 kg a.i. ha^{-1}	39.15	55.28	87.56
T_5	Topramezone @ 0.04 kg a.i. ha^{-1} + atrazine @ 0.25 kg a.i.ha^{-1}	38.12	54.57	85.52
T_6	Acetochor @ 2.25 kg a.i. ha^{-1}	34.76	51.84	80.94
T_7	Alachlor @ 0.5 kg a.i. ha^{-1}	39.90	56.84	86.54
T_8	2,4-Diethyl ester @ 0.6 kg a.i. ha^{-1}	51.97	63.88	96.77
T_9	Acetochlor @ 4.5 kg a.i. ha^{-1}	51.28	62.31	95.61
T_{10}	SEm±	39.54	55.71	82.90
	CD (P=0.05)	1.60	1.08	1.57
	Initial value	4.75	3.21	4.66
	Weedy check	53.54		

At 45 days after sowing, among herbicide treatments, the lowest fungal population was recorded under topramezone @ 0.04 kg a.i. ha^{-1}+atrazine @ 0.25 kg a.i. ha^{-1} (T_6), followed by Pendimethalin @ 0.5 kg a.i.ha^{-1} + atrazine @ 0.5 kg a.i. ha^{-1} (T_5) and atrazine @ 1.0 kg a.i. ha^{-1} (T_4). The highest fungi population was found under alachlor @ 0.5 kg a.i. ha^{-1} (T_8) which was almost similar to 2, 4-Diethyl ester @ 0.6 kg a.i. ha^{-1} (T_9).

At 75 days after sowing, among herbicide treatments, the lowest fungi population was recorded from topramezone @ 0.04 kg a.i. ha^{-1} + atrazine @ 0.25 kg a.i. ha^{-1} (T_6) which was at par with Pendimethalin @ 0.5 kg a.i.ha^{-1} + atrazine @ 0.5 kg a.i. ha^{-1} (T_5). The highest fungi population was recorded under alachlor @ 0.5 kg a.i. ha^{-1} (T_8) which was close to 2, 4-Diethyl ester @ 0.6 kg a.i. ha^{-1} (T_9).

At harvest, among herbicide treatments, the lowest fungi population was observed from topramezone @ 0.04 kg a.i. ha^{-1}+ atrazine @ 0.25 kg a.i. ha^{-1} (T_6) which was at par with acetochlor @ 4.5 kg a.i. ha^{-1} (T_{10}) and Pendimethalin @ 0.5 kg a.i.ha^{-1} + atrazine @ 0.5 kg a.i. ha^{-1} (T_5). The highest fungi population was found under alachlor @ 0.5 kg a.i. ha^{-1} (T_8) which was significantly superior over rest of the treatments among herbicide treatments.

Ramesh and Nadanassababady (2005) found that significant differences in population of soil fungi was noticed shortly after application of herbicides i.e. 5 days after sowing as compared to their population before herbicide application which was in conformity with the results of Gopalswamy *et al.* (1994). Sandor (2007) reported that herbicides decreased the number of total microscopic fungi. So far as the physiological process of microorganisms was concerned, the enzymatic activities increased with herbicides use.

Kulashrestha *et al.* (1976) stated that atrazine @ 0.5, 1.0 and 2.0 kg ha^{-1} did not leave any herbicide residues. Sharma and Angiras (1997) reported that atrazine @ 1.5 kg ha^{-1} as pre-emergence and atrazine @ 1.5 kg ha^{-1} as broadcast persisted up to 47 days in silty clay loam soil. Saikia *et al.* (2000) reported that atrazine showed initial slow rate of loss of atrazine in sandy loam soil up to 20 days and thereafter faster dissipation and at maize harvest (90 days), no detectable residue was found. They also reported that atrazine @ 1.0 to 2.0 kg a.i ha^{-1} in maize did not leave any detectable residues. Saikia and Pandey (2001) stated that atrazine was biologically active in sandy loam soil up to 90 days and its biological activity was well pronounced at 2.0 kg a.i ha^{-1}. Ayansina and Oso (2006) concluded that higher concentrations of atrazine herbicide resulted in much lower microbial counts as compared to recommended herbicide dose. Herbicides also exhibited the elimination of some microbial species. Olabode *et al.* (2010) reported that response of soil microorganisms to atrazine doses varied depending upon herbicides. Pozo *et al.* (1994) reported that the presence of alachlor @ 2.0-10.0 kg ha^{-1} in soil increased the population of fungi. Sahid and Kasim (1994) reported that fungal populations in soil also declined in the presence of either alachlor or metolachlor herbicides at higher concentrations.

Cal *et al.* (1993) reported that atrazine and alachlor herbicides decreased fungal populations. Konstantinovic *et al.* (1999) reported that alachlor/atrazine herbicides increased the population of fungi. Alachlor was generally more inhibiting towards the microbes as compared to atrazine. Increased herbicide doses increased the inhibitory effect, which was best exhibited at the beginning of the growing period. Das *et al.* (2002) noted that alachlor and atrazine herbicide had stimulatory effect on soil microbial population. Reddy A. (2003) observed that atrazine at 0.25 to 0.5 kg ha^{1} as pre-emergence and pendimethalin @ 0.5 kg a.i ha^{-1} as pre-emergence in maize did not leave any significant residue. Nikolova *et al.* (2004) indicated acetochlor decreased the growth of soil microorganisms.

Li *et al.* (2005) revealed that acetochlor at high concentration of 150 and 250 mg kg^{-1} had an acute and chronic toxicity on both soil fungal population and total fungal biomass, but at low concentration of 50 mg kg^{-1} had stimulating effect that was stronger with total fungal biomass than with soil fungal population. Jing *et al.* (2010) reported that fungi population decreased at 14 days after applying acteochlor, but then recovered at 30th day and was stimulated at 60th day.

Zhen *et al.* (2013) reported that dissipation half lives of acetochlor were 2.8 and 3.4 days in rhizosphere and bulk soil, respectively. As compared to bulk soil, microbial communities in rhizospheric soil were inclined to be affected by acetochlor. Fungal growth was prone to be inhibited. Soil microbial community was significantly affected by acetochlor at its early 15 days stage.

Soil bacteria counts (CFU x 10^{6} g^{-1} soil)

Data on population of bacteria in soil at different growth stages of the crop is presented in Table 2. All the herbicide treatments showed significant influence on the population of total bacteria in rhizospheric soil of winter maize indicating in lower range with increasing herbicide doses. Reduction in their population occurred in all herbicide treated plots up to that period over weed free and weedy check. Thereafter, bacteria population was gradually increasing at different time intervals and at harvest, their population increased considerably in herbicidal treated plots though weed free and weedy check showed higher bacteria population than other herbicide treated plots. Initially the bacteria population in weed free plot (T_2) was lower than weedy check (T_1), however, it remain continued for rest of the time intervals and harvest. But at harvest, the data showed that their population increased considerably in herbicide treated plots and higher than initial population of bacteria (Table 2).

Table 2: Bacteria population in soil as influenced by different weed control treatments

	Treatment	Bacteria population (CFU x 106 g^{-1} Soil)		
		45 DAS	75 DAS	Harvest
T_1	Weedy check	59.55	76.39	116.80
T_2	Weed free check	51.37	74.27	112.75
T_3	Acetochlor @ 1.125 kg a.i. ha^{-1}	45.08	68.73	102.64
T_4	Atrazine @ 1.0 kg a.i. ha^{-1}	39.13	61.67	93.03
T_5	Pendimethalin @ 0.5 kg a.i.ha^{-1} + atrazine @ 0.5 kg a.i. ha-1	41.33	64.86	93.16
T_6	Topramezone @ 0.04 kg a.i. ha^{-1} + atrazine @ 0.25 kg a.i.ha^{-1}	38.18	61.67	90.33
T_7	Acetochor @ 2.25 kg a.i. ha^{-1}	39.08	64.82	95.28
T_8	Alachlor @ 0.5 kg a.i. ha^{-1}	47.27	70.23	104.82
T_9	2,4-Diethyl ester @ 0.6 kg a.i. ha^{-1}	43.67	66.13	97.75
T_{10}	Acetochlor @ 4.5 kg a.i. ha^{-1}	39.03	53.72	87.91
	SEm±	2.03	1.01	1.67
	CD (P=0.05)	6.05	3.02	4.98
	Initial value		34.53	

At 45 days after sowing, among herbicide treatments, the lowest total bacteria population was recorded under topramezone @ 0.04 kg a.i. ha^{-1} + atrazine @ 0.25 kg a.i. ha^{-1} (T_6) which was statistically at par with rest of the herbicide treatments except alachlor @ 0.5 kg a.i. ha^{-1} (T_8) and acetochlor @ 1.125 kg a.i. ha^{-1} (T_3) which indicated more number of total bacteria counts and exhibited statistically parity with each other.

At 75 days after sowing, among herbicide treatments, application of acetochlor @ 4.5 kg a.i. ha^{-1} (T_{10}) registered the lowest total bacteria population which was significantly lower than rest of the herbicide treatments. The highest total bacteria population was found under alachlor @ 0.5 kg a.i. ha^{-1} (T_8) which was at par with acetochlor @ 1.125 kg a.i. ha^{-1} (T_3).

At harvest, among herbicide treatments, the lowest total bacteria population was recorded under acetochlor @ 4.5 kg a.i. ha^{-1} (T_{10}) which showed significantly lower over rest of the herbicide treatments except topramezone @ 0.04 kg a.i. ha^{-1} + atrazine @ 0.25 kg a.i. ha^{-1} (T_6) and acetochlor @ 1.125 kg a.i. ha^{-1} (T_3). Moreover, alachlor @ 0.5 kg a.i. ha^{-1} (T_8) recorded the highest total bacteria population among all the herbicide treatments except acetochlor 1.125 kg a.i. ha^{-1} (T_3).

Ramesh and Nadanassababady (2005) found that significant differences in population of soil bacteria was noticed shortly after application of herbicides i.e. 5 days after sowing as compared to their population before herbicide application which was in conformity with the results of Gopalswamy *et al.* (1994). Sandor (2007) reported that herbicides decreased the number of total viable bacteria. The population of nitrifying bacteria and cellulose degrading bacteria increased significantly. Olabode *et al.* (2010) reported that bacterial population was inversely related to atrazine doses with the highest value for control (290 x 10^6 cfu g^{-1} soil) and the least in 100% recommended dose (29 x 10^6 cfu g^{-1} soil). Pozo *et al.* (1994) reported that the presence of alachlor @ 2.0-10.0 kg ha^{-1} in soil increased the population of bacteria. Sahid and Kasim (1994) reported that bacterial populations in soil also declined in presence of either alachlor or metolachlor herbicides at higher concentration.

Konstantinovic *et al.* (1999) reported that alachlor/atrazine herbicides reduced the population of bacteria. Das *et al.* (2002) noted that alachlor and atrazine herbicides were not always inhibitory in action and stimulatory effect on important microbial counts was observed.

Jing *et al.* (2010) reported that number of bacteria increased two weeks after applying acetochlor, then inhibited by acetochlor @ 30 mg kg^{-1} at 30th day. After that, actinomycetes population recovered while bacteria population was still inhibited till 60th day. Zhen *et al.* (2013) reported that as compared to bulk soil, microbial communities in rhizospheric soil were inclined to be affected by acetochlor. Bacterial growth was most likely increased. Residual acetochlor did not confer long term impairment on viable bacterial counts in the rhizosphere and bulk soil.

Soil actinomycetes counts (CFU x 10^5 g^{-1} soil)

Data on the population of actinomycetes in soil at different intervals of growth stages of the crop is presented in Table 3. All the herbicide treatments showed significant influence on the population of actinomycetes in rhizospheric soil of winter maize indicating in lower range with increasing herbicide doses. Significant differences were recorded between herbicide treated plots and the weed free treatment and weedy check after application of herbicide up to 45 days after sowing. Thereafter, at harvest the population of actinomycetes increased to a considerable level (Table 3).

At 45 days after sowing, among herbicide treatments, significantly actinomycetes population was recorded the lowest under acetochlor @ 4.5 kg a.i. ha^{-1} (T_{10}) which showed statistical parity with topramezone @ 0.04 kg a.i. ha^{-1} + atrazine @ 0.25 kg a.i. ha^{-1} (T_6), acetochor @ 2.25 kg a.i. ha^{-1} (T_7), Pendimethalin @ 0.5 kg a.i.ha^{-1} + atrazine @ 0.5 kg a.i. ha^{-1} (T_5) and atrazine @ 1.0 kg a.i. ha^{-1}

(T_4) and actinomycetes population was observed highest under alachlor @ 0.5 kg a.i. ha^{-1} (T_8) which was almost similar to acetochlor @ 1.125 kg a.i. ha^{-1} (T_3) and 2,4-Diethyl ester @ 0.6 kg a.i. ha^{-1} (T_9). Similarly, at 75 days after sowing, among herbicide treatments acetochlor @ 4.5 kg a.i. ha^{-1} (T_{10}) registered significantly lowest actinomycetes population which was superior over rest of the herbicide treatments except acetochor @ 2.25 kg a.i. ha^{-1}. Moreover, actinomycetes population was found significantly highest under alachlor @ 0.5 kg a.i. ha^{-1} (T_8) which was almost similar to acetochlor @ 1.125 kg a.i. ha^{-1} (T_3).

At harvest, among herbicide treatments significantly lowest actinomycetes population was obtained from pendimethalin 0.5 kg a.i ha^{-1} + atrazine @ 0.5 kg a.i. ha^{-1} each (T_5) which was at par with topramezone @ 0.04 kg a.i. ha^{-1} + atrazine @ 0.25 kg a.i. ha^{-1} (T_6), atrazine @ 1.0 kg a.i. ha^{-1} (T_4) and 2,4-Diethyl ester @ 0.6 kg ha^{-1} (T_9). However, acetochlor @ 4.5 kg a.i. ha^{-1} (T_{10}) recorded highest actinomycetes population, followed by alachlor @ 0.5 kg a.i. ha^{-1} (T_8) and acetochlor @ 1.125 kg a.i. ha^{-1} (T_3).

Ramesh and Nadanassababady (2005) found that significant differences in population of soil actinomycetes was noticed shortly after application of herbicides i.e. 5 days after sowing as compared to their population before herbicide application which was in conformity with Gopalswamy *et al.* (1994). Olabode *et al.* (2010) reported that bacterial population was inversely related to atrazine doses noted highest for control and least in 100% recommended dose. However, actinomycetes showed a reverse trend. Konstantinovic *et al.* (1999) reported that alachlor/atrazine herbicides increased the population of actinomycetes. Jing *et al.* (2010) reported that number of actinomycetes increased two weeks after applying acetochlor, then inhibited by acetochlor @ 30 mg kg^{-1} at 30th day. After that, actinomycetes population recovered.

All the herbicides showed significant adverse effect on the population of fungi and bacteria in rhizosphere soil of winter maize up to 45 days after sowing. Reduction in their population occurred in all the herbicide treated plots up to that period over weed free and weedy check. Thereafter, fungi and bacteria population was gradually increasing at different time intervals and at harvest, their population increased considerably in herbicide treated plots though the weed free and weedy check showed higher value of fungi and bacteria population than other herbicide treated plots. Initially the fungi and bacteria population in weed free plot was lower over weedy check, however, it remain continued for rest of time intervals and harvest. But at harvest, the data showed the population increased considerably in herbicide treated plots and higher than the initial population of the fungi and bacteria.

Like bacteria and fungi, significant differences were recorded between herbicide treated plots and weed free and weedy check after application of herbicides up to 45 days after sowing. Thereafter, at harvest, the population of actinomycetes increased to a considerable level. Soil actinomycetes population was found lower with increasing herbicide doses.

Conclusion might be drawn that soil microbial population (total bacteria, fungi and actinomycetes) did not vary considerably initially in herbicidal treated plots but after herbicide application, they differed significantly for a short period of time i.e. 45 days after sowing. At harvest, the population increased considerably in each case and was higher than that of initial population justifying no long term adverse effect of herbicides on the beneficial soil micro-flora.

Table 3: Actinomycetes population in soil as influenced by weed control treatments

	Treatment	Actinomycetes population (CFU x 10^5 g^{-1} soil)		
		45 DAS	75 DAS	Harvest
T_1	Weedy check	61.56	72.75	106.54
T_2	Weed free check	56.33	67.18	84.26
T_3	Acetochlor @ 1.125 kg a.i. ha^{-1}	48.23	58.54	95.05
T_4	Atrazine @ 1.0 kg a.i. ha^{-1}	45.28	54.84	75.15
T_5	Pendimethalin @ 0.5 kg a.i. ha^{-1} + atrazine @ 0.5 kg a.i. ha^{-1}	44.61	54.76	73.83
T_6	Topramezone @ 0.04 kg a.i. ha^{-1} + atrazine @ 0.25 kg a.i.$haha^{-1}$	41.06	52.15	75.01
T_7	Acetochor @ 2.25 kg a.i. ha^{-1}	42.25	50.36	89.77
T_8	Alachlor @ 0.5 kg a.i. ha^{-1}	52.70	63.11	97.68
T_9	2,4-Diethyl ester @ 0.6 kg a.i. ha^{-1}	46.95	56.27	78.72
T_{10}	Acetochlor @ 4.5 kg a.i. ha^{-1}	38.30	45.08	98.93
	SEm±	2.45	1.90	2.57
	CD (P=0.05)	7.28	5.66	7.65
	Initial value		42.14	

References

Anonymous, (2010-11). Bihar Agricultural Statistics at a Glance. Directorate of Statistics and Evaluation, Bihar.

Ayansina, A.D.V. and Oso, B.A. (2006). Effect of two commonly used herbicides on soil microflora at two different concentrations. *African J. of Biotec.* 5 (2): 129-132.

Bouyoucos, G. J. (1962). Hydrometer method for making particle size analysis of soil. *Agronomy Journal* 54: 464-465.

Cal, A., Tadeo, J. L., Obrador, A., Melgarejo, P. and Pascual, S. (1993). Effects of atrazine and alachlor herbicides on the soil microflora of a maize monoculture. Investigation Agraria, Production & Protection Vegetables, 8 (1): 97-108.

Cochran, W. G and Cox, G. M. (1963). Experimental design. John Willy and Sons, New Delhi.

Das, S. K., Pahwa, M. R. and Yadava, R. B. (2002). Soil dehydrogenase activity in relation to atrazine and alachlor application. *Range Management and Agroforestry* 23 (2): 126-129.

Fisher, R.A. (1935). Statistical methods for research workers. Oliver and Boyd, Edinburg London Publication.

Gopalasamy, G., Anthoni, R.S. and Kareem, A. (1994). Interaction of herbicides with azolla and soil microbial. *Indian Journal of Weed Science* 26 (3-4): 28-34.

Grossbard. E. 1976. In: Herbicides-Physiology, Biochemistry, Ecology (Audus, J.J. Ed.). Academic Press. London. p. 99.

Jackson, M. L. (1973). Soil Chemical Analysis, PHI Pvt. Ltd. New Delhi.

Jing R.Y., Wang, L.Y., Wang, Y., Tan, H.B., Mu, G.Q. and Wang, W.D. (2010). Effect of acetochlor application on soil microorganism number and enzymes activities. *Chinese Journal of Eco Agriculture* 18 (6): 1302-1305.

Konstantinovic, B., Govedarica, M., Jarak, M. and Milosevic, N. (1999). Herbicide efficiency and their impact on microbiological activity in soil. *China Research Progress in Plant Protection and Plant Nutrition* p. 228-232.

Kulshrestha, G., Mani, V. S. and Dewan, R. S. (1976). Effect of simazine and atrazine on maize and their residual effects on succeeding *rabi* crops. *Indian Journal of Agronomy* 20 (2): 201-202.

Li, X.Y., Zhang, H.W., Zhou, Q. X., Su, Z.C. and Zhang, C. G. (2005). Effects of acetochlor and methamidophos on fungal communities in black soils. *Pedosphere* 15 (5): 646-652.

Nikolova, V., Dowson, I. and Baeva, G. (2004). Effect of acetochlor on the weeds of maize plantation and soil biological activity. *Herbologia* 5 (1): 23-29.

Oerke, E. C. and Dehne, H. W. (2004). Safeguarding production—losses in major crops and the role of crop protection. *Crop Protection* 23: 275–285.

Olabode, O. S., Adesina, G. O. and Babajide, P. A. (2010). Weed control efficiency of reduced atrazine doses and its effect on soil organisms in maize (*Zea Mays* L.) fields of south western Nigeria. *Journal of Tropical Agriculture* 48: 52-54.

Olsen, S.R., Cole, C.V., Watanabe, F. S. and Dean, L.A. (1954). Estimation of available phosphorus in soils by extraction with sodium bicarbonate. U.S. Department of Agriculture, Washington, D.C. Circular 939.

Patel, V. J., Upadhyay, P.N., Patel, J. B. and Meisuriya, M.I. (2006). Effect of herbicide mixture on weeds in kharif maize (*Zea mays* L.) under middle Gujarat conditions. *Indian Journal of Weed Science* 38 (1 & 2): 54-57.

Porwal, M. K. (2000). Economics of weed control measures in winter maize (*Zea mays* L.). *Indian Journal of Agronomy* 45 (2): 344-347.

Pozo, C., Salmeron, V., Rodelas, B., Martinez-Toledo, M. V. and Gonzalez-Lopez (1994). Effects of the herbicide alachlor on soil microbial activities. *Journal of Eco-toxicology* 3 (1): 4-10.

Ramesh, G. and Nadanassababady, T. (2005). Impact of herbicides on weeds and soil ecosystem of rainfed maize (*Zea mays* L.). *Indian Journal of Agricultural Research* 39 (1): 31-36.

Reddy, Audi, D. (2003). M.Sc. (Ag.) Thesis, Tamil Nadu Agricultural University, Coimbatore.

Sahid, I. and Kasim, Z. (1994). Effects of high rate of alachlor and metolachlor on microbial activities in soil. *Pertanika Journal of Tropical Agricultural Science* 17 (1): 43-47.

Saikia, T. P., Pandey, J. and Kulshrestha, G. (2000). Investigation on residue of atrazine and fluchloralin in maize (*Zea mays*)-chickpea (*Cicer arietinum*) and maize (*Zea mays*)-Indian mustard (*Brassica juncea*) cropping sequences. *Indian Journal of Agronomy* 45 (4): 653-657.

Saikia, T.P. and Pandey, P (2001). Atrazine persistance in maize field. *Annals of Agricultural Research* 22 (1): 169-170.

Sandor, Z. (2007). The effect of some herbicides on microbes and their activity in soil. *Cereal Research Communications* 34 (1): 275-278.

Sharma, N. and Angiras, N.N. (1997). Studies on persistence of herbicides applied in maize by bioassay technique. *World Weeds* 4 (1/2): 37-39.

Shivashankar, K., Shantharam, S., Krishnamurthy, K. and Rao, B. V. V. (1981). Effect of fertilizer and herbicidal interactions on soil microbial population and nutrient uptake by soybeans. Proceedings of the Eighth Asian-Pacific Weed Science Society Conference, Bangalore, Vol. II, 1981, p. 137-142.

Zhen, B., Hui, J. X., Hong, B. H., Li, C. Z. and Xu, D. Z. (2013). Alterations of microbial populations and composition in the rhizosphere and bulk soil as affected by residual acetochlor. *Environmental Science and Pollution Research* 20 (1): 369-379.

10

Evaluation of Fungicides on Management of Spot Blotch Disease Causing *Bipolaris sorokiniana* of Wheat

Vinay Kumar, C. S. Azad, G. Chand and A. Kumar

Department of Plant Pathology, Bihar Agricultural University Sabour-813 210 Bhagalpur, Bihar, India

Abstract

Spot blotch of wheat is devastating disease as one of the yield limiting factor especially in north eastern plains zone and also in north western plains zone of India. Chemical fungicides play an important role in controlling the spot blotch in India due to non availability of spot blotch resistant commercial varieties. To identify the suitable chemicals method and time of application, various fungicides thiram 37.5% WP, carboxin 37.5% WP +, propiconazole 25% EC, tebuconazole 25% EC and mancozeb 75% WP) were evaluated either as seed treatment or foliar sprays or in combination under artificial epiphytotic in vivo *conditions for two crop seasons. Seed treatment (ST) by thiram + carboxin @ 2.5 g/kg of seed along with Foliar spray (FS) of propiconazole @ 0.1% at boot leaf stage on Flag-1 leaf followed by second spray at 20 days interval (two sprays) resulted in best management of spot blotch in severe conditions. It was found that the fungicide treatment not only reduced the spot blotch disease but also increases the grain yield.*

Keywords: *Bipolaris sorokiniana*, spot blotch, wheat and management.

1. Introduction

Wheat (*Triticum aestivum* L.) is considered as one of the most widely grown and consumed food crop of the world. Presently, it provides 20 per cent of food calories to mankind in the world and it is staple food for nearly 40 per cent of world population (Pingali, 1999). During In India, wheat is cultivated in an area of 27.20 million hectare producing about 73.20 million tonnes of grain with productivity being 2690 kg/ha (FAOSTAT, 2016).

There are several constraints to the world production of wheat. The crops suffers from at least 17 different diseases in the country (Ahmed and Hossain, 1985), twelve of them are caused by fungi. Among the fungal diseases six are considered to be economically important because of their damaging nature and wide distribution throughout the wheat growing areas of the country. These are spot blotch, foliar leaf blight, seedling blight, leaf rust, foot and root rot and black point of wheat, of which spot blotch is economically most important one (Ahmed and Hossain, 2005).

Spot blotch is caused by *Bipolaris sorokiniana* (Syn. *Cochliobolus sativus*) is the major and devastating disease of wheat in India (Hossain and Azad, 1992). The pathogen is considered to contribute significantly in lowering average yield under favourable conditions ranging from 20-80% (Duveiller and Gilchrist, 1994). In addition to yield losses, the grain quality also deteriorates depending on the level of susceptibility of a cultivar to the pathogen.

Unfortunately not a single cultivar in India is found to free from this disease (Hossain and Azad, 1992). Since spot blotch occurs in all the wheat growing agro-climatic zones, deployment of resistant cultivars remains the most effective strategy for the management of disease. The resistance source is not easily available and is not stable due to development and the appearance of new/more virulent races of pathogens (Katasntones *et al*., 2007).

Management methods like host resistance, biological and chemical control are suggested for the spot blotch of wheat but, farmers tend to use chemicals frequently as it is a fast acting remedy. Quick and ensured effectiveness of chemical pesticides on pathogens gives an edge over other methods of management. The pathogen *Bipolaris sorokiniana* mainly survives as conidia on seeds, infected plant debris, collateral hosts and in the soil (Reis, 1991). The management practices will be accomplished through both seed treatment and foliar spray to reduce the primary as well as secondary spread of inoculums.

Evaluation of new and nonhazardous fungicide is required for effective management of spot blotch pathogen. Therefore in this experiment, the efficacy of fungicides as seed treatment as well as foliar spray alone or both was evaluated.

Materials and Methods

Experimental site

A field trial was carried out during Rabi season of the years 2017 at Bihar Agricultural University, Sabour, Farm, Bhagalpur (Bihar) in randomized block design with three replication. The variety Agra local was used for this study. Recommended agronomical package and practices were followed for all the treatments. For each treatment, there were three rows of five meter length with row to row distance of 25 cm along with 1.25 m gap between replications and 75 cm gap between plots. The seed rate @ 125 kg ha^{-1} (per plot approx. 110 g) was adopted and sown on 20th Nov. 2017. The NPK fertilizer (120:60:40 $kgha^{-1}$) and FYM @ 2 tha^{-1} were applied. Three irrigations were assured at 20, 50 and 80 days and standard agronomic practices were followed. Untreated seed without any fungicide spraying was maintained as check. For maintaining uniform disease pressure in the field, the inoculum of *Bipolaris sorokiniana* was artificially multiplied on sterilized wheat grains. Twenty days after inoculation, the conidial suspensions ($1x10^6$ conidia per ml) were sprayed on standing crop to ensure high disease severity for proper evaluation of fungicidal efficacy.

Fungicides used

To study the efficacy of different fungicides under field condition, five different fungicides viz. Thiram, carboxin, propiconazole, tebuconazole and control were used against spot blotch of wheat. Fungicide spray was made by knapsack sprayer of 15 litre capacity fitted with a hallow cone triple action nozzle. The suspension of each fungicide was prepared separately by adding required quantity of respective fungicides in required amount of water. First spray was given just after the appearance of the disease symptoms followed by second foliar sprays at 20 days interval.

Observations

The disease data was recorded in three stages (flowering, dough and hard dough) from randomly selected 25 plants from each plot tagged. So 25 plants plot -1 were tagged for disease rating using the double digit scale (0-9) developed (Zadok *et al.*, 1974)

Table 1: Double digit (DD) rating scale for spot blotch disease of wheat (Zadok's scale)

Percentage leaf area covered	Severity scale
0 (No disease)	0
1-10%	1
11-20%	2
21-30%	3
31-40%	4
41-50%	5
51-60%	6
61-70%	7
70-80%	8
>80%	9

The spot blotch severity is taken in per cent leaf area covered separately for flag (F) and one leaf below flag (F-l) and the rating is done as follows

Disease incidence of spot blotch was taken on plot basis by given formula.

$$\text{Percent disease incidence} = \frac{\text{Number of diseased plants}}{\text{Total number of plants}} \times 100$$

Statistical analysis

The data was analysed statistically by Randomized Block Design (RBD) using statistical software STPR developed by G. B. Pant University of Agriculture and Technology, Pantnagar. Data recorded were compared by the means of critical differences at five per cent level of significance in field studies.

Results and Discussion

Effect of fungicides on seed germination and disease incidence.

Relative performance of different fungicides on seed germination and disease incidence is presented in Table 2. All the fungicides reduced the disease incidence and enhancing seed germination significantly in comparison to untreated control irrespective of their mode of applications. The average seed germination at 20 days after sowing (DAS) ranged from 80-96 per cent. Minimum seed germination (80.00%) was observed in control while maximum seed germination per cent (96.00%) was recorded in three treatments *viz.,* ST by thiram + carboxin @ 2.5 g/kg of seed, ST by thiram + carboxin @ 2.5 g/kg of seed + FS sprays of propiconazole @ 0.1% (one) at boot leaf stage on flag-1 leaf and ST by thiram + carboxin @ 2.5 g/kg of seed + FS of propiconazole @ 0.1% at boot leaf stage on flag-1 leaf followed by second spray at 20 days interval (two sprays) followed (93 %) by ST by thiram @ 3 g/kg of seed.

Table 2: Effect of fungicides on disease incidence and seed germination at 20 DAS.

	Treatments	Seed germination (%)	Disease incidence (%)
T1	ST by thiram @ 3 g/kg of seed	93	11
T2	ST by thiram + carboxin @ 2.5 g/kg of seed	96	6
T3	ST by thiram + carboxin @ 2.5 g/kg of seed + FS sprays of propiconazole @ 0.1% (one) at boot leaf stage on Flag-1 leaf	96	6
T4	ST by thiram + carboxin @ 2.5 g/kg of seed + FS of propiconazole @ 0.1% at boot leaf stage on Flag-1 leaf followed by second spray at 20 days interval (two sprays)	96	5
T5	FS of propiconazole @ 0.1% at boot leaf stage on Flag-1 leaf	91	9
T6	FS of propiconazole @ 0.1% at boot leaf stage on Flag-1 leaf followed by second spray at 20 days interval (two sprays)	91	9
T7	FS of tebuconazole @ 0.1% at boot leaf stage on Flag-1 leaf	91	9
T8	FS of tebuconazole @ 0.1% at boot leaf stage on Flag-1 leaf followed by second spray at 20 days interval (two spray)	91	9
T9	Three FS of mancozeb @ 0.25% at boot leaf stage on Flag-2 leaf followed by second and third spray at 10 days intervals each (three spray)	91	10
T10	Control	80	14
	CD @ 5%	-	2.56
	CV	-	17.15
	SEM±	-	0.86

Means of three replication
ST = Seet treatment
FS = Folia spray

Disease incidence at 20 days after sowing (DAS) ranged from 5-14 per cent. Maximum disease incidence (14%) was recorded in control while minimum disease incidence (5%) was recorded in ST by thiram + carboxin @ 2.5 g/kg of seed + FS of propiconazole @ 0.1% at boot leaf stage on flag-1 leaf followed by second spray at 20 days interval (two sprays) which was followed by 6% in case of ST by thiram + carboxin @ 2.5 g/kg of seed (6%) and ST by thiram + carboxin @ 2.5 g/kg of seed + FS sprays of propiconazole @ 0.1% (one) at boot leaf stage on flag-1 leaf.

This is due to suppression or elimination of seed and soil borne pathogens and favoring the beneficial microorganisms surrounding the seeds in soil. Goulart *et al.* (1995) observed that spraying with tebuconazole, propiconazole 25 EC and Flutriafol on above ground parts of wheat controlled the leaf blight incidence of *B. sorokiniana*.

Effect of fungicides on spot blotch severity at Flowering, Dough and Hard Dough stage.

Severity of spot blotch per plot was screened under field conditions against *B. sorokiniana.* The disease was scored on 0-9 dd scale. The progress of the disease in susceptible variety Agra local was monitored from 2nd fortnight of March and disease severity at flowering, dough and hard dough stage during 2016-17 crop seasons (Table 3).

At flowering stage disease severity ranged from 12-36 in dd scale. Minimum spot blotch severity (12) in dd scale was recorded in three treatments like ST by thiram + carboxin @ 2.5 g/kg of seed, ST by thiram + carboxin @ 2.5 g/kg of seed FS sprays of propiconazole @ 0.1% (one) at boot leaf stage on flag-1 leaf and ST by thiram + carboxin @ 2.5 g/kg of seed + FS of propiconazole @ 0.1% at boot leaf stage on flag-1 leaf followed by second spray at 20 days interval (two sprays) which was followed by FS of propiconazole @ 0.1% at boot leaf stage on flag-1 leaf whereas maximum leaf blight/blotch were recorded in control i.e. 36 in dd scale.

At dough stage spot blotch severity ranged from 23 to 47 in dd scale. Minimum spot blotch severity (23) was recorded in ST by thiram + carboxin @ 2.5 g/kg of seed + FS of propiconazole @ 0.1% at boot leaf stage on flag-1 leaf followed by second spray at 20 days interval (two sprays) which was at par with ST by thiram + carboxin @ 2.5 g/kg of seed and ST by thiram + carboxin @ 2.5 g/kg of seed + FS sprays of propiconazole @ 0.1% at boot leaf stage on flag-1 leaf i.e. 24 in dd scale whereas maximum spot blotch severity (47) were recorded in control.

At hard dough stage spot blotch severity ranged from 34 to 69 in dd scale. Minimum spot blotch severity (34) was recorded in ST by thiram + carboxin @

Table 3: Evaluation of fungicidal on spot blotch severity of wheat

	Treatments	Flowering	Dough	Hard dough
T1	ST by thiram @ 3 g/kg of seed	23	34	57
T2	ST by thiram + carboxin @ 2.5 g/kg of seed	12	24	46
T3	ST by thiram + carboxin @ 2.5 g/kg of seed + FS sprays of propiconazole @ 0.1% (one) at boot leaf stage on Flag-1 leaf	12	24	35
T4	ST by thiram + carboxin @ 2.5 g/kg of seed + FS of propiconazole @ 0.1% at boot leaf stage on Flag-1 leaf followed by second spray at 20 days interval (two sprays)	12	23	34
T5	FS of propiconazole @ 0.1% at boot leaf stage on Flag-1 leaf	23	34	47
T6	FS of propiconazole @ 0.1% at boot leaf stage on Flag-1 leaf followed by second spray at 20 days interval (two sprays)	23	34	46
T7	FS of tebuconazole @ 0.1% at boot leaf stage on Flag-1 leaf	24	35	47
T8	FS of tebuconazole @ 0.1% at boot leaf stage on Flag-1 leaf followed by second spray at 20 days interval (two spray)	23	34	46
T9	Three FS of mancozeb @ 0.25% at boot leaf stage on Flag-2 leaf followed by second and third spray at 10 days intervals each (three spray)	23	35	57
T10	Control	36	47	69
	CD @ 5%	1.04	0.56	0.87
	CV	2.84	1.01	1.04
	SEM±	0.35	0.24	0.29

Means of three replication

ST = Seed treatment

FS = Foliar spray

2.5 g/kg of seed+ FS of propiconazole @ 0.1% at boot leaf stage on flag-1 leaf followed by second spray at 20 days' interval (two sprays) which was at par with ST by thiram + carboxin @ 2.5 g/kg of seed + FS of propiconazole @ 0.1% at boot leaf stage on flag-1 leaf i.e. 35 in dd scale whereas maximum spot blotch severity (69) were recorded in control.

The same result was observed by Singh *et al.* (2011) on wheat variety HD 2329 with propiconazole 25 EC and tebuconazole 25 EC @ 0.1% under field conditions to control the spot blotch (65.80%). Although foliar sprayings alone also had better effects than the untreated control but they are not as effective as that of ST along with foliar spraying of propiconazole 25 EC. Aminuzzaman and Hossain (2007) also observed that the fungicides benzothiodiazole, propiconazole 25 EC and azoxystrobin controlled leaf blight either alone or in their combinations significantly.

Seed weight/plot (Kg) and 1000 grain weight (g)

The effect of different fungicides also reflected on yield attributes like grain yield as well as 1000 grain weight. Data pertaining to Seed weight/plot (Kg) and 1000 grain weight (gm) presented in Table 4.

All the treatments showed increase in the yield attributes as compared to control. Seed weight/plot varied from 2.91-4.48 kg. Maximum Seed weight/plot (4.48 kg) was recorded in ST by thiram + carboxin @ 2.5 g/kg of seed + FS of propiconazole @ 0.1% at boot leaf stage on flag-1 leaf followed by second spray at 20 days' interval (two sprays) which was at par with FS of propiconazole @ 0.1% at boot leaf stage on flag-1 leaf (4.07 kg) whereas minimum Seed weight/plot (2.91 kg) was recorded in control. Same trend was observed in case of 1000 grains weight per plot. 1000 grains weight per plot varied from 41.38-47.03 g. Maximum1000 grains weight per plot (47.03 g) was observed ST by thiram + carboxin @ 2.5 g/kg of seed + FS of propiconazole @ 0.1% at boot leaf stage on flag-1 leaf followed by second spray at 20 days' interval (two sprays) which was followed by FS of propiconazole @ 0.1% @ 0.25% at boot leaf stage on flag-1 leaf followed by second spray at 20 days' intervals (two sprays). While 1000 grains weight (41.38 g) was recorded in control.

The same results were obtained by Alam *et al.* (1995) while spraying with propiconazole 25 EC @ 0.04% on wheat to control the leaf blight pathogen. Kabir and Hossain (2000) also observed the effect of different combinations of macronutrients (N, P, K, S) micronutrients (B, Cu, Zn), irrigation and tilt (2 sprays) in controlling Bipolaris leaf blight (BPLB), caused by *Bipolaris sorokiniana* (*Cochliobolus sativus*), in wheat cv. Kanchan.

Table 4: Effect of fungicide on yield of wheat

	Treatments	Seed weight/plot (kg)	1000 grains weight (gm)
T1	ST by thiram @ 3 g/kg of seed	3.12	42.53
T2	ST by thiram + carboxin @ 2.5 g/kg of seed	3.55	43.80
T3	ST by thiram + carboxin @ 2.5 g/kg of seed + FS sprays of propiconazole @ 0.1% (one) at boot leaf stage on Flag-1 leaf	4.03	44.71
T4	ST by thiram + carboxin @ 2.5 g/kg of seed + FS of propiconazole @ 0.1% at boot leaf stage on Flag-1 leaf followed by second spray at 20 days interval (two sprays)	4.48	47.03
T5	FS of propiconazole @ 0.1% at boot leaf stage on Flag-1 leaf	3.90	44.00
T6	FS of propiconazole @ 0.1% at boot leaf stage on Flag-1 leaf followed by second spray at 20 days interval (two sprays)	4.07	44.95
T7	FS of tebuconazole @ 0.1% at boot leaf stage on Flag-1 leaf	3.90	44.21
T8	FS of tebuconazole @ 0.1% at boot leaf stage on Flag-1 leaf followed by second spray at 20 days interval (two spray)	4.01	45.12
T9	Three FS of mancozeb @ 0.25% at boot leaf stage on Flag-2 leaf followed by second and third spray at 10 days intervals each (three spray)	3.70	44.28
T10	Control	2.91	41.38
	CD @ 5%	0.24	0.32
	CV	3.76	0.42
	SEM±	0.82	0.10

Means of three replication
ST = Seed treatment
FS = Foliar spray

Conclusion

Most of the fungicides have good control over spot blotch of wheat. Thus fungicides used for managing the wheat disease play an important role towards the management of wheat diseases. Therefore ST by thiram + carboxin @ 2.5 g/kg of seed + FS of propiconazole @ 0.1% at boot leaf stage on Flag-1 leaf followed by second spray at 20 days interval (two sprays) which have better control over disease can be recommended for chemical control of wheat.

References

Ahmed F, Hossain I (2005) Effect of pathotypes of *Bipolaris sorokiniana* on leaf blight and grain yield of wheat C V. Kanchan inoculated at maximum tillering stage under field condition. *Bangladesh Journal of Seed Science and Technology*, 9: 1-4.

Ahmed H U, Hossain M M (1985) Final Report (1982-1985). Crop diseases survey and Establishment of Herbarium at BARI. Plant Pathology Division. BARI Joydebpur, Gazipur. 107pp.

Alam KB, Malaker PK, Shaheed MA, Ahmed MU, Ahmed F and Haque MS (1995). Yield loss assessment of wheat due to Bipolaris leaf blight in Bangladesh. *Bangladesh Journal of Plant Pathology* 11: 35-38.

Aminuzzaman FM and Hossain I (2007). Evaluation of plant activator and chemical fungicides on leaf blight (*Bipolaris sorokiniana*) development and yield of wheat. *Pakistan Journal of Biological Sciences* 10:1797-803.

Duveiller E and Gilchrist L (1994). Production constraints due to *Bipolaris sorokiniana* in wheat: Current situation and future prospects. p. 343–352. In D.A. Saunders and G.P. Hettel (ed.) Wheat in heat-stressed environments: Irrigated, dry areas and rice-wheat farming systems. CIMMYT, Mexico, D.F.

FAO STAT (2016) Production-crops. Food and Agriculture organization of the United Nation. 2011 http:// faostat.fao.org/site/339/defalt.asps.

Goulart ACP, Paiva FA and Andrade PJM (1995). Effect of fungicide spraying on above ground parts of wheat and incidence of *Bipolaris sorokiniana* and *Pyricularia grisea* associated with seeds. *Fitopatologia- Brasileira* 20: 628-632.

Hossain I, Azad A K (1992) *Bipolaris sorokiniana*, its reaction and effect on yield of wheat. *Progressive Agriculture*, 5(2):63-69.

Kabir MS and Hossain I (2000). Integrated management of Bipolaris leaf blight of wheat. *Bangladesh Journal of Plant Pathology* 16: 9-12.

Katasntones G, Koutrovbas SD, Ntanos DA and Lupoho E (2007). A comparison of three experimental designs for the field assessment of resistance to rice brown leaf spot of rice disease (*Bipolaris oryzae*). *Journal of Phytopathology* 155: 204-210.

Pingali P L (1999) CIMMYT 1998-99 World Wheat Facts and Trends. Global Wheat Research in a Changing World: Challenges and Achievements. CIMMYT, Mexico. *Plant Disease Research,* 16(1):113-115.

Reis EM (1991). Integrated disease management: The changing concept of controlling head blight and spot blotch. In: Saunders DA, Hettel GP (eds) Wheat in Heat-Stressed Environments: Irrigated, Dry Areas and Rice- Wheat Systems. CIMMYT, Mexico DF, pp 165-177

Singh SK, Srivastava KD, Aggarwal R and Singh VB (2011). Control of spot blotch (*Bipolaris sorokiniana*) of wheat using systemic fungicides. *Indian Phytopathology* 64: 82-84.

Zadoks J C, Chang T T, Konzak C F (1974). A decimal code for the growth stages of cereals. *Weeds Research,* 14: 415.

11

Genetic Studies for Yield and Yellow Vein Mosaic Virus Resistance in Okra (*Abelmoschus Esculentus* L. Moench)

Randhir Kumar[1], P K Patel[1], S S Solankey[1], Hemant Kumar Singh[2] and Gireesh Chand[3]

[1]*Department of Horticulture (Vegetable & Floriculture), Bihar Agricultural University, Sabour (Bhagalpur), Bihar-813210, India*
[2]*Farm Science Centre, Kishanganj, Bihar-855107, India*
[3]*Department of Plant Pathology, Bihar Agricultural University, Sabour (Bhagalpur), Bihar – 813210, India*

Abstract

The present investigation was carried out in okra consisting of 11 diverse genotypes (8 lines & 3 testers) and their 24 F1 hybrids. Phenotypic and genotypic correlation indicated positive association of average fruit length with average fruit weight while negative association between days taken to first flower with number of fruits per plant. The maximum positive direct effect on yield was due to number of fruits per plant followed by average fruit weight. The F_1 hybrid VRO-6 × Parbhani Kranti exhibits highest negative heterobeltiosis for days taken to 1st flowering while D-1-87-5 × Pusa A-4 and Arka Abhay × Parbhani Kranti are earliest heterobeltiotic hybrids for days taken to 1st harvest. The hybrid Arka Abhay × Pusa A-4 represents highest heterobeltiosis for average fruit length, number of fruits/ plant and average yield. Among all parents, only Akra Abhay exhibits better GCA effect. The highest SCA effect for average yield observed in VRO-6 × Arka Anamika, while VRO-6 × Pusa A-4 for per cent infestation of YVMV. The cross Arka Abhay × Pusa A-4 incurred the highest net returns/ ha and B: C ratio (3.21) followed by that of D-1-87-5 × Parbhani Kranti and the parent Hisar Unnat gave the higher net returns/ ha with B: C ratio of 2.02 among the parents. These *elite hybrids may be tested for yield and other quality traits under different agro-climatic conditions for commercial exploitation of hybrid vigour.*

Keywords: Okra, correlation, path analysis, heterosis, combining ability, YVMV, B: C ratio

Introduction

Okra is an important vegetable crop in the tropical and subtropical region of the world belongs to the family Malvaceae. It's grown throughout the tropical and subtropical part of world. It is widely grown all over India both in summer and rainy season. India is the largest producer of okra in the world with total area of 0.49 million hectares and production 5.78 million tones green pods, whereas productivity of the crop is 11.6 MT/ ha (Anonymous, 2017). Hence, an attempt has been made to study the 'line × tester' analysis (Kempthorne, 1957), to know the heterobeltiosis (heterosis over better parent), relative heterosis (heterosis over mid parent) and economic heterosis (heterosis over check variety) for interested traits in okra (Singh *et al.*, 2009). Heterosis is a special genetic mechanism wherein the distant genotypes are brought together in a specific pattern to express their ability to make a dramatic shift in the magnitude of a particular trait. The genetical studies revealed that yield and its components is most assessing in nature and magnitude of gene effect is important for increasing the yield potential. Exploitation of heterosis and hybrid vigour has been reported for increase in yield and other yield related traits. Okra has suffered major cultivation problem in India due to lack of yielding varieties along with hybrids with resistance to one of the most severe problem i.e. yellow vein mosaic virus (YVMV). Various approaches being used to overcome this problem one of them considered as heterosis breeding for exploitation of heterosis breeding. Moreover, okra which is categorized under often-cross-pollinated group showed easy emasculation and high number of seed production in single pollination. It should be kept in mind that due to high chromosome number and polygenic control of major economic traits, 100 % homozygosity in the parents is difficult to achieve (Dhankar and Mishra, 2006). In okra insufficient work has been done in estimating the heterosis effects in different environments. Therefore, the present investigation has been undertaken to estimation of the heterosis over better parents in different seasons for fruit yield and related traits in okra.

Materials and Methods

The present investigation was carried out in line × tester mating design in okra consisting of 11 diverse genotypes (8 lines & 3 testers) and their 24 F1 hybrids was evaluated in a complete randomized block design (CRBD) with three replications at the research farm of the Department of Horticulture (Vegetable & Floriculture), Bihar Agricultural College, Sabour, Bhagalpur (Bihar) during 2010 – 12. The parental materials comprised of 8 lines viz., D-1-87-5, Nirmal-303, Hisar Unnat, Arka Abhay, Indam- 9821, Ankur-40, Varsha Uphar, VRO-6 and 3 testers i.e., Pusa-A-4, Arka Anamika and Parbhani Kranti (Table 1).

Table 1: Genotypes of okra employed in the investigation.

Sl.No.	Genotypes	Specific traits	Source
1.	D-1-87-5	High yielding, long poded, early variety.	IARI, New Delhi
2.	Nirmal 303	Long poded, high yielding variety.	Nirmal Seeds Pvt. Ltd., Pachora, Maharashtra
3.	Hisar Unnat	Light green pods, early, high yielding and resistant to YVMV.	CCSHAU, Hisar, Hariyana
4.	Indam- 9821	Light green and long poded, high yielding variety.	Indo American Hybrid Seeds (India) Pvt. Ltd., Bangalore, Karnataka
5.	Ankur-40	Smooth pods with attractive green colour, high yielding variety.	Ankur Seeds Pvt. Ltd., Nagpur, Maharashtra
6.	*VRO-6	Resistant to YVMV, high yielding and better for Kharif season.	IIVR, Varanasi, Uttar Pradesh
7.	Varsha Uphar	Early harvesting, pods are medium in size and dark green colour.	CCSHAU, Hisar, Hariyana
8.	Arka Abhay	Wider adaptable variety and resistant to YVMV.	IIHR, Bangalore, Karnataka
9.	Arka Anamika	Moderately resistant to YVMV, high yielding variety.	IIHR, Banglore, Karnataka
10.	Pusa A-4	Resistant to YVMV, high yielding and good for fresh fruit export.	IARI, New Delhi
11.	Parbhani Kranti	YVMV resistant variety.	MPKV, Rahuri, Maharashtra

*Standard check variety – VRO-6

The recommended agronomic practices were adopted for raising a good okra crop. Observations were recorded on 10 economically important traits *viz.*, Plant height (m), number of branches/ plant, days to 1st flowering, days to 1st harvest, average fruit length (cm) average fruit weight (g), number of fruits/ plant, number of seeds per pod, average yield (q/ ha) and per cent infestation of YVMV. The soil of the plot was sandy loam in texture having good fertility properly leveled and well drained. The pH of the soil under study was 6.8 (Table 2).

Table 2. Soil test results of experimental plot.

Sl. No	Content	Result	
1.	pH	7.95	Slightly Basic
2.	E.C. (Desi/m)	0.117	Normal
3.	Organic Carbon (%)	0.42	Low
4.	Available P_2O_5 (kg/ha)	41.04	Medium
5.	Potash (kg/ha)	91.12	Low

The heterosis of F_1.s over the better parent (BPH) and mid parent (MPH) was calculated by using the formula:

$$\text{Per cent heterosis over better parent (BPH)} = \frac{F_1 - BP}{BP} \times 100$$

$$\text{Per cent heterosis over mid parent (MPH)} = \frac{F_1 - MP}{MP} \times 100$$

$$\text{Per cent heterosis over standard parent (SPH)} = \frac{F_1 - SP}{SP} \times 100$$

Where, F_1 =Mean value of F_1s, BP= Mean of better parent, MP= mean of mid parent value and SP= mean of standard parent value.

Analysis of combining ability was carried out as recommended by Kempthorne, 1957. The genetic parameters, such as phenotypic, genotypic, and environmental coefficients of variation (GCV, PCV and ECV), heritability in broad sense (h^2b), genetic advance and correlation coefficients for each character were estimated as suggested by Tsegaye *et al.* 2007.

Scoring of YVMV disease incidence was scored on 0 – 4 scale (Table 1) at the 15 days intervals (30 day, 45 day, 60 day and 75 days) after sowing and PDI and CI value was calculated by the procedure coined by Banerjee and Kaloo, 1987.

$$\text{PDI (\%)} = \frac{\text{Number of infected plants}}{\text{Total number of plants observed}} \times 100$$

$$\text{CI} = \text{RV} \times \text{PDI}$$

Where

RV = Response value

PDI = per cent disease infection.

Table 3: Scale for classifying disease reaction in okra to YVMV disease.

Symptoms	Severity grade	Response value	Coefficient of infection	Reaction
Symptoms absent	0	0	0 – 4	HR
Very mild symptoms up to 25% leaves	1	0.25	4.1 – 9	R
Appearance of disease between 26-50% leaves	2	0.50	9.1 – 19	MR
Symptom between 51-75% leaves	3	0.75	19.1 – 39	MS
Severe disease infection at 75% leaves	4	1.00	39.1 – 69	S
Above 75% leaves	>4	>1.00	69.1 – 100	HS

Note, R = Resistant, S = Susceptible, H R = Highly resistant, H S = Highly susceptible, M R = Moderately resistant, M S = Moderately susceptible.

Results and Discussion

The analysis of variance of the experiment indicated significant difference among the treatments for all the characters except per cent infestation of YVMV (Table 4). Parent vs. crosses were highly significant for the characters like days taken to first harvest, average fruit length (cm) number of fruits/ plant and average yield (q/ha).

The highest genotypic coefficient of variation (Table 5) was noticed for average yield (22.52) followed by number of fruits/ plant (19.20) and plant height (12.33). The maximum phenotypic coefficient of variation was observed for average fruit yield (24.74) followed by percent infestation of YVMV (24.24) and number of fruits/ plant (24.17). The highest broad sense heritability (h^2b) was obtained for average yield (82.89 %) followed by number of fruits/ plant (63.11 %) and number of branches/ plant (62.47 %). The genetic advance expressed as percentage of mean was the highest for average yield (42.24 %) followed by number of fruits/ plant (31.42 %) and number of branches per plant (19.31 %). Existence of high variability for yield per plant in okra was also reported by Adiger *et al.*, 2013.

In general, genotypic correlations were higher than phenotypic correlations (Table 6). Phenotypic and genotypic correlations of average yield (q/ha) with number of fruits/ plant (G=0.914, P=0.784) were significantly positive, whereas, it was negatively correlated with days taken to 1st flowering (G=-0.588, P=-0.491). Phenotypic and genotypic correlation indicated significant negative association for days taken to first flower with number of fruits per plant (G=-0.503, P=-0.385) and average yield (G=-0.588, P=-0.490). Similar pattern of correlation was also reported by Dhankar and Dhankar 2002.

To study the cause and effects of relationship the whole system of variables was represented in the form of path coefficient. The maximum positive direct effect on yield (Table 7 & Fig. 1) was due to number of fruits per plant (0.820)

Table 4. Analysis of Variance (ANOVA) for Line × Tester analysis and its combining ability for ten quantitative traits in okra.

Sources	d.f	Plant height (m)	Number of branches per plant	Days taken to first flower	Days taken to first harvest	Average fruit length (cm)	Average Fruit weight (g)	Number of fruits/ plant	Number of seeds per pod	Average Yield (q/ha)	Per cent infestation of YVMV
Replication	2	0.089	0.619	11.063	9.867	1.048	10.016	1.416	133.039	276.459	656.363
Treatment	34	0.070**	1.056**	12.904**	5.633	2.540**	4.392**	42.395**	93.467**	1844.807**	39.906
Parent	10	0.092**	0.543**	11.496**	1.685	3.704**	10.462**	21.908**	72.745*	415.354**	39.250
F_1	23	0.064**	1.324**	14.059**	3.753**	1.324**	1.861	50.388**	106.211**	2171.681**	38.967
Parent Vs F_1	1	0.002	0.031	0.387	88.356**	18.864**	1.824	63.416**	7.568	8621.247**	0.0587
Error	68	0.024	0.176	3.542	1.602	0.526	1.310	6.914	31.707	118.728	37.352

*,** Significant at 5% and 1%, respectively.

Table 5. Mean, range, genotypic and phenotypic coefficient of variation heritability and genetic advance in okra.

Sl No.	Characters	Mean	Range			Coefficient of variation		h^2b (%)	GA as % of Mean
			Line	Tester	Crosses	GCV	PCV		
1.	Plan height (m)	1.01	0.85-1.31	0.85-1.03	0.78-1.32	12.33	19.70	39.18	15.90
2.	Number of branches/ plant	4.56	3.63-5.20	4.43-4.90	3.63-5.77	11.86	15.00	62.47	19.31
3.	Days taken to 1st flowering	40.02	36.99-42.34	41.17-42.46	34.82-44.33	4.41	6.45	46.84	6.22
4.	Days taken to 1st Harvest	46.52	46.33-48.67	47.33-48.67	44.67-49.33	2.49	3.69	45.62	3.47
5.	Average fruit length (cm)	15.36	13.06-17.64	14.34-15.13	14.63-17.14	7.46	11.25	43.95	10.18
6.	Average fruit weight (g)	13.59	11.49-14.24	11.03-18.21	11.46-15.71	5.33	7.12	56.09	8.23
7.	Number of fruits/ plant	17.91	13.62-20.29	13.72-21.24	9.29-24.92	7.31	11.65	39.37	9.45
8.	Number of seeds per pod	62.08	57.66-68.11	53.88-65.89	49.33-73.44	19.20	24.17	63.11	31.42
9.	Average yield (q/ha)	106.51	78.50-112.04	80.58-83.53	59.03-156.36	22.52	24.74	82.89	42.24
10.	Percent infestation of YVMV	25.28	20.26-31.45	23.18-29.20	16.56-32.93	1.70	24.24	49.00	25.00

Table 6: Phenotypic and genotypic correlation coefficient in okra.

Characters		Plant height	Days taken to first flower	Average fruit length	Average fruit weight	Number of fruits/plant	Average yield
Plant height (m)	G	1.0000	-0.2436	0.5525**	0.1017	0.2186	0.2533
	P	1.0000	-0.2079	0.3267	-0.0150	0.1299	0.1522
Days taken to 1st flowering	G		1.0000	-0.0369	-0.1898	-0.5032**	-0.5889**
	P		1.0000	-0.1201	-0.139	-0.3852*	-0.4909**
Average fruit length (cm)	G			1.0000	0.4470	0.2217	0.3556*
	P			1.0000	0.1553	0.1596	0.2784
Average fruit weight(g)	G				1.0000	0.0878	0.4102*
	P				1.0000	0.0272	0.2782
Number of fruits/ plant	G					1.0000	0.9144**
	P					1.0000	0.7841**

G = Genotypic correlation coefficient, P = Phenotypic correlation coefficient, *,** Significant at 5% and 1%, respectively.

Table 7: Genotypic direct and indirect effects in okra.

Traits	Plant height (m)	Days taken to 1st flower	Days taken to 1st harvest	Average fruit weight (g)	Number of fruits/ plant	Yield(q/ ha)
Plant height (m)	-0.0079	0.0292	0.0223	0.0303	0.1794	0.2533
Days taken to1st flowering	0.0019	-0.1198	-0.0015	-0.0566	-0.4130	-0.5889
Average fruit length (cm)	-0.0044	0.0044	0.0403	0.1333	0.1819	0.3556
Average Fruit Weight (g)	-0.0008	0.0227	0.0180	0.2981	0.0721	0.4102
Number of Fruit/ Plant	-0.0017	-0.0265	0.0957	0.0262	0.8208	0.9144

*Bold lines indicate direct effects, R^2 =0.9557, Residual effect = 0.2104

Table 8: Best three heterotic F_1s and GCA and SCA effects for ten characters in okra.

Characters	Hybrids (F_1)	MP (%)	BP (%)	SP (%)	Parents	GCA	Hybrids (F_1)	SCA
Plan height (m)	V-6 × A.An.	54.90*	54.30**	28.25*	VRO-6	0.1851	A-40 × P.K.	0.2422 **
	V-6 × P-4	46.04	34.25*	10.71	Nirmal -303	0.0751	H.U. × A.An.	0.1464
	H.U. × A.An.	21.09	21.09	0.65	Parbhani Kranti	0.0486	V.U × A.An.	0.1381
Number of branches / plant	H.U. × A.An.	24.90*	22.56**	11.64	Arka Abhay	0.4875	A- 40 × P-4	1.0722 **
	A-40 × A.An.	22.14*	20.30**	9.59	Arka Anamika	0.1542	N-303 × P-4	0.9097 **
	N-303 × A.An.	15.44*	12.95	7.53	Pusa-A-4	0.1208	I - 9821 × P-4	0.8167 **
Days taken to 1st flowering	V-6 × P.K.	-11.79*	-17.03**	-17.03**	VRO-6	-2.4240	H.U. × P.K	-3.6225**
	A.Ab. × P-4	-13.20*	-13.38**	-15.03**	Hisar Unnat	-1.6618	A.Ab. × P-4	-2.7764*
	H.U. × P-4	-5.32	-8.98*	-10.72**	Pusa-A-4	-0.9831	H.U. × P-4	-2.2236*
Days taken to 1st Harvest	D-1 × P-4	-7.27**	-8.22**	-8.22**	Hisar Unnat	-0.6806	D-1 × P-4	-1.7347*
	A.Ab. × P.K	-6.94**	-8.22**	-8.22**	Pusa-A-4	-0.5694	V-6 × A.An.	-1.1597
	A.Ab. × P-4	-5.96**	-6.29**	-8.22**	Arka Abhay	-0.3472	A.Ab. × P.K.	-0.9375
Average fruit length (cm)	A.Ab. × P-4	18.07*	16.97**	19.53**	Nirmal -303	0.8107	H.U. × A.An.	0.9053 *
	A.Ab. × P.K.	12.70*	12.85**	12.85**	Hisar Unnat	0.2651	V.U. × P.K.	0.8036
	A-40 × P.K.	12.29*	12.12**	12.46**	Varsha Uphar.	0.1751	A-40 × P.K.	0.7956
Average fruit weight (g)	V.U. × P.K.	22.39*	19.92*	24.96**	Nirmal -303	0.6844	I - 9821 × P-4	1.2200
	D-1 × P.K.	20.13*	10.9	31.04**	Arka Abhay	0.6278	D-1 × P.K.	1.1197
	H.U. × P-4	14.62*	10.52	36.20**	VRO-6	0.3589	H.U. × A.An.	0.6719
Number of fruits/plant	A.Ab. × P-4	71.39*	65.51**	17.33	Arka Abhay	4.1369	H.U. × P-4	5.1608 **
	N-303 × P-4	51.00*	48.76**	8.68	Nirmal -303	1.9714	V-6 × A.An.	4.9747 **
	N-303 × A.An.	56.00*	46.98**	7.38	Pusa-A-4	1.7235	A- 40 × P-4	3.8967 *
Number of seeds per pod	V-6 × A.An.	25.54*	21.50**	11.46	I -9821	5.2465	A.Ab. × P.K.	9.0258 **
	H.U. × P-4	22.91*	18.89*	4.05	VRO-6	3.8010	A-40 × A.An.	7.3744 *
	I- 9821 × P-4	14.89*	17.01*	5.57	Ankur-40	2.2088	D-1 × P.K.	5.8575
Average Yield (q/ha)	A.Ab. × P-4	93.00*	87.18**	94.12**	Arka Abhay	26.6579*	V-6 × A.An.	41.0658 **
	D-1 × P.K.	88.65*	86.78**	86.78**	VRO-6	12.2401	H.U. × P-4	27.9386 **
	H.U. × P-4	49.05*	30.09**	80.95**	Pusa-A-4	9.1710	D-1 × P.K.	26.2042 **
Percent infestation of YVMV	A.Ab. × A.An.	-29.37	-33.23	-28.03	Arka Abhay	-4.8620	V-6 × P-4	-3.7773
	A-40 × P.K.	-5.77	-11.62	-11.62	Ankur-40	-1.6878	A.Ab. × P-4	-3.5786
	D-1 × P-4	-20.1	-27.52	-8.52	D-1 -87-5	-0.9046	I-9821 × P-4	-3.2105

Where, D-1 = D-1 -87-5, N-303 = Nirmal -303, H.U. = Hisar Unnat, I - 9821 = INDAM -9821, A-40 = Ankur-40, V- 6 = VRO – 6, V.U. = Varsha Uphar, A.Ab. = Arka Abhay, P-4 = Pusa A-4, A.An. = Arka Anamika, P.K. = Parbhani Kranti. *,** Significant at 5% and 1%, respectively.

followed by average fruit weight (0.298) and average fruit length (0.040) while, other variable had negative direct effects. The maximum negative direct effect on yield was due to days to first flowering (-0.119) and plant height (-0.008). The maximum positive indirect effect for yield was due to average fruit length with number of fruits per pant (0.182) followed by plant height with number of fruits per plant (0.179). The maximum negative indirect effect on yield was due to days taken to 1st flowering with number of fruits per plant (-0.413). Similar trend were also found by Hazra and Basu 2000 and Reddy *et al.* 2013.

The cross VRO-6 × Arka Anamika exhibited highest positive heterobeltiosis (Table 8) for plant height (54.30%) and number of seeds/ pod (25.54%) however, Hisar Unnat × Arka Anamika (22.56%) represent highest positive heterobeltiosis for number of branches/ plant. The F_1 hybrid VRO-6 × Parbhani Kranti (-17.03%) exhibit highest negative heterobeltiosis for days taken to 1st flowering while, D-1-87-5 × Pusa A-4 and Arka Abhay × Parbhani Kranti is earliest better parent heterotic hybrids for days taken to 1st harvest (-8.22 %). The hybrid Arka Abhay × Pusa A-4 represents highest heterobeltiosis for average fruit length (16.97%), number of fruits/ plant (65.51%) and average yield (87.18%) moreover; Varsa Uphar × Parbhani Kranti (19.92%) retained highest heterobeltiosis for average fruit weight. The hybrid Arka Abhay × Arka Anamika represent highest negative better and standard parent heterosis (-33.23%, -29.37%, respectively) that showed resistant response against this most severe viral disease of okra. Significant negative heterosis for this character in okra has been reported earlier by Adiger *et al.* 2013, Kumar *et al.* 2013 and Solankey *et al.* 2016. Evidently manifestation of heterosis for yield and yield components may be due to non additive gene effects in the parents. However, present study revealed manifestation and considerable amount of heterosis for yield per plant in okra and indicates large scope for heterosis breeding for further improvement in yield.

Considering the GCA effect of different characters (Table 8) it was found non-significant for all the genotypes except Akra Abhay for average yield (q/ ha). The results of SCA effect indicated that the crosses Ankur-40 × Parbhani Kranti (0.24) for plant height (m), Ankur-40 × Pusa A-4 (1.07m) for number of branches/ plant, Hisar Unnat × Pusa A-4 (-3.62) for days taken to 1st flowering, D-1-87-5 × Pusa A-4 (-1.73) for days taken to 1st harvest, Hisar Unnat × Arka Anamika (0.90) for average fruit length (cm), Indam- 9821 × Pusa A-4 (1.22) for average fruit weight (g), Hisar Unnat × Pusa A-4 (5.16) for number of fruits/ plant, Arka Abhay × Parbhani Kranti (9.02) number of seeds/ pod, VRO-6 × Arka Anamika (41.06) for average yield (q/ha) and VRO-6 × Pusa A-4 (-3.77) for per cent infestation of YVMV exhibited high value of SCA effect. The SCA effect of all the characters showed significant value except average fruit weight and per cent infestation of YVMV. This is in accordance with

Khatik *et al.*,2012, Indu Rani and Veeraragavathatham,2013 Kumar *et al.* 2013 and Solankey *et al.* 2016. These high SCA effects could therefore be useful to predict or identify heterotic responsive hybrids in okra.

The incidence to YVMV indicates (Fig. 2) that out of 24 F1 hybrids only ten hybrids have resistance response against YVMV in which Arka Abhay × Arka Anamika (PDI = 16.65%, CI = 4.16) followed by Ankur-40 × Parbhani Kranti (PDI = 20.45%, CI = 5.11) and Arka Abhay × Pusa A-4 (PDI = 20.91%, CI = 5.23) are most resistant hybrids. The resistant response of these hybrids is due to the presence of resistant gene from their parents. Similar findings were reported by Reddy *et al.*, 2012 and Ali *et al.*, 2012.

The maximum net return and B: C ratio was obtained due to heterosis among various heterotic combinations. The cross Arka Abhay × Pusa A-4 incurred the highest net returns i.e. Rs.143113.00/ ha and B: C ratio (3.21) followed by that of D-1-87-5 × Parbhani Kranti (Rs. 136013.00/ ha, B: C ratio 3.05) and the parent Hisar Unnat gave the highest net return of Rs. 89929.00/ ha with B: C ratio of 2.02 among the parents.

In the present study based on per se performance, heterosis and SCA effects, the hybrids Arka Abhay × Pusa A-4, VRO-6 × Arka Anamika and VRO-6 × Pusa A-4 were found superior hybrids for yield and yield attributing traits. The three short listed hybrids may be tested for yield and other quality traits under different agro-climatic conditions for commercial exploitation of hybrid vigour.

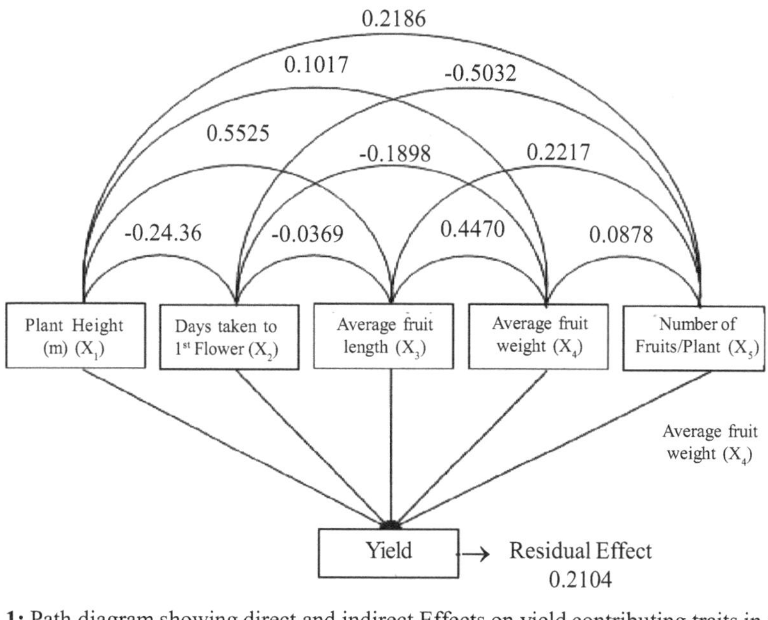

Fig. 1: Path diagram showing direct and indirect Effects on yield contributing traits in okra.

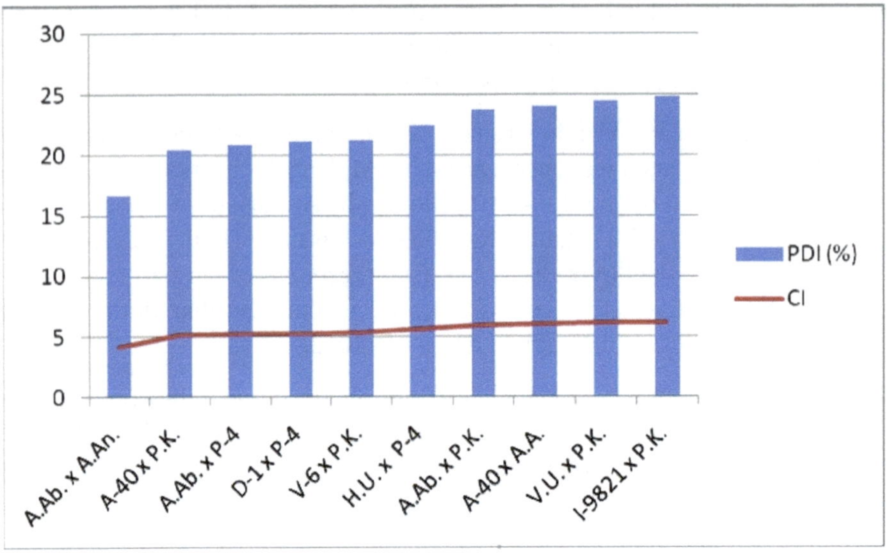

Fig. 2: Best ten resistant F_1 hybrids of okra.
Where, D-1 = D-1 -87-5, N-303 = Nirmal -303, H.U. = Hisar Unnat, I - 9821 = INDAM - 9821, A-40 = Ankur-40, V- 6 = VRO – 6, V.U. = Varsha Uphar, A.Ab. = Arka Abhay, P-4 = Pusa A-4, A.An. = Arka Anamika, P.K. = Parbhani Kranti.

Acknowledgements

Authors express their gratitude to Department of Horticulture (Vegetable & Floriculture), Bihar Agricultural University, Sabour for providing research facility and bottle gourd genotypes.

References

Adiger S, Shanthkumar G, Gangashetti PI and Salimath PM (2013) Heterosis for fruit yield and its component traits in double cross derived inbred lines of okra [*Abelmoschus esculentus* (L.) Moench]. *Ind. J. of Genet.* 73 (1): 116-19.

Ali MI, Khan MA, Rashid A, Ehetisham-ul-haq M, Javed MT and Sajid M (2012) Epidemiology of okra yellow vein mosaic virus (OYVMV) and Its Management through Tracer, Mycotal and Imidacloprid. *Amr. J. of Plant Sci.* 3: 1741-45.

Anonymous (2017) Indian Horticulture Database. National Horticulture Board, Ministry of Agriculture, Government of India, pp 4-5.

Banerjee MK and Kalloo G (1987) Sources and inheritance of resistance to leaf curl virus in *Lycopersicon* spp. *Theor. and Appl. Genet.* 73: 707-10.

Dhankar BS and Dhankar SK (2002) Genetic variability, correlation and path analysis in okra (*Abelmoschus esculentus* (L.) Moench). *Veg. Sci.* 29 (1): 63-8.

Dhankar BS and Mishra JP (2006) Objectives of okra breeding (In) Hybrid Vegetable Development, IBDC, New Delhi, p. 203.

Hazra P and Basu D (2000) Genetic variability, correlation and path analysis in okra. *Annals of Agril. Res.* 21 (3): 452-53.

Indu Rani C and Veeraragavathatham D (2013) Heterosis for yield and yield components in okra. *Ind. J. of Hort.* 70 (2): 290-92.

Kempthorne O (1957) An introduction to genetical statistics. John Wiley and Sons (Eds.), New York, pp 458-70.

Khatik, K.R., Chaudhary, R. and Khatik, C.L. 2012. Heterosis studies in okra [*Abelmoschus esculentus* (L.) Moench]. *Annals of Hort.* 5(2): 213-18.

Kumar A, Baranwal DK, Aparna J and Srivastava K (2013) Combining Ability and Heterosis for yield and its contributing characters in okra (*Abelmoschus esculantus* (L.) Moench). *Madras Agril. J.* 100 (1-3): 30-35.

Reddy MT, Babu KH, Ganesh M, Reddy KC, Begum H, Reddy RSK and Babu JD (2013) Correlation and path coefficient analysis of quantitative characters in okra (*Abelmoschus esculentus* (L.) Moench). Songklanakarin *J. of Sci. and Tech.* 35 (3): 243-50.

Reddy MT, Haribabu K, Ganesh M, Reddy KC, Begum H, Reddy RSK and Babu JD (2012) Genetic analysis for yield and its components in okra (*Abelmoschus esculentus* (L.) Moench). *Songklanakarin J. of Sci. and Tech.* 34 (2): 133-41.

Singh B, Kumar D, Singh KV and Chaudhary V (2009) Heterobeltiosis and inbreeding depression in okra [*Abelmoschus esculentus* (L.) Moench]. *Adv. in Plant Sci.* 22 (1): 273–5.

Solankey SS, Singh AK and Singh RK (2013) heterosis of okra resistance sources for okra yellow vein mosaic virus in okra., *Indian J of Agricultural Sciences* 86 (11): 1460–5.

Tsegaye E, Dechassa N and Sastry D, (2007) Genetic variability for yield and other agronomic traits in sweet potato. *J. of Agron.* 6 (1): 94-99.

12

Modulation of Mango Malformation Disease Management Strategy

Gireesh Chand, D.K. Chakrabarti*, Hemant Kumar and Santosh Kumar**

Department of Plant Pathology, Bihar Agricultural University, Sabour-813210 Bhagalpur, Bihar, India
**Department of Plant Pathology, N.D. University of Agriculture and Technology, Faizabad-242229, Uttar Pradesh, India*
***T.N. Post Graduate Degree College, Tanda-224196, India*

Abstract

The agricultural scientists particularly those who are in advisory service, irrespective of specialization, are often approached by the farmers with diseased samples of their crops and sought advice on plant protection strategy. The strategy includes components of control measures, doses, mode and time of application. In the present article different steps of formulation of plant disease control strategy are discussed. To further elaborate the contents, examples from integrated management strategy of mango malformation disease is cited.

Keyword: Mango Malformation

Introduction

Mango malformation, disease was first time reported from Darbhanga District of Bihar State in 1891 by G. Watt. The disease is currently prevalent in almost all the mango growing country and is thus designated as the plant disease of International importance and previously considered to be a serious problem in the northern parts of the country, has now started to appear in central India too in severe form. It is well known, the mango malformation is the most serious disease, rendering mango cultivation non-lucrative in subcontinent and other regions of the world (Ahmad *et al.,* 2002; Ploetz, 2001). Mango malformation caused by fungus *Fusarium moniliforme var.* Subglutinans, are proved (Freeman 1999; Zheng and Ploetz, 2002). Recently, these isolates were described as members of a new species, *F. mangiferae* Britz, Wingfield and Marasas sp nov. (Britz *et al.,* 2002). The casual organism of mango malformation grows well at lower temperature and higher relative humidity. The disease is quite common in both grafted and the seedling plants (Kumar and Chakrabarti, 1997). The symptoms manifest as bunchy top (BT) in 4-5 month old seedlings in the nursery, vegetative malformation (VM) of twigs arising from axillary buds and malformation of inflorescence (MF). Normally floral malformation is more prevalent in bearing trees than vegetative malformation. Flowers in the malformed panicle are much enlarged and crowded with hypertrophied axes of the panicle. Malformed inflorescences/ panicle of different varieties were variable in respect of their shapes, sizes, growth and compactness, depending upon the cellular structure and physiology under environmental factors (Chakrabarti *et al.,* 1990). Generally malformed inflorescences produce no fruit, or abort already stages (Schloser, 1971) and is directly responsible for reduction in yield (Kumar *et al.*, 1993 and Singh *et al.,* 1998). In the present study the incidence of Floral malformation on a large number of mango cultivars was recorded over a period of 5 years with a view to identify the entries of future resistant breeding programme.

Materials and Methods

The experiment was conducted at the Farmers mango orchards under the judiciary of N.D. University of Agriculture and Technology, Faizabad-242229, India. The bearing plants of 10 mango germplasms were selected for the study. The soil was silty loam, lightly compact, with range from 0.40-0.63% organic matter and pH range from 6.5-7.8. The Trees spaced at 12 m between rows and plants were 5 to 8 m high depending upon the genotype. There were three general fungicide-insecticide sprays per year (first prior to blooming , second post fruit setting and third after fruit harvesting) for plant protection but no pruning of malformed panicles was practiced in the progeny orchard during, prior year and study period to allow sufficient amount of inoculums under natural conditions. Observations were recorded 100 randomly selected panicles from all the four sides on the middle height of the canopy of the test plants. The plants were 20-25 years old. For each cultivar 4 replications were maintained. The percentage of malformed panicles counted. The data for the five years were pooled and analysed using a Complete Randomized Block Design.

Results and Discussion

Symptom based control strategy: Usually there is a tendency to diagnose plant diseases only by visual symptoms and prescribe control measures accordingly. Such types of practices are adopted when laboratory facilities are lacking; but often become misleading. For example, various factors only on the basis of the visual symptoms were attributed to cause mango malformation diseases. Thus, for a long time the cause of mango malformation was debated and various hypotheses on etiology of mango malformation were proposed (Table 1).

Table 1: Different factors suggested as the cause of malformation disease in mango.

Symptoms	Inference
Dwarfing of shoots and panicles	Nutrient deficiency
Leaves reduced to leaflets and phyllody	Virus
Excess flowering	High C/N ratio
Sterile pollen	High gibberellins content
Less hermaphrodite flowers	Low auxin content

It is obvious that control measures based only on assumption are destined to fail. However, it may work if one has long field experience and the disease is well known.

Pathogen based control strategy: Scientists having comparatively better facilities try to identify microorganisms associated with the diseases plant parts and depending upon the nature of the organism prescribe chemical or other control measures. Sometimes they ignore to confirm pathogenicity of the suspected organism. It happened initially with malformation disease of mango. Scientists observing fast nature of spread of the disease concluded that it might be caused by a living organism and isolated eriophyse mite and a fungus, *Fusarium moniliforme* var. *subglutinans* from malformed panicles and shoots. As no virus could be isolated from malformed cells, the involvement of virus was ruled out. Although the range of suspects was narrowed down to mites and the *Fusarium*, the actual inducer of the malformation was yet to be pin pointed. This prompted to confirm the pathogenicity by artificially inoculating a healthy plant with the suspected organism and produce similar symptoms. Efforts in this direction were continued for a long time but due to faulty methods results were erratic and that created more confusion about the cause of the disease. The ambiguity was removed long after when appropriate inoculation technique to reproduce the disease symptoms was developed and thus, *F.moniliforme* var. *subglutinans* was established as the inducer of the disease.

Physiology of pathogenesis based control strategy: Usually pathogens produce disease symptoms by their direct action over the host. Such diseases can be controlled by killing the pathogens. But efforts to control the malformation by eliminating the *Fusarium* or the mites did not give desired results. It urged to delineate the role of the *Fusarium* and eriophyse mite and investigate the mechanism of disease development by the pathogen (physiology of pathogenesis). Role of mite was found to be restricted as the vector that helped the fungus to transmit and enter into the host cells by causing mechanical injuries over developing buds. Investigation on role of *F. moniliforme* var. *subglutinans* revealed that the fusarial invasion stimulated the host to produce and accumulate a phenolic compound, mangiferin, at the site of infection to fight the pathogen. Mangiferin checked the ingress of the fungus deep into the host cells and later killed it in the colonized cells. But mangiferin had many attendant side effects. It upset the biochemical equilibrium and the physiology of the host, which subsequently manifested as disease symptoms. Besides, production of normal steroidal compounds of the host was affected and impaired the development of reproductive organs. This is a unique example of disease manifestation by the pathogen through altered mechanism of host physiology. So far the direct effects are concerned; the pathogen secreted some toxic compounds inside the host that contributed to produce the symptoms. Hence, once the abnormal metabolites were produced inside the host, mere killing of the pathogen could not arrest the symptom manifestation. The above information suggested that the disease could have been controlled if the pathogen was prevented prior to infection and the plant parts with abnormal metabolites were removed. The identification of the pathogen and its mode of action help to select the management components. But the strategy to select the right time and mode of striking the pathogen can be framed only after studying the epidemiology of the disease.

Epidemiology based control strategy: The Fig. 1 depicts that the pathogen multiplied over dead necrotic malformed panicles and spread to the developing buds immediately after rainy season. Hence, malformed panicles and shoots were recommended to be removed before rainy season preferably after harvesting of fruits. One should be vigilant particularly if the climatic factors are favourable as shown in the figure. The fungal spores were disseminated by the mites. Therefore, spraying of acaracide was suggested. The conidia germinated over young buds under a particular climatic condition. Hence, the buds should have a prophylactic spray when such climatic conditions prevailed. Up to this stage the pathogen was influenced mainly by climatic factors. But once it entered the host through mechanical injuries created by mites, the host metabolites also affected the pathogen in colonizing the cells and in manifestation of the disease symptoms. Mild temperature and high humidity promoted the disease development while it was arrested at high temperature. Hence, in the epidemic prone area late flowering cultivars are preferred. Similarly regular bearing cultivars as compared with alternate bearers are more vulnerable. The alternate bearing cultivars suffered maximum during on years. Hence, during on years extra precaution should be taken. It was also noticed that more was the number of malformed shoots on a plant during October (time of flower bud initiation), the greater was the incidence of floral malformation in the following crop season. Thus malformed shoots in October should thoroughly be pruned. Pruning resulted into high degree of disease control in the next crop season. But thereafter the infection rate increased rapidly and in the second year the disease recorded high incidence. Therefore pruning should be carried out systemically every year. But effects of spraying of fungicides like carbendazim were evident in the second year of the spray. It was also important to determine the number of spray required. Captan, a fungicide, was reported to effectively control the development of vegetative malformation. Captan was sprayed over emerging buds of a mango tree in an infected orchard. Seven days after of the spray, the buds were harvested and cultured on growth media. Three days after of incubation the fungal colonies developed over 8% buds. But within next 6 days (after 15 days of spraying) the fungal growth was recorded over more (64%) buds. As captan is not systemic in action could not kill the pathogen colonized inside the cells. Initially due to presence of captan, the fungus remained suppressed and could not grow on bud surface. But after 15 days when efficacy of captan was over, it came out and grew over the buds. This indicated that only one spray was not adequate to check the infection. Hence, the spray of captan was repeated for the second time after 15 days. This time the incidence was comparatively less (40%). But satisfactory control (9%) was achieved only after third spray. On the basis of the above results 3 prophylactic sprays of captan at 15 days interval were recommended to check vegetative malformation. Thus, a successful management strategy requires the correct identification of the causal organism, mechanism of the symptom production and complete information of the effects of environmental and host parameters and mode of action of the management components. To make it field effective and acceptable to farmers, the strategy should be developed with active participation of the beneficiaries.

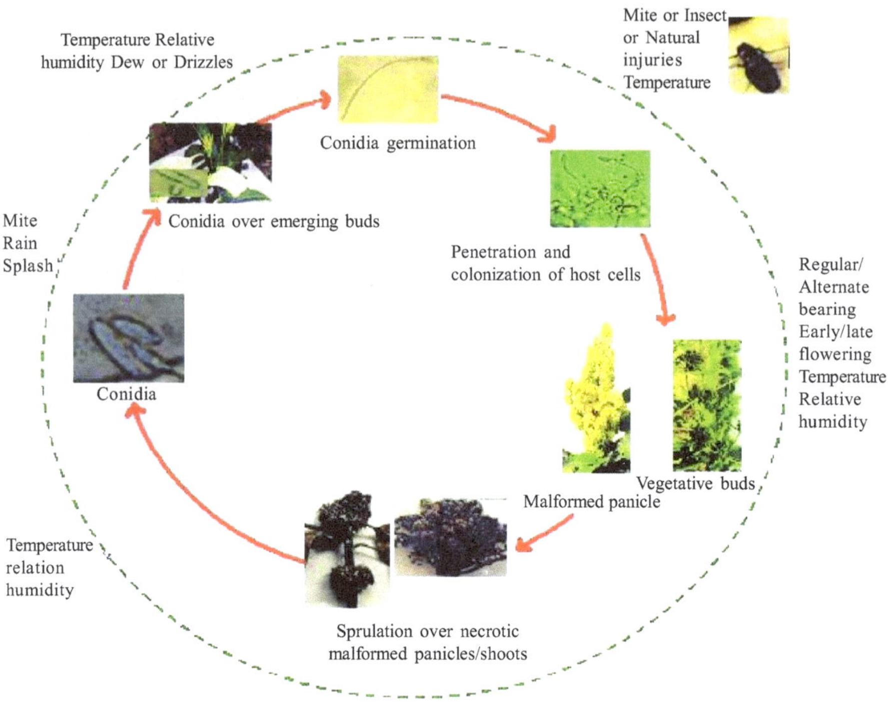

Fig. 1: Schematic diagram depicting the dynamics of mango malformation

Future control strategy: The future control strategy has been designed not to directly challenge the pathogen. Instead the host immunity against the pathogenic invasion will be enhanced by treating with biotic and abiotic components. The other approach is to attack the pathogen by its natural enemies (antagonist). For example, to control mango malformation we have identified one pathogencity related protein that is capable to induce natural resistance of mango plants against malformation. Besides a natural antagonist (*Aspergillus niger*) of *F. moniliforme* var. *subglutinans* has also been identified that reduced the population of the pathogen over the host surface.

References

Chakrabarti, D. K. 1996. Etiology and remedy of mango malformation. In *Disease Scenario in Crop Plants* Vol. 1 (Eds. V. P. Agnihotri, Om Prakash, Ram Krishna and A. K. Mishra), International Books & Periodicals Supply Service, Delhi, pp. 49-59.

Chakrabarti, D.K. and R. Kumar. 2002. Mango malformation: present status and future strategy. In *IPM System in Agriculture*, Vol.8, (Eds. R.K. Upadhyay, D.K. Arora and O.P. Dubey), Aditya Books Pvt. Ltd., N. Delhi, pp. 237-255

Chakrabarti, D.K. and R. Kumar. 2004. Status of mango malformation disease in West Bengal. In *Plant Pathology: Problems & Perspectives* (Eds. S.K.Raj, S.K.Pan and S.B. Chattopadhyay), B.C.Krishi Viswavidyalaya, Mohanpur, W. Bengal, pp. 147-149.

Chakrabarti, D.K, Mukesh K. Pandey, Gireesh, Chand, Rajesh Kumar, Ved Prakash and K. Singh. 2009. Mango malformation: epidemiology and principles of management. In *Diseases of Fruit Trees and their Eco-friendly Management* (Eds. A. Arya and C. Monaco), pp.58-69.

13

Substrates and Supplements for Sustainable Cultivation of Oyster Mushroom

Santosh Kumar[1], Gireesh Chand[1], Deepak Kumar Patel[3]
Anita Kumari[2], Umesh Singh[4]

[1]*Department of Plant Pathology, Bihar Agricultural University Sabour-813210, Bihar, India*
[2]*Department of Extension Education, Bihar Agricultural University Sabour-813210, Bihar, India*
[3]*KVK, Sabour, Bhagalpur (Bihar Agricultural University, Sabour-813210 Bihar, India*
[4]*Department of Soil Science and Agriculture Chemistry, MBAC Agwanpur, Saharsa, Bihar, India*

Abstract

Mushroom production is emerging as an added dimension in agriculture diversity; its cultivation lies on the utilization of agricultural wastes rich in proteinaceous materials. Five different substrates such as wheat straw, maize cob, paddy straw, banana pseudo stem, and lentil straw were used with suitable supplements to evaluate the average period of spawn run, pin head initiation, time taken for harvesting of flushes, fruit yield during both crop season 2014 and 2015. In 2014, highest fruit yield (380.3 g/ 500g) were recorded when wheat straw supplemented with rice bran (2% of the substrate weight), corn flour @ 25 g/kg prepared straw and gypsum @ 20 g/kg straw among various used substrates. This treatment also resulted better in respect of time taken for spawn run (9.3 days), pin head initiation (11.7 days), time taken for harvesting of flushes (Ist flush- 20.5, IInd flush- 26.7, IIIrd flush- 32.9). The second best treatment was paddy straw when supplemented with rice bran (2% of the substrate weight), corn flour @ 25 g/kg prepared straw, and gypsum @ 20 g/kg. The lowest fruit yield (193.6 g/500g), time taken for spawn run (15.9 days), pin head initiation (22.4 days), time taken for harvesting of flushes (Ist flush- 27.9, IInd flush-

37.1, IIIrd flush- 44.7) were recorded with banana pseudostem (chopped) when supplemented with rice bran (2 % of the substrate weight), corn flour @ 25 g/kg prepared straw and $CaCO_3$ gypsum @ 20 g/kg straw. The same experiment was repeated during the year crop season 2015. Surprisingly wheat straw supplemented with rice bran (2% of the substrate weight), corn flour @ 25 g/kg prepared straw and gypsum @ 20 g/kg prepared straw was found again superior over other treatments with more or less similar performance. Similarly more or less same performances were resulted in rest of the treatment too. The incidence of mould infection in mushroom was also noticed in accordance with the kinds of substrates used during both crop season 2014 and 2015. Lowest incidence of mould i.e. green mould (5.13 %), black mould (3.10 %) and blue mould (2.42%) was observed on wheat straw when supplemented with rice bran (2% of the substrate weight), corn flour @ 25 g/kg prepared straw and gypsum @ 20 g/kg straw, green mold (3.13 %), black mold (3.10 %) and blue mold (2.42 %). Similarly more or less same pattern of mould incidence was reported in the crop season 2015.

Keywords: Substrates and Supplements, Oyster

Introduction

Mushroom production is emerging as an added dimension in agriculture diversity; its cultivation lies on the utilization of agricultural wastes rich in proteinaceous materials. This is being considered as one of the profitable and eco-friendly technology, and is most pertinent for converting wastes into wealth. (Biswas *et al*, 1997; Cohen *et al*, 2002). Mushroom cultivation is being an indoor cultivation, low costing, labour intensive, high profit venture and suitable for rural areas as it can provide employment to small farmers, landless labourers, women, unemployed youth and even retired or in-service personnel in rural areas to a an extent (Das, 2015). Its relevance in the present scenario can be examined from the fact that the agricultural land is decreasing day by day due to industrialization, population pressure and escalating wasteland due to intensive agriculture. The mushroom can be cultivated in air and the entire cultivation is an indoor affair, so women friendly in nature. Keeping above facts in view, the experiment designed on **"Substrates and supplements for sustainable cultivation of oyster mushroom in Bihar"** had been carried out for two consecutive years, 2014 and 2015 and the result is encouraging. Simultaneously, this research study will help to Bihar state for improving the socioeconomic conditions of landless farmers to a few extents.

Materials and Methods

The present studies were conducted at the mushroom production unit, Department of Plant Pathology, BAU, Sabour during two consecutive years 2014 and 2015. Locally available substrates like wheat straw, maize cob, paddy straw, banana pseudostem, and lentil straw were evaluated for cultivation of oyster mushroom. These substrates were cut approximately 4 cm lengths except only wheat. The chopped substrates were soaked in fresh water for 12 hours followed by hot water treatment at 60° C for 30 minutes. Excess water was decanted on sloppy cemented floor and was dried in shed for two hours to retain 65-70 % moisture. Three supplements namely rice bran (2% of the substrate weight), corn flour @ 25 g/kg prepared straw, and $CaCO_3$ gypsum @ 20 g/kg prepared straw are mixed at the end of prepared straw, aim to early mycelia colonization, pin head initiation and fruit development. This does not only reduces the duration of production but also enhances the quality of mushroom fruit and benefit/cost ratio. Spawning was done with grain based spawn @ 3 % (dry weight basis) of straw by thorough mixing. The thorough spawning technique was used to enhance mycelia growth where the spawn was completely mixed with the substrate. The prepared substrates with supplements were placed in a clean sterilized room and 100 g of mushroom spawn were mixed into each 3 kg prepared substrates to making a 3 % spawn. Spawned substrate were filled in polypropylene bag (Size-35 x 50 cm, 80 gauges) are tied on the top with the help of sterilized cotton wool which was fixed with a rubber band. The prepared bag with making holes with the help of sterilized glass rod of about 1 cm diameter at the distance of 10-15 cm across the surface for free diffusion of gases and heat generated inside. Each treatment were replicated three times. The bags were kept in cropping room at 26–28‴ C for about 15–17 days in a well-ventilated room and bags were transferred to the growing house for fruiting when mycelia had fully grown, polythene bags were removed. The beds were moistened by repeating sprinkling water thrice a day and stopping just a day before harvesting.

Observation and data collection

The fruiting bodies are harvested by hand by grabbing from the base and performing a twisting motion. The number of mushroom and its fresh weight were recorded every six days for 6 consecutive weeks. Observation regarding time taken for spawn run (days), initiation of pin head formation (days), time taken for harvesting of flushes (days), and yield of each bag (g/500g) of the mushrooms were calculated after the cropping period. The cost benefit ration was calculated using the formula;

$$\text{Cost : Benifit ratio} = \frac{\text{Total input cost}}{\text{Total output cost}}$$

The incidence of mold infection in mushroom was also noticed in accordance with the kinds of substrates used during both crop season 2014 and 2015. Disease (mould) incidence was scored based on a 0-5 rating scale with 0= disease free, 1= 1-20 % area covered by disease, 2= 21-40 % area covered by disease, 3= 41-60 % area covered by disease, 4 = 61-80 % area covered by disease and 5 = 81-100 % area covered by the disease.

Results and Discussion

The average period of spawn run, pin head initiation, time taken for harvesting of flushes, and fruit yield of oyster mushroom greatly varied in accordance with the kinds of substrates used (Table 1 and 2). Five different substrates such as wheat straw, maize cob, paddy straw, banana pseudo stem, and lentil straw were used with suitable supplements during both crop season 2014 and 2015. In 2014, highest fruit yield (380.3 g/500g) were recorded when wheat straw supplemented with rice bran (2% of the substrate weight), corn flour @ 25 g/kg prepared straw and gypsum @ 20 g/kg straw among various used substrates. This treatment also resulted better in respect of time taken for spawn run (9.3 days), pin head initiation (11.7 days), time taken for harvesting of flushes (Ist flush- 20.5, IInd flush- 26.7, IIIrd flush- 32.9). The second best treatment was paddy straw when supplemented with rice bran (2% of the substrate weight), corn flour @ 25 g/kg prepared straw, and gypsum @ 20 g/kg. This treatment resulted in time taken for spawn run (10.4 days), pin head initiation (13.4 days), time taken for harvesting of flushes (Ist flush- 23.7, IInd flush- 32.9, IIIrd flush- 37.4), and fruit yield 320.3 g/500g. The lowest fruit yield (193.6 g/500g), time taken for spawn run (15.9 days), pin head initiation (22.4 days), time taken for harvesting of flushes (Ist flush- 27.9, IInd flush- 37.1, IIIrd flush- 44.7) were recorded with banana pseudostem (chopped) when supplemented with rice bran (2 % of the substrate weight), corn flour @ 25 g/kg prepared straw and $CaCO_3$ gypsum @ 20 g/kg straw. The same experiment was repeated during the year crop season 2015. Surprisingly wheat straw supplemented with rice bran (2% of the substrate weight), corn flour @ 25 g/kg prepared straw and gypsum @ 20 g/kg prepared straw was found again superior over other treatments with more or less similar performance; highest fruit yield (381.9 g/ 500g), time taken for spawn run (9.9 days), pin head initiation (12.0 days), time taken for harvesting of flushes (Ist flush- 21.6, IInd flush- 27.4, IIIrd flush- 33.6). Similarly more or less same performances were resulted in rest of the treatment too.

The incidence of mould infection in mushroom was also noticed in accordance with the kinds of substrates used during both crop season 2014 and 2015. (Table 3). Lowest incidence of mould i.e. green mould (5.13 %), black mould (3.10 %) and blue mould (2.42%) was observed on wheat straw when supplemented with rice bran (2% of the substrate weight), corn flour @ 25 g/kg prepared straw and gypsum @ 20 g/kg straw, green mold (3.13 %), black mold (3.10 %) and blue mold (2.42 %). Second lowest incidence of mould incidence i.e. green mold (7.70 %), black mold (5.93 %) and blue mold (5.04 %) was recorded in case of paddy straw supplemented with rice bran (2 % of the substrate weight), corn flour @ 25 g/kg prepared straw and gypsum @ 20 g/kg straw. Similarly more or less same pattern of mould incidence was reported in the crop season 2015.

Cost benefit analysis

Cost of technology/bag: (Size-35 x 50 cm, 80 gauges)**:** Wheat straw substrate

Input cost:

i) Spawn: Rs.10.00

ii) Substrate: Rs.12.00

iii) Supplements: Rs. 20.00

  a. rice bran

  b. corn flour

  c. Gypsum

iii) PP Bag: Rs. 01.00

vi) Management: Rs. 05.00

vii) Miscellaneous: Rs. 05.00

Total input cost: Rs. 53.00

Product cost: Rs. 150.00

Benefit cost: Rs. 97.00

Cost : Benefit: 1 : 1.8

Likely outcome of technology

- Recommendation for oyster mushroom production.
- Highly economic, easily adoptable and productive technology.

Table 1: Influence of different substrates and supplements for production of oyster mushroom during crop season 2014.

Substrates	Spawn run (Days)	Initiation of pin head formation (Days)	Time taken for harvesting of flushes			Yield (g/500g) dry substrate
			Ist flush (Days)	IInd flush (Days)	IIIrd flush (Days)	
T1=Wheat straw + rice bran (2 % of the substrate weight) + corn flour @ 25 g/kg prepared straw + gypsum @ 20 g/kg prepared straw.	9.3	11.7	20.5	26.7	32.9	380.3
T2=Maize cob (chopped) + rice bran (2 % of the substrate weight) + corn flour @ 25 g/kg prepared straw+ gypsum @ 20 g/kg of prepared straw.	10.9	17.3	27.0	35.8	42.5	216.2
T3=Paddy straw + rice bran (2 % of the substrate weight) + corn flour @ 25 g/kg prepared straw + gypsum @ 20 g/kg of prepared straw.	10.4	13.4	23.7	32.9	37.4	320.3
T4=Banana pseudostem (Chopped) + rice bran (2 % of the substrate weight) corn flour @ 25 g/kg prepared straw + gypsum @ 20 g/kg straw.	15.9	22.4	27.9	37.1	44.7	193.6
T5=Lentil straw + rice bran (2 % of the substrate weight) corn flour @ 25 g/kg prepared straw + gypsum @ 20 g/kg straw.	14.8	19.6	30.4	39.4	45.9	240.7
T5=Wheat straw (Farmer practice)	13.6	16.2	26.4	35.0	40.7	266.6
CD (P = 0.05)	0.8	0.6	1.6	1.3	1.5	5.3
SE(m)	0.3	0.2	0.5	0.4	0.5	1.7
C.V. (%)	3.5	1.9	3.4	2.1	2.0	1.1

Table 2: Influence of different substrates and supplements for production of oyster mushroom during crop season 2015

Substrates	Spawn run (Days)	Initiation of pin head formation (Days)	Time taken for harvesting of flushes			Yield (g/500g) dry substrate
			I[st] flush (Days)	IInd flush (Days)	IIIrd flush (Days)	
T1=Wheat straw + rice bran (2 % of the substrate weight) + corn flour @ 25 g/kg prepared straw + gypsum @ 20 g/kg prepared straw	9.9	12.0	21.6	27.4	33.6	381.9
T2=Maize cob (Chopped) + rice bran (2 % of the substrate weight) + corn flour @ 25 g/kg prepared straw + gypsum @ 20 g/kg of prepared straw	11.7	16.2	27.6	36.7	43.5	213.8
T3=Paddy straw + rice bran (2 % of the substrate weight)+ corn flour @ 25 g/kg prepared straw + gypsum @ 20 g/kg of prepared straw	11.0	14.0	24.2	32.1	38.1	322.3
T4=Banana pseudostem (chopped)+ rice bran (2 % of the substrate weight) corn flour @ 25 g/kg prepared straw + gypsum @ 20 g/kg straw	16.7	21.4	29.1	36.9	45.4	195.2
T5=Lentil straw + rice bran (2 % of the substrate weight) corn flour @ 25 g/kg prepared straw + gypsum) @ 20 g/kg straw	15.3	20.5	29.9	39.4	45.9	245.1
T6=Wheat straw (Farmer practice)	12.5	16.2	24.9	35.6	41.4	264.5
CD (P = 0.05)	1.1	0.7	1.5	0.4	1.3	4.2
SE(m)	0.3	0.2	0.5	0.1	0.4	1.3
C.V. (%)	4.6	2.4	3.0	0.6	1.8	0.8

Table 3: Per cent incidence of mould infection on different substrates.

Substrates	Mould infection (%)					
	2014			2015		
	Green mold	Black mold	Blue mold	Green mold	Black mold	Blue mold
T1=Wheat straw + rice bran (2 % of the substrate weight) + corn flour @ 25 g/kg prepared straw + gypsum @ 20 g/kg prepared straw.	3.13	3.10	2.42	3.80	3.03	2.89
T2=Maize cob (chopped) + rice bran (2 % of the substrate weight) + corn flour @ 25 g/kg prepared straw+ gypsum @ 20 g/kg of prepared straw.	9.23	8.23	8.23	9.04	7.48	7.19
T3=Paddy straw + rice bran (2% of the substrate weight) + corn flour @ 25 g/kg prepared straw + gypsum @ 20 g/kg of prepared straw.	6.56	5.93	5.04	6.58	4.85	5.00
T4=Banana pseudostem (Chopped) + rice bran (2 % of the substrate weight) corn flour @ 25 g/kg prepared straw + gypsum @ 20 g/kg straw.	22.21	17.54	15.68	23.00	16.08	17.35
T5=Lentil straw + rice bran (2 % of the substrate weight) corn flour @ 25 g/kg prepared straw + gypsum @ 20 g/kg straw.	12.00	12.33	12.33	10.67	11.52	13.67
T5=Wheat straw (Farmer practice)	7.70	6.61	7.87	6.94	5.08	7.03
CD (P = 0.05)	1.16	1.38	1.21	1.02	1.06	0.34
SE(m)	0.36	0.43	0.37	0.32	0.33	0.10
C.V. (%)	5.85	8.08	6.95	5.53	6.90	2.06

- Helpful for proper utilization of agro waste materials and in the maintenance of ecological balance.
- Suitable for Bihar, where agro waste is easily available due to extensive agricultural based economy.

How the new technology will make impact the income of the farmers' and its benefits over conventional technologies

- This technology is superior over conventional technology, because it requires less time and give more benefits in terms of cost.
- This technology is superior over conventional technology because it reduces the duration of production, enhances the quality of mushroom fruit and more chance to reduce mold infection.
- This proposed technology does not involve chemicals required for substrate treatment; therefore it is better in terms of lower input cost and food bio-safety.
- The addition of supplements in the substrates resulting in early mycelia colonization, pin head initiation and fruit development that reduces the duration of production.
- It is not only reduced the duration of production but also enhances the quality of mushroom fruit and also reduced the chances of mold infection during mycelial growth.

Acknowledgements

The authors are highly grateful to the Directorate of Extension education, Bihar Agricultural University (BAU), Sabour and Rastriya Krishi Vikash Yojna (RKVY), Government of Bihar, for providing financial support under project entitled "Development of improved technology for commercial production of mushroom in rural area of Bihar". This manuscript bears BAU communication No. 509/2018.

References

Biswas, M.K., Shukla, C.S. and Kumar, S.M. 1997. Method for increasing biological efficiency of oyster mushroom (*Pleurotus florida*) in Madhya Pradesh. *Advance in Plant Sciences*, 10 (1), 69-74.

Cohen, R., Persky, L. and Hadar, Y. 2002. Biotechnological applications and potential of wood-degrading mushrooms of the genus *Pleurotus*. *Applied Microbiology and Biotechnology*, 58, 582-594.

Das, D. 2015. Commercial utilization of mushroom cultivation, *International Journal in Management and Social Science*, 12b (2): 58-66.

14

Effect of Certain Fungicides and Botanicals Against Late Blight of Potato (*Phytophthora infestans*)

P.K. Ray[1] and R.B. Verma[2]

[1]*Subject Matter Specialist (Horticulture), Krishi Vigyan Kendra, Saharsa Bihar, India*

[2]*Associate Professor, Bihar Agricultural University, Bhagalpur, Bihar, India*

Abstract

Potato (Solanum tuberosum L.*), an important cash crop of India, is prone to many diseases and amongest these, late blight [*Phytophthora infestans *(Mont) de-Bary] is one of the highly destructive diseases and a major constraint in the profitable cultivation of potato. After realizing the significance of controlling the devastating disease for the sustainability in potato production and thus ensuring more profitability, the present investigation has been conducted with an objective to select the most effective fungicides and botanicals for the management of the disease. The present study was carried out by KVK, Saharsa during rabi season for consecutive two years (2015-16 and 2016-17) as On-Farm Trial mode at farmers fields of an adopted village of Saharsa district in Bihar. In each trial, there were four treatments including one control i.e. farmers' practice. The study concludes that the best treatment option to combat late blight disease is Seed treatment with* Trichoderma viride *@ 5g per kg of seed and spray of Ridomil @ 2g per litre of water starting from 30 DAP alternating with Dimethomorph 1g + ridomil 2g per litre of water at 10 days intervals. The results of economic analysis reveal that the net return as well as benefit cost ratio was also highest in Seed treatment with* Trichoderma viride *@ 5g per kg of seed and spray of Ridomil @ 2g per litre of water starting from 30 DAP alternating with Dimethomorph 1g + ridomil 2g per litre of water at 10 days intervals.*

Keywords: Late blight, Potato, Chemicals, Trichoderma, Yield and Economics

Introduction

Late blight of potato caused by *Phytophthora infestans* (Mont.) de Bary, is one of the most important and devastating diseases affecting potato crops (*Solanum tuberosum* L.) in different countries of the world (Fernandez-Northcote *et al.*, 2000; Namanda *et al.*, 2004). Historically, the disease has often resulted in destructive consequences and the most documented event is the great famine caused by this disease in Ireland (1845) when almost half of the potato crop was destroyed (Fernandez-Northcote *et al.*, 2000). Almost one million people died in the great famine and another million had to emigrate to United State and other regions (Arneson 1998; Fernandez-Northcote *et al.*, 2000). Late blight continues to be one of the main limiting factors for potato production in the world and if the disease is not controlled, losses can reach 100% (Ghorbani *et al.*, 2004) and even with low infection levels, the crop may be unsuitable for storage (Fernandez-Northcote *et al.*, 2000).

The first sign of infected tissue is brown spots on the leaves often surrounded by a halo of chlorotic (yellowed) tissue, later on covered the entire foliage with cottony white fungal growth and great impact when stem are infected because all tissue above this point will die. This disease is favored by wet conditions with high humidity greater than 90% but this fungus has great ability to adopt to variety of environments (Ahmad and Mirza, 1995) that is why it is found in temperate as well as in subtropical regions. During moist weather, whole plants may be killed in a short time (George and Preston, 2004) and it spread very rapidly if kept unchecked (Khan *et al.*, 2003).

Management of late blight requires aggressive measures that include combined use of cultural, scouting, sanitation and most importantly the combination of host plant resistance with application of fungicides (Johnson *et al.*, 1998; Kirk *et al.,* 2005; Namanda *et al.*, 2004). The use of protectant and systemic fungicides for managing late blight has perhaps been the most studied aspect of this disease management in temperate countries (Olanya *et al.,* 2001). Preventive fungicides principally inhibit spore germination and penetration, but once the pathogen enters the leaves, these fungicides become ineffective. The aim of this study was to test the efficacies of common fungicides for management of late blight and establish the appropriate spray interval for control of late blight on potato under natural conditions

Materials and Methods

The experiment was conducted at the farmers' field of Saharsa district, Bihar as 'On Farm Trial' mode for two years during 2015-16 and 2016-17 in *Rabi* season when there was severe incidence of this late blight disease. The planting was done during 2nd week of November and the variety *Kufri Pukhraj* is used for this experiment. The experiment was conducted in a Randomized Block Design with 3 replication and 4 treatments with recommended agronomic practices. The plot size of each treatment was 5m x 5m and spacing was maintained 60cm x 20cm each for row to row and plant to plant. The crop was harvested during last week of February. The details of technologies assessment/ refinement, farming situation, area of intervention and technology option was presented in Table-1.

To record the late blight incidence, ten plants per plot were randomly selected and disease scoring was done with the help of disease scoring scale (0-9 scale) (Mc Kinney, 1923).

$$\text{PDI} = \frac{\text{Sum of all numerical ratings}}{\text{Total no. of plant examined x maximum rating scale}} \times 100$$

Percent Increase in Yield (PIY) over control was calculated based on the following formula

$$\text{PIY} = \frac{\text{Treatment yield - Control yield}}{\text{Control yield}} \times 100$$

Yield obtained was recorded plot wise and incremental C:B ratio of different treatment was worked out by dividing the net returns from total cost of fungicides.

Table 1: Technology option assessed during 2015-16 and 2016-17

Problem area	Important cause	Production system	Micro farming situation
Low productivity of Potato	High infestation of late blight	Rice based	Irrigated medium land with clay to sandy clay loam soil

Intervention plan	
Farmers' practice – I	Spray of Mancozeb @ 2.5 gram per litre of water starting from onset of the disease
Technology option – II	Spray of Copper oxychloride @ 3 gram per litre of water starting from 30 DAP alternating with Metalaxyl-Mancozeb @ 2.5g gram per litre of water at 10 days intervals
Technology option – III	Seed treatment with Carbendazim @ 3g per kg of seed and spray of Carbendazim @ 3g per litre of water starting from 30 DAP alternating with Cymoxanil- Carbendazim 3g per litre of water at 10 days intervals.
Technology option – IV	Seed treatment with *Trichoderma viride* @ 5g per kg of seed and spray of ridomil @ 2g per litre of water starting from 30 DAP alternating with Dimethomorph 1g + ridomil 2g per litre of water at 10 days intervals

Results and Discussion

Effect of different fungicides on disease severity (PDI)

Application of different plant protection chemicals used in the experiment had significant effect on disease severity of late blight. The crop which was practiced by farmers himself as his own choice suffers severely from this disease. The results (Table 2) indicated that the lowest percent disease index (19.28%) was recorded in Technology options –IV these findings are also similar to that of the observations of (El-Naggar *et al,* 2016; Chowdappa *et al*, 2013; Wilson *et al*, 2008a) throughout the crop season. While the maximum percent disease index (93.78%) was found in Farmers' Practice followed by Technology options-II (42.20%) and Technology options-III (24.60%). The results corroborated with the findings of Wilson *et al*, 2008a. Seed treatment plays a vital role for prevent the initial appearance of the disease. These findings are also in line with earlier observation (De and Sengupta, 1988 and 1991).

Effect of different fungicides on yield of potato

All the treatment of fungicides proved significantly superior in increasing the yield of potato (Table-2) by effectively controlling the late blight disease in comparison to Farmers' Practice. The highest yield of potato was recorded in Technology option – IV (323.5 q/ha) which is 55.38% more than Farmers' practice (208 q/ha) followed by Technology option – III (306.0 q/ha) and Technology option –I (239.0 q/ha). These results are in agreement with the findings of Shikha and Harsha., 2014; Yuan Hang *et al*., 2014; Harman *et al*., 2004). The significant increase in yield in Technology option –II might be due to effective control of late blight disease starting from seed treatment with Mancozeb which prevent the pathogen to attack at initial stage and later alternate spray schedule of two fungicides can check the spread of the disease by suppressing the growth and sporulation of the pathogen. By this way plant remains healthy and resulting more yield.

Economics and incremental Cost Benefit (C:B) ratio of different treatments

The Cost Benefit ratio was worked out by dividing the net returns from total cost of cultivation (Table-2). The highest net return was recorded from the treatment of Technology option –IV Rs. 2,85,200 per ha followed by Technology option –III Rs. 2,63,400 per ha. The lowest gross return was obtained in Farmers' Practice plot Rs. 1,68,600 per ha. The incremental C:B ratio of different treatments showed that maximum C:B ratio of 3.13 was obtained from the Technology option-IV and Technology option- III 15.73. Thus looking to the economics of different treatments it can be concluded that the severe late

Table 2: PDI, Yield, Net profit and benefit cost (B:C) ratio under different treatments

Treatments	PDI %	Yield (q/ha)	Yield % increase over control	Cost ofcultivation (Rs./ha)	Gross returns (Rs./ha)	Net returns (Rs./ha)	B:Cratio
T_1	93.78	208.0	-	75000	243600	168600	2.25
T_2	42.20	239.0	14.80	87000	298800	211800	2.43
T_3	24.60	306.0	47.11	93000	356400	263400	2.83
T_4	19.28	323.5	55.38	91000	376200	285200	3.13
SEm+	0.63	0.49	-	-	-	-	-
CD(P=0.05)	1.86	1.15	-	-	-	-	-

blight disease can effectively controlled by adopting proper fungicides with prophylactic measures like Seed treatment with *Trichoderma viride* @ 5g per kg of seed and spray of ridomil @ 2g per litre of water starting from 30 DAP alternating with Dimethomorph 1g + ridomil 2g per litre of water at 10 days intervals (Technology option-IV) recorded low disease severity, higher yield, net return and incremental C:B ratio. In Farmers' practice recorded highest disease severity, lower yield, net return and incremental C:B ratio was found to be less effective for the control of late blight of potato.

Conclusion

On the basis of result obtained from On Farm Trials, it can be concluded that Seed treatment with *Trichoderma viride* @ 5g per kg of seed and spray of Ridomil @ 2g per litre of water starting from 30 DAP alternating with Dimethomorph 1g + ridomil 2g per litre of water at 10 days intervals was found more feasible and economically viable and superior over farmers practice. It was suggested that such participatory approach involving extension works and farmers in demonstration of research emanated proven technology may go a long way to curtail losses due to pest /disease incidences.

References

Ahmad, I. and J. I. Mirza. (1995). Occurrence of A2 mating type of *Phytophthora infestans* in Pakistan. Nat. Sem. on Res. & Dev. of Potato Prod. In Pakistan, Apr. 23-25, NARC/ PSPDP/PARC, Islamabad.

Arneson, P. A. (1998). Late blight. Cornell Univ. Ithaca. New York. pp - 99.

Baider, A. and Colen, Y. (2003). Synergistic interaction between BABA and Mancozeb in controlling *Phytophthora infestans* in potato and tomato and *Pseudoperenospora cubensis* in cucumber. *Phytoparasitica.* 31: 399.

Chowdappa, P., Mohan Kumar, S.P., Jyothi Lakshmi, M. and Upreti, K.K. (2013). Growth stimulation and induction of systemic resistance in tomato against early and late blight by Bacillus subtilis OTPB1 or *Trichoderma harzianum* OTPB3. *Biological Cont.*, 65: 109–117

De, B. K. and Sengupta, P. C. (1988). Studies on spray schedule of fungicides against late blight disease of potato caused *Phytophthora Infestans. Indian. Agril.,* 32:1-17.

De, B. K. and Sengupta. P. C. (1991). Evaluation of fungicides against late blight of potato in plains of West Bengal. *J. Indian Potato Assoc.,* 18:176-77.

El-Naggar, M. A., Abouleid, H. Z., El-Deeb, H.M., Abd-ElKareem, F, and Elshahawy, I. E. (2016). Biological control of potato late blight by means of induction systemic resistance and antagonism. *R.J.P.B.C.S.* 13: 1338-1348

Fernández-Northcote, E .N., O, Navia. and A. Gandarillas. (2000). Basis of strategies for chemical control of potato late blight developed by PROINPA in Bolivia. *Fitopatol*, 35(3): 137-149.

George, K. and S. Preston. (2004). Organic alternatives for late blight control in potatoes. Nat. Sustainable Agric. Info. Serv. U.S. Deptt. Agric. USDA USA.

Ghorbani, R., S. J. Wilcockson., C, Giotis. and C, Leifert. (2004). Potato late blight management in organic agriculture. *Pest Manag. J.* 9: 11-15.

Harman G. E., C. R. Howell., A. Viterbo., I, Chet. and M, Lorito. (2004). Trichoderma species - Opportunistic, avirulent plant symbionts. *Nature Reviews Microbiology* 2(1): 43–56.

Johnson, D. A., J. R. Alldredge and P. B. Hamm. (1998). Expansion of potato late blight forecasting models for the Colombian Basin of Washington and Oregon. *Plant Dis.*, 82: 642-645.

Khan, M. A., A. Rashid., Q, Ullah. and M. J. Iqbal. (2003). Control of Late Blight of Potato by Foliar Application of Fungicides. *Int. J. Agric. Biol.*, 5(4): 540-542.

Kirk, W. W., F. M. Abu-El Samen., J. B. Muhinyuza., R. Hammerschmidt., D. S. Douches., C. A. Thillc., H. Groza and A. L. Thompson. (2005). Evaluation of potato late blight management utilizing host plant resistance and reduced rates and frequencies of fungicide applications Crop Prot., 24: 961-970.

Mc Kinney, H. H. (1923). Influence of soil temperature and moisture on infection of wheat seedlings by *Heminthosporium. sativum. J. Agril. Sci.,* 26:195-218.

Namanda, S., O. M. Olanya., E. Adipala., J. J. Hakiza., R. E. Bedewy., A. S. Baghsari. and P. Ewell. (2004). Fungicide application and host resistance for potato late blight management: benefits assessment from on-farm studies in S.W.Uganda. *Crop Prot.*, 23(11): 1075-1083.

Olanya, O. M., E. Adipala., J. J. Hakiza., J. C. Kedera., P. Ojiambo., J. M. Mukalazi., G. Forbes, and R. Nelson. (2001). Epidemiology and population dynamics of *Phytophthora infestans* in sub-Saharan Africa: progress and constraints. *Afr. Crop Sci. J.* 9: 181-193.

Shikha T, Harsh NSK. (2014). Phylloplane fungi as biocontrol agent against Alternaria leaf spot disease of (Akarkara) Spilanthes oleracea. *Bioscience Discovery*, 5:139- 144.

Wilson, P. S., P. M. Ahvenniemi., M. J. Lehtonen., M. Kukkonen., H, Rita. and J. P. T. Valkonen. (2008a). Biological and chemical control and their combined use to control different stages of the Rhizoctonia disease complex on potato through the growing season. *Annals of Applied Biology*, 153(3), 307–320.

Yuan Hang, Q. U., Qi. W., Yan Po, Y., Zhen Lin, H. and Yan, L. (2014). Antagonistic Trichoderma isolates against potato late blight caused by *Phytophthora infestans*. *Mycosystema*, 33:1231 1241.

15

Characterization and Utilization of Fungi as Bio-Control Agents

Alka Kushwaha[1], Udit Narain[2], Gireesh Chand[3] and Vandana Krishna[4]

[1]*Department of Botany, D.A-V. College, Kanpur, Uttar Pradesh, India*
[2]*Department of Plant Pathology, C.S. Azad University of Agriculture & Technology, Kanpur, Uttar Pradesh, India*
[3]*Department of Plant Pathology, Bihar Agriculture University, Sabour Bhagalpur, Bihar, India*
[4]*Department of Botany, D.A.V. College, Dehradun, Uttarakhand, India*

Introduction

The term biological control was first used in scientific literature in 1914. Baker and Cook (1974) described biological control as "reduction of inoculum density or disease producing activities of a pathogen or parasite in its active or dormant state, by one or more organisms, accomplished naturally or thoroughly manipulation of environment, host, or antagonists or by mass introduction of one or more antagonists."

Certain genera of fungi have greater potential for being effective bio-control agents eg. *Trichoderma, Gliocladium, Chaetomium;* entomogenous fungi as *Entomophthora, Beauveria, Metarrhizium, Hirsutella;* Nematophagous *viz.*, *Catenaria, Zoopage, Stylopage, Paecilomyces* and predaceaus fungi like *Arthrobotrys, Dictylella, Dactylaria* and *Nematoctonus* (Narain, 2018). Biopesticide formulations based on these fungi are also called as "Microbial pesticides".

The morphological characters of the most of the fungal bio control agents are based on the monograph on fungi Imperfecti by Barnett and Hunter (1972).

Bio-Agents

1. *Trichoderma* Pers. ex Fr. : *Trichoderma* (Teliomorph *Hypocrea*) is a fungal genus found in many eco-systems. *Trichoderma* as biological control agent has been widely used against many plant pathogens, such as fungi, bacteria, viruses, nematodes and higher parasitic plants. The significance of *Trichoderma* in control of plant diseases that results in improvements in sustainable agriculture has to be emphasized (Al-Ani, 2018) as the global bio-pesticides market is blooming with a major share of various commercial formulations of *Trichoderma*. This filamentous fungus has given more attention because of its effectiveness against several plant pathogens (Dubey and Tripathi, 2018). Some strains have the ability to reduce the severity of plant diseases by inhibiting plant pathogens, mainly in the soil or on plant roots, through their high antagonistic and mycoparasitic potential. The presence of fungal prey and the availability of root derived nutrients have been major attractors for ancestors of *Trichoderma* to establish them in the rhizosphere and to facilitate the evolution of positive interaction with plants. Among the fungal antagonists, *Trichoderma* has gained the maximum popularity as bio-control agent.

Morphology of *Trichoderma* spp. is a key identification characteristics such as colony morphology, colony edge, reverse colour, alongwith, colour, shape, size of conidia and their formation and phialides. Credit goes to Rifai (1969) who laid down the foundation of the taxonomy of this interesting group of fungi.

The colour of mycelium remains yellow green to dark green after 2-3 days. No characteristic odour. Conidial production uniform with green conidia distributed throughout. Reverse of the Petri-plates lemon yellow in colour with no concentric ring. Phialides long, swollen in middle, slender and horn shaped, frequently bend towards the apex of the bearer. Phialospores (conidia) are usually globose or obovoid often, perfectly smooth walled (Rifai, 1969).

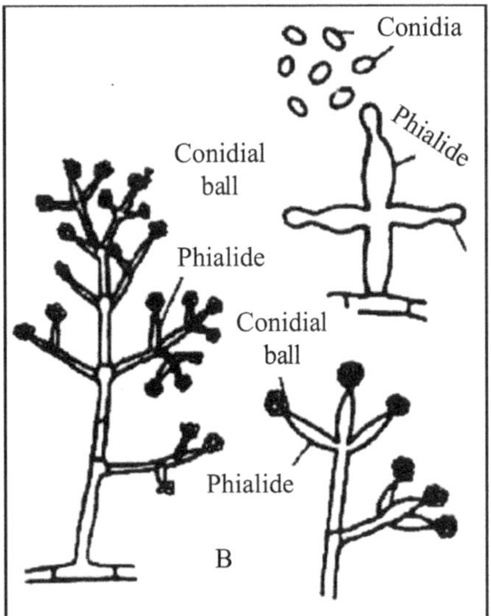

Trichoderma viride

Various *Trichoderma* spp. have been widely used as antagonistic fungal agents against several pests as well as plant growth enhancers. Prospects of biological control of soil-borne plant pathogens using the genus *Trichoderma*, as one of the promising bio-control agents, has been described from many parts of the world. *Trichoderma* spp. as biological control agents have been widely used against many plant pathogens such as viruses, bacteria, fungi, nematodes and also higher parasitic plants. Species of *Trichoderma* alone or in combination with fungicides proved effective against several seed and soil borne diseases (Dubey and Tripathi, 2018). These are free-living, saprophytic fungi and are highly interactive in root, soil and foliar environments. They can also compete with other microorganisms; for example, they compete for key exudates from seeds that stimulate the germination of propagules of plant- pathogenic fungi in soil and, more generally, compete with soil microorganisms for nutrients and/ or space.

The genus *Trichoderma* has been described for successful reductions of Fusarium wilt in many crops with application of different species. Faster metabolic rates, anti-microbial metabolites, and physiological conformation are key factors which chiefly contribute to antagonism of these fungi. Mycoparasitism, spatial and nutrient competition, antibiosis by enzymes and secondary metabolites, and induction of plant defence system are the typical biocontrol actions of these fungi.

2. *Gliocladium* Corda : *Gliocladium* is an asexual fungal genus in the Hypocreaceae. Certain other species including *Gliocladium virens* were recently transferred to the genus *Trichoderma* and *G. roseum* became *Clonostachys rosea* f.sp. *rosa* in the Bionecteriaceae. *Gliocladium* is a mitosporic, filamentous fungus. Species of *Gliocladium* rarely produce a sexual state. Species of *Gliocladium* are considered to have pathogenic potential against phytopathogens although they are not commonly thought of as a disease causing agent in humans and animals. Gliotoxin is a metabolite of *G. deliquescens* (now *Trichoderma*). The significance of gliotoxin has not yet been determined. Microscopically, *Gliocladium* species produces hyphae, conidiophores, and 1-celled conidia borne from hyaline phialides. The conidiophores are erect, dense, and have a brush-like structure which produce tapering, slimy phialides. *G. deliquescence* is an important species, a saprophytic soil borne fungus having the pathogenic potential (Morquer *et al.,* 1963).

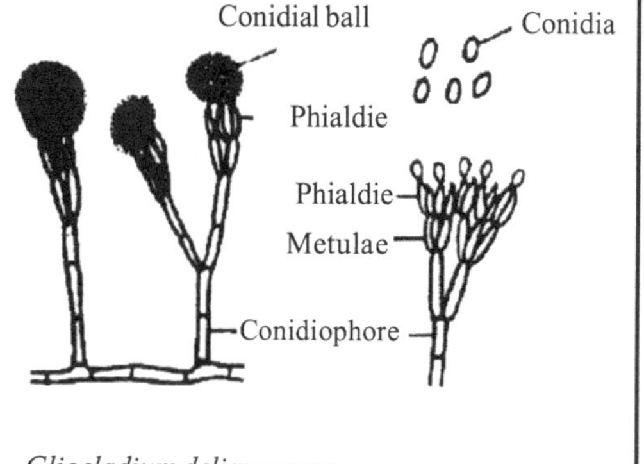

Gliocladium deliquescens

3. *Chaetomium* Kunz ex Fr. : It is a well-known genus of the family Chaetomiaceae with several species. It includes the species, which are found on straw, cloths, waste products etc. Sometimes they cause severe damage to them. Perithecia are superficial, ostiolate provided with greatly elongated beak like structures. Loose, tightly coiled hair like appendages on the body and on beak. Perithecial wall thin and paraphyses lacking. The ascal wall disappears at maturity and asci have thin, gelatinous wall, which may dissolve before the ascospore matures. The ascospores at maturity are embedded in a jelly and often come out in cirrhus, which is ribbon-like slender of spores held together by mucous and coming out through ostioles. Asci are club-shaped and thin walled. Ascospores are mostly lemon shaped, dark-coloured and one-celled. The genus is named on the character (chaite = hair).

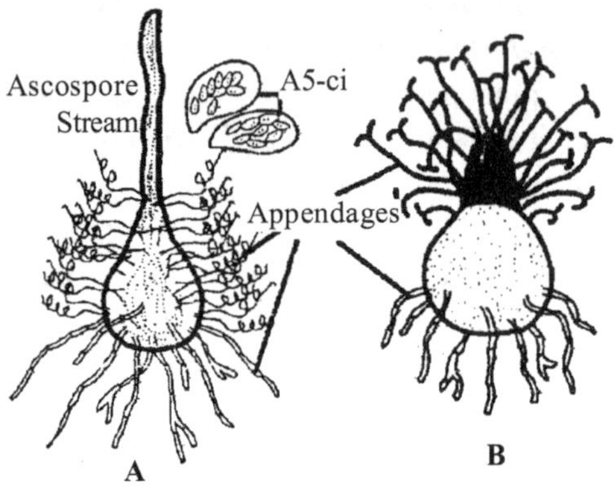

Chaetomlum: *C. globosum* **(A)**
C. thermophile **(B)**

Chaetomium is one of the extremely familiar genera of Pyrenomycetes (Ascomycotina) encountered on various agricultural commodities. The genus contains more than 200 species, all characterized by dark coloured perithecia with short necks which are clothed with irregularly coiled or tightly spiraled hairs. It is a common colonizer of soil and cellulose containing substates. Globosurn has been reported effective in reducing damage caused by seed rot and damping off, several seed borne and soil borne plant pathogens like *Pythium ultimum, Alternaira raphani, A. brassicicola, Fusarium* spp. and its antifungal metabolites have been reported (Biswas *et al.,* 2011) and resistance to wheat spot blotch induced by its crude extract (Biswas *et al.,* 2012). Seed coatings with selected isolates of *C. globosum* protect corn, oat and barley from seedling blight caused by *Fusarium* spp. and *Drechslera sorokiniana*. Increased field stands of maize hybrids were noticed when the seeds were coated with *C. globosum* ascospores. Seed treatment with ascospores of *C. globosum* reduces damping off of sugarbeet caused by seed borne *Phoma betae* and soil borne *Pythium ultimum* or *Rhizoctonia solani.*

4. *Kalisena* : *Aspergillus niger* van Tiegh. is commonly called as "black mould" and is a common contaminant in laboratories. The mycelium is scanty, hyaline to white or light yellow. Conidiophores arise from the "foot cell" and terminate in an inflated apex upon which radiating phialides are formed. Conidial heads appear globose. They are black, globose, or radiate. Conidia are produced in chains on the sterigmata. They are single-celled, pale to dark brown, more or less globose, with low to prominent ridges and echinulations that are with rough or echinulate surfaces. *A. niger* has been utilized to form *Kalisena* by Vineeta Sen (1999).

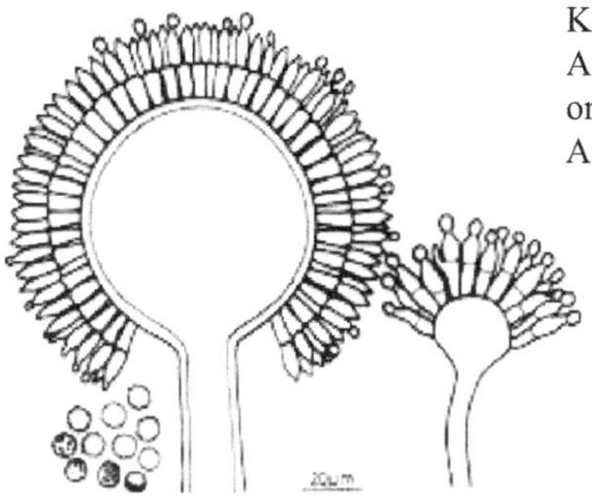

Aspergilus niger

Biofungicide (kalisena) Larger Image

Kalisena: (Aspergillus niger AN27)
A effective Biofungicide as well as biofertilizer, Based on the technology developed by IARI, New Delhi
Advantage of Use:

1. A Biofungicide and controls *Fusarium* spp., *Pythium* spp., *Rhizoctonia* spp., *Macrophormina* spp. and *Sclerotinia* spp.
2. Can work under diverse abiotic conditions (Temperature ranging from 0-45°C, no specific humidity and pH range from 3-10)
3. Excellent biofertilizer cum growth promoter.
4. Enhance seed germination percentage, speed up initial plant growth.

Entomongenous Fungi

Most of the fungal species invading insects belong to Hyphomycetes and Entomophthorales. Entopathogenic fungi infect their hosts by contgact as well as penetrating the insect cuticle and are pathogenic to both soft and hard bodies insects.

1. *Beauveria* Vuill. : Mycelium white or slightly coloured with a white fluffy to powdery appearance; conidiophores single, irregularly grouped or in verticillate cluster; in some species inflated at the base, tapering to a slender spore bearing portion which appears zigzag on which several spores are produced; conidia hyaline, rounded to ovoid, 1-celled, dry, borne singly on small sterigmata; parasitic on insects. Important species is *B. bassiana*, most widely used as biopesticide for control of many insect pests of crop plants (Benham and Miranda, 1953).

Beauveria bassiana named after the Italian entomologist, Agostino Bassi, who discovered it in 1815 as the cause of the muscardine disease, which then led to carrier transmitting it by airborne means. It was formerly also known as *Tritirachium shiotae*. The name, *B. bassiana* has long been used to describe a species complex of morphologically similar and closely related isolates. *B. bassiana* consists of many distinct lineages that should be recognized as distinct phylogenetic species and the genus *Beauveria* was redescribed with a proposed type for *B. bassiana*. In light of this work and the known existence of cryptic species, it is important to characterise isolates used to develop biological insecticides.

Beauveria bassiana can be used as a biological insecticide to control a number of pests such as termites, whiteflies, aphids, thrips, grasshoppers, locusts and many other insects. As an insecticide, the spores are sprayed on affected crops as an emulsified suspension or wettable powder or applied to mosquito nets as a mosquito control agent. Another species, *B. brongniartii* has been employed for the control of harmful insect pests.

Beauveria bassiana parasitizes a very wide range of arthropod hosts. However, different strains vary in their host ranges, some having rather narrow ranges, like strain Bba 5653 that is very virulent to the larvae of the diamondback moth and kills only few other types of caterpillars. Some strains do have a wide host range and should therefore be considered non-selective biological insecticides. These should not be applied to flowers visited by pollinating insects.

(A) *B. bassiana* is parasitic on adult beetles of :

(i) *Lachnosterma consagunea* (Rao and Vijaylakshmi, 1959).

(ii) Caterpillars of *Plusia* sp. (Rama Raje Urs *et al.,* 1965).

(iii) Banana leaf beetle (*Nodostromoa subconstatum*) (Roy and Pujari, 1979).

(B) *B. bassiana* strain *globulifera* on *Monoscrosporium ellipsosporium* (Chowdhry *et al.,* 1979).

(C) *B. tenella* on caterpillar (Rahalkar and Thirumalachar, 1974).

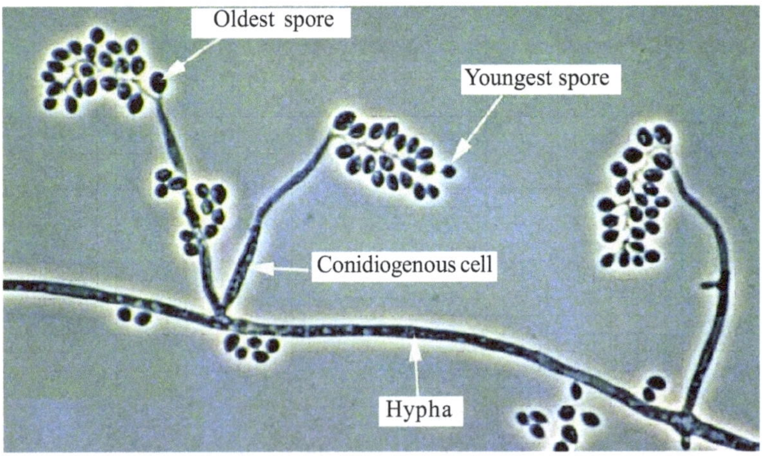

Morphology of *B. bassiana*

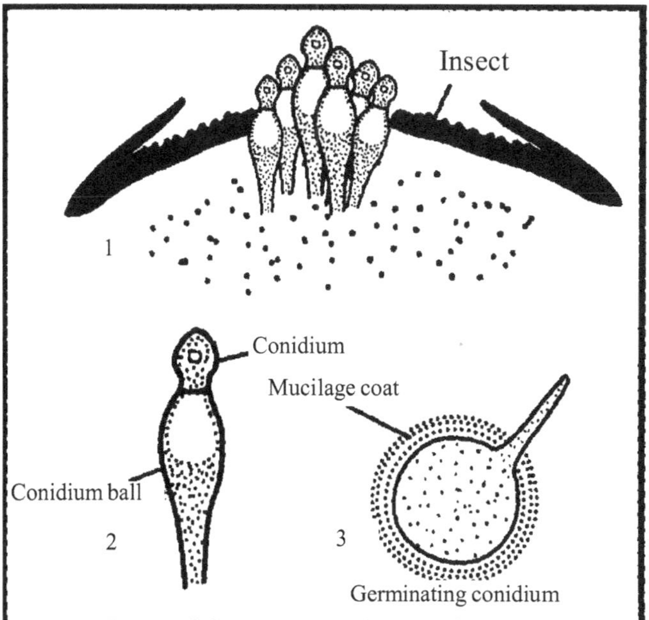

Entomophthora muscae: 1-3, Asexual stage

2. *Entomophthora* Fries : It includes fungi which are chiefly parasitic on insects. The most familiar species is *Entomophthora muscae*, commonly called as "fly fungus", which is often found on the bodies of houseflies. Innumerable conidia come out which have been shot off the conidiophores growing out of the body of the fly. This forcible ejection of the conidia is a prominent characteristics of *Entomophthora.*

The mycelium has a definite tendency to form septa and then to fragment into portions which are called as hyphal bodies. Such bodies multiply by division or budding, and each eventually produces a conidiophore bearing a conidium at its tip. In some species, such as *Entomophthora fumosa* and *E. fresenii,* hyphal bodies copulate and develop zygospores. Some of the saprobic species have a well-developed mycelium which persists as such. Few of the Entomophthoras have been grown in culture.

Entomophthora reproduces asexually by means of sporangia, functioning as conidia, which are borne on simple or branched conidiophores. The conidia are forcibly discharged from the conidiophores, and, in most species, germinate by producing germ tubes. The conidia of the *Entomophthora* are covered by a mucilaginous substance which adheres to any object against which the conidium is catapulted. In *Entomophthora muscae* and other species, if the conidium lands on a substratum suitable for its growth, it germinates and forms mycelium; otherwise it produces a secondary conidium.

Zygospores are formed in several species, but their further development is unknown. It is probable that they germinate by means of germ tubes. In principle, zygospore formation in most Entomophthorales investigated is similar to that in the Mucorales, but the details are somewhat different and characteristics.

Entomophthora spp. parasitic on insects are :

(i) *E. aphidis* on *Aphis* sp. of *Pisum sativum* (Butler and Bisby, 1931).

(ii) *E. coranata* on *Myzus persicae* (Ramaseshaiah, 1967).

(iii) *E. fumosa* on rice brown plant hoppers (*Nilaparvata lugens*) (Sawal *et al.,* 1978).

(iv) *E. muscae* on housefly (*Musca domestica*) (Kapoor and Chowdhry, 1996).

(v) *Entomophthora* sp. on Bihar hairy caterpillar (Thontadarya *et al.,* 1973).

3. *Metarrhizium* Sorok. : Conidiophores forming a sporulating layer; phialides single, in pairs or in whorls; conidia (phialospores) produced in basipetal chains, compacted into columns, long-ovoid to cylindrical, 1-celled, hyaline or slightly pigmented, olive-green in mass; parasitic on soil inhabiting insects, or saprophytic in soil (Speare, 1920; Petch, 1930).

M. anisopliae is an entopathogenic fungus, which is utilized against the pathogenic pests like black vine weevil, spittle bugs, cockroaches and termites (Rama Raje Urs and Govindu, 1971, Deshpandey *et al.*, 1974). This species has been reported on Pyrilla of sugarcane (Kamat and Dhande, 1952; Jagatap, 1973; Rao and Vijaylakshmi, 1959; Prasad, 1961) on brinjal mealy bug (Chowdhry, 1976).

4. *Vertricillium* Nees : Conidiophores slender, branched, at least some of the branches verticillate (in whorls), conidia (phialospores) ovoid to ellipsoid, hyaline, 1-celled, borne singly or in small moist clusters apically. Vascular parasites causing wilts of higher plants, parasitic on other fungi (Buckley *et al.*, 1969; Isaac, 1953) and on aphids (Nagaich, 1973), mango leaf hopper (Nirwan and Upadhyay, 1976). Mycoparasitic on *Oidium tingtanium* (Raghvendra Rao

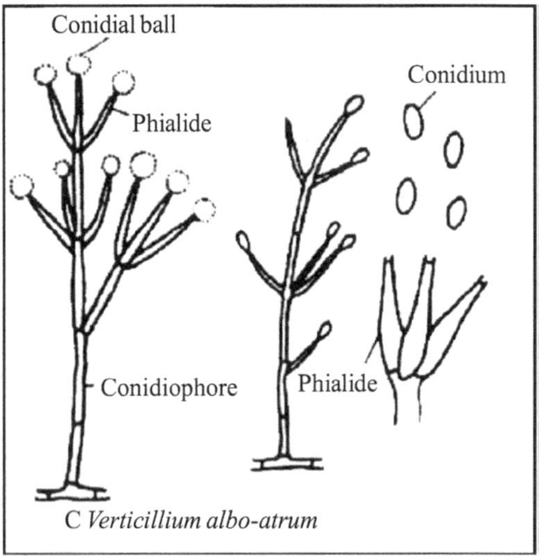

C *Verticillium albo-atrum*

and Pavgi, 1977). *Verticillium chlamydosporium* has been proved as a potential biological control agent for root knot nematodes (De Leij and Kerry, 1991).

5. *Hirsutella* Pat. : Synnemata simple with numerous branches arising nearly at right angles (some species lack synnemata), phialides arising laterally on synnemata or from mycelium on host, hyaline, inflated below, abruptly or gradually narrowing to long slender sterigmata; conidia hyaline, 1-celled, oblong to cylindrical, covered with mucus; parasitic on insects (Fisher, 1950; Mains, 1951; Morris, 1963). Important species is *H. saussurei* (Speare, 1920), parasitic on sugarcane leaf hopper (Prasad, 1961).

6. Nomurea Maubl. : *N. rileyi* (Farlow) Samson has been reported parasitic on leaf eating catterpillars (*Sopodoptera exigu* and *S. litura* by Rao and Phadake 1977 and Phadke *et al.,* 1978).

Nematophagous Fungi

Plant parasitic nematodes form an important nitch in agro-system. They feed on plant organs as ectoparasites, semi-endoparasites and endoparasites and cause reduced plant productivity.

The microorganisms that parasitize or prey on nematodes, fungi hold an important position and some of them have shown great potential as bio-control agent (Tribe, 1980). Many species of fungi have been found associated with nematodes but only few of them are successful bio-control agents (Bandopadhyay *et al.,* 2001; Singh, 2012).

The fungi involved in the biological control of nematodes are grouped into: Endoparasitic fungi, Predacious fungi and Opportunistic fungi.

(A) Endoparasitic fungi : They do not produce extensive mycelium but exist in the environment as conidia, which infect nematodes by either adhering to the surface of the nematodes or being ingested. The spores rapidly germinate and invade the entire nematode, with assimilate hyphae absorbing all the body contents. Two zoosporic fungi, *Catenaria auxiliaris* and *Nematophthora gynophila,* have a role in regulating population of *Heterodera* spp. Some other endoparasites which have some role in bio-control are *Acrostaiagmus*, and *Nematoctonus* etc. (Singh and Gupta, 1986; Singh *et al.,* 1993; Kumar and Singh, 2006). Some species of endo parasitic fungi have been presented to reduce the damage caused by cyst nematodes and root knot nematodes (Jatala *et al.*, 1979).

(1) ***Nematoctonus* Drechsler :** Mycelium not extensive, provided with clamp connections; assimilative hyphae developing within minute animal; conidia (blastospores) mostly hyaline, 1-celled, produced singly on short, simple or

forked sterigmata; chiefly attacking nematodes in soil. Important species is *N. haptocladus* which is parasitic and predacious on nematode (Drechsler, 1946) and also *N. robustus,* parasitic on mematodes (Jones, 1964).

(B) Predacious fungi :- There are certain species of predacious fungi which capture and kill nematodes in soils. With age, these fungi exhibit reduction in nematode-trapping efficiency. Predatory fungi produce extensive hyphal network in the environment and produce trapping devices at intervals along with each hypha. The traps capture nematodes either mechanically or by adhesion, allowing fungus to penetrate the nematode rapidly and digest the body contents. Predatory fungi form different types of traps, such as unmodified adhesive hyphae (*Stylopage* and *Zoopage* spp.), adhesive nets (*Arthrobotrys* spp.), adhesive knobs (*Dactylella* spp.), constricting rings (*A. dactyloides* and *Dactylaria brochopaga*) and non-constricting rings (*Dactylaria candida*) to capture the nematodes. *Arthrobotrys* isolate gives good protection against root-knot nematodes on tomato. These results have better hope for their use in bio-control of nematodes.

(1) ***Arthrobotrys* Corda :** Conidiophorers long, slender, simple, septate, hyaline, slightly enlarged at apex and spore bearing regions. New growing points formed sympodially; conidia hyaline, 2-celled, ovate oblong, borne on peglike denticles in loose dry cluster; saprophytic or parasitic on nematodes (Cooke and Godjrey, 1964; Haard, 1968).

(2) ***Stylopage* Drechsler :** Mycelium slender, non-septate, sparsely branched, conidia hyaline, borne singly or successively on erect, simple conidiophores; occurring on decaying plant material and capturing and consuming amoebae or small nematodes, eg. *S. lepte* (Drechsler, 1935).

(3) ***Zoopage* Drechsler :** Mycelium sparse, slender, sparingly branched, non-septate; conidia hyaline, elongated, single or catenulate; occurring in leaf mould and subsisting amoaebae and small nematodes, eg. *Z. mistospora* (Drechsler, 1938).

(4) ***Dactylella* Grove :** Conidiophores tall, slender, simple, hyaline, conidia hyaline, several celled, ellipsoid, fusoid or cylindrical, borne singly at apex or in a loose cluster on prominent denticles, saprophytic or parasitic on nematodes (Drechsler, 1950; Cooke and Godfrey, 1964; Cooke and Dickinson, 1965).

(5) ***Dactylaria* Saccardo :** Conidiophores more or less erect, simple, short, sometimes little differentiated from the mycelium hyaline, septate, denticulate and sometimes enlarged at the apex, conidia hyaline, 2-to several called, cylindrical or clavate, sometimes longer and single at apex; saprophytic or parasitic on nematodes (Drechsler, 1950; Cooke and Godfrey, 1964).

Another genus, *Monacrosporium* related to *Dactylaria* is found parasitic on nematode (Cooke and Dickson, 1965). Subramaniam (1953) has reported *M. lysipagum* (*Dactylaria lysipaga*) and (Sachidanand and Ramakrishnan 1971) *M. endermatrum* for capturing and killing many species of nematodes.

(C) Opportunistic fungi : Nematodes belonging to Heteroderid group (*Heterodera* and *Meloidogyne*) at the sedentary stages of their life-cycle are vulnerable to attack by these fungi either within the roots or when exposed on the root surface or in the soil (Jatala *et al.*, 1979; Kerry, 1988). Once in contact with cysts and egg masses, these fungi grow rapidly and eventually parasitize all eggs that are in early embryonic developmental stages. Wide range of opportunistic fungi parasitize eggs and cysts of nematodes. *Trichoderma harzianum, Trichoderma virens, Aspergillus niger, Paecilomyces lilacinus, Verticillium chlamydosporium* are found promising bio-control agents.

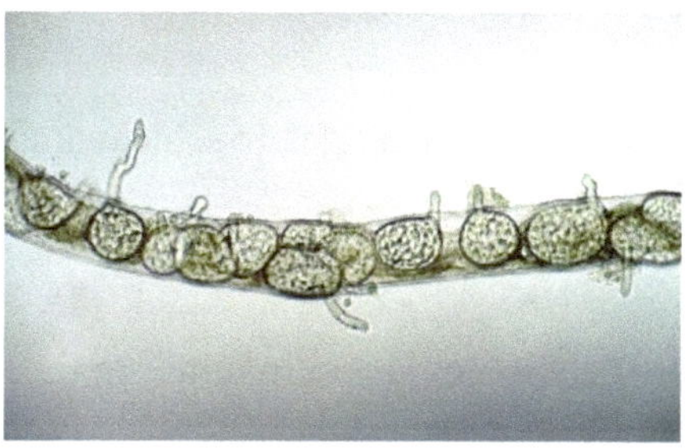

Catenaria

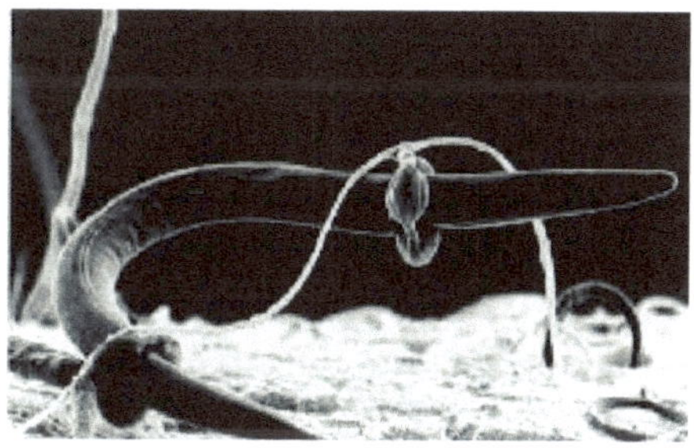

Trapping of nematode

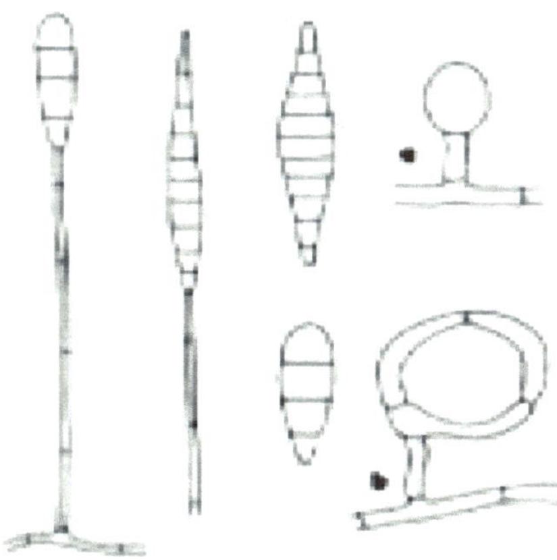

Dactylella

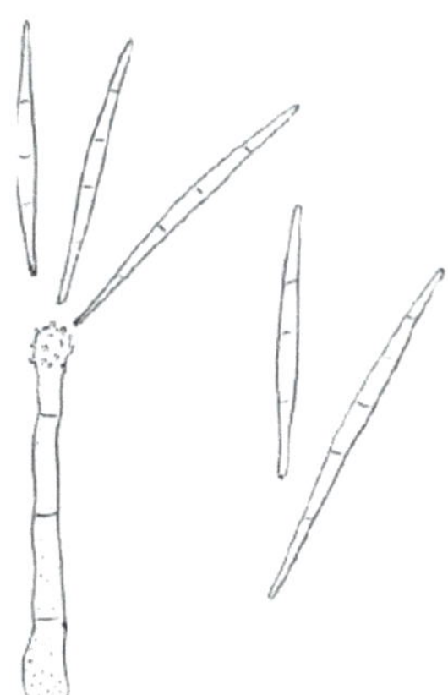

Dactylaria

Paecilomyces Bainier

Conidiophores and branches are more divergent than in *Penicillium*; conidia (phialospores) in dry basipetal chains, 1-celled, ovoid to fusiod, hyaline, saprophyte (Brown and Smith, 1957; Onions and Barron, 1967). *P. fumosoroseue* and *P. lilacinus* are pathogenic to white flies, thrips, aphids and to nematodes also (Cannayane and Sivakumar, 2001). Sharma and Trivedi (1989) reported that *P. lilacinus* penetrated the eggs of *Meloidogyne incognita* nematode and fed upon the internal contents leaving empty shells.

Some fungi killing and capturing of nematodes :

(i) *Arthrobotrys conoides* and *A. oligospora* on *Acroboles* sp., *Cephalobus* sp. and *Plectus* sp. (Sachidananda and Ramakrishnan, 1971).

(ii) *Catenaria vermicola* parasitic on larvae and eggs of *Heterodera avenae* (Chowdhry and Dhawan, 1984)

(iii) *Dactylaria brochopaga* on *Diplogaster* sp., *Cephalobus* sp. and *Rhabdilis* sp. and *D. psychrophilis* : (Sachidananda and Swarup, 1966, 1967)

(iv) *Dactylella asthenophaga* on some parasitic nematodes (Sachidananda and Ramakrishnan, 1971)

Hyperparasites

Hyperparastes are those fungi which grow on another parasitic fungi. In their mode of action, they check the growth and development of such fungi.

1. ***Ampelomyces* Ces.** (*Cicinnobolus* Ehrenb): Pycnidia dark, rounded, clavate or fusoid, developing inside conidiophores of powdery mildew fungi (Erysiphaceae), without ostiole; conidia hyaline or sub-hyaline to dark, 1-celled, ovoid to oblong; parasitic on Erysiphaceae. Important species, *A. quisqualis* (Linnemann, 1968) which is found parasitic on *Acrosporium* sp. (fungus) as reported by Narendra and Rao (1972) and as hyperparasite (Belsare *et al.* (1980 & 1981) and on powdery mildew fungus (*Oidium cyperissiae* (Patil, 1974).

2. **Coniothyrium Sacc.:** Pycnidia black, globose, separate erumpent, ostiolate; conidiophores short, simple, conidia dark, small, 1-celled, ovoid or ellipsoid; parasitic or saprophytic. Important species is *C. hyperparasiticum* which has been reported to be hyperparasitic on pycnidia of *Stauronema spinifexii* (Subhedar and Rao, 1975 and 1979).

Some of the fungi used for production of biopesticidies

(Singh *et al.*, 2016)

Gliocladium spp.
Beauveria basiana
Verticillium lecanii
Verticillium chlamydosporium
Candida oleophila (yeast)
Nomuraea rileyi
Coniothyrium minitans
Phlebia gigantean
Paecilomyces lilacinus
Chaetomium globosum

Trichoderma spp.
Metarrhizium anisopliae
Hirsutella species
Ampelomyces quisqualis
Fusarium oxysporium (non-pathogenic)
Pythium oligrandum
Penicillium islanindicum
Aspergillus niger-strain AN27
Myrothecium verrucaria
Piriformospora indica

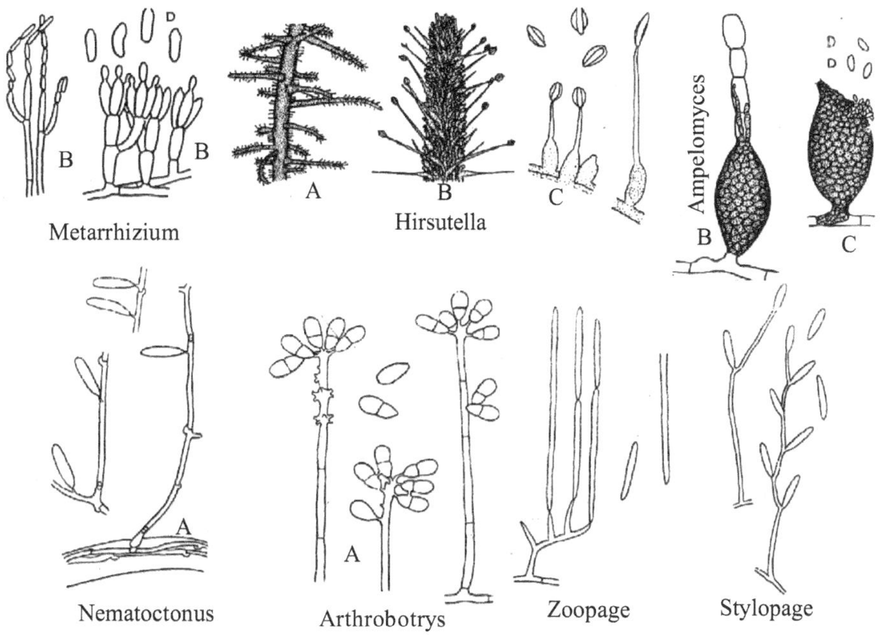

Morphological features of bio-control agents

Metarrhizum B & C Conidiophores with conidia, D. Conidia; *Hirsutella* : A.&B. Portion of synnemata, C. Phialides and conidia; *Ampelomyces:* B&C. Pycnidia, D. conidia; *Nematoctonus:* A. Mycelium in dead nematode, B. Hypha bearing conidia and clamp connections; *Arthrobotrys:* A. conidiophore bearing conidia, B. conidia; *Zoopage & Stylopage :* Conidiophores bearing conidia (From Illustrated genera of imperfect fungi (Barnet & Hunder, 1972).

References

Al-A, L.K.T. (2018). *Trichoderma :* Beneficial role in sustainable agriculture by plant disease management. In : Egamberdieva, D. and Ahmad, D. (Eds.). *Plant microbiome* : Stress response. Micro organisms for sustainability. Vol. 5 Springer, Singapore.

Baker, KF. Cook, RJ (1974). *Biological control* of *plant pathogens.* W.H. Freeman, Francisco, U.S.A., 433 pp.

Balsare SW, Moniz L, Deo VB (1980). Some new host records of the hyperparasite, *Ampelomyces quisqualis* Ces. from India. *Biovigyanam,* 5 : 77-78.

Balsare, SW, Moniz L, Deo VB (1981). The hyperparasite, *Ampelomyces quisqualis* Ces. from Maharashtra, India. *Biovigyanam,* 6 : 173-176.

Bandopadhyay P, Kumar D, Singh VK, Singh KP (2001). Eco-friendly management of root-knot nematode of tomato by *Arthrobotrys oligospora* and *Dactylaria brochopaga. Indian J. Nematology,* 31 : 153-156.

Barnett HL, Hunter BB (1972). *Illustrated genera of Imperfeat Fungi.* Bergess Publishing Company, Minneopolis, USA., 241 pp.

Benham RW, Miranda JL (1953). The genus *Beauveria* : Morphological and taxonomic studies of several species and two strains from wharf-piling borers. *Mycologia,* 45 : 727-746.

Biswas SK, Aggarwal R, Srivastava KD, Gupta S, Dureja P (2011). Characterization of antifungal metabolites of *Chaetomium globosum* and their antagonism against fungal plant pathogens. *J. Biological Control,* 26 (1) : 70-74.

Biswas SK, Srivastava K, Biswas C (2012). Resistance to wheat spot blotch induced by crude extract of *Chaetomium globosum* and mildly virulent strain of *Drechslera sorokiniana. J. Mycopathol. Res.,* 50 (2) : 267-271.

Brown AHS, Smith G (1957). The genus *Paecilomyces* Bainier and its perfect stage *Byssochlamys* Westling. *Trans. Br. mycol. Soc.,* 40: 17-89.

Buckley PM, Wyllie TD, DeVay JE (1969). Fine structure of conidia and conidium formation in *Verticillium alboatrum* and *V. nigrescens. Mycologia,* 61 : 240-250.

Butler EJ, Bisby GR (1931). The fungi of India. *Imp. Council Agric. Res. Indian Sci. Monogr. I.,* XVIII + 237 pp.

Cannayane I, Sivakumar CK (2001). Nematode egg-parasitic fungus-I. *Paecilomyces lilacinus* - A review. *Agricultural Review,* 22 (2) : 79-86.

Chowdhry PN, Dhawan SC (1984). *Catenaria vermicola* in *Heterodera avenae* nematode. *Curr. Sci.,* 53 : 96.

Chowdhry S (1976). *Metarrhizium anisopliae* (Meteh) Sorokin on brinjal mealy bug and its use in biological control of pest. *Curr. Sci.,* 45 : 34.

Cooke RC, Dickinson CH (1965). Nematode-trapping species of *Dactylella* and *Monacrosporium. Trans. Br. mycol. Soc.,* 48 : 621-629.

Cooke RC, Godfrey BES (1964). A. key to nematode - destroying fungi. *Trans. Br. mycol. Soc.,* 47 : 61-74.

De Leij FAAM, Kerry BR (1991). The nematophagous fungus, *Verticillium chlamydosporium,* as a potential biological control agent for *Meloidogyne arenaria. Revue Nematol.,* 14: 157-164.

Deshpandey RS, Vishwanath S, Anil Kumar TB, Siddappaji, C (1976). Two additional insect hosts of *Metarrhizium anisopliae. Indian Phytopath.,* 27 : 415-416.

Dreshsler C (1935). Some non-catenulate conidial Phycomycetes preying on terricolous amoebae. *Mycologia,* 27 : 176-205.

Dreshsler C (1938). New Zoopagaceae capturing and consuming soil amoebae. *Mycologia,* 30 : 137-157.

Drechsler C (1946). A clamp bearing fungus parasitic and predaceous on nematodes. *Mycologia,* 38 : 1-23.

Drechsler C (1950). Several species of *Dactylella* and *Dactylaria* that capture free-living nematodes. *Mycologia,* 42 : 1-79.

Dubey SC, Tripathi A (2018). Development of *Trichoderma* formulations and their applications for plant disease management. In : *Microbial based interventions for sustainable pest management and improving soil health.* Eds. Kumar, K., Singh, B., Mishra, R.K., Bandi, SM Singh, N.P. I.I.P.R., Kanpur, pp. 26-31.

Fisher FE (1950). Two new species of *Hirsutalla* Patouillard. *Mycologia,* 42 : 290-297.

Haard K (1968). Taxonomic studies on the genus *Arthrobotrys* Corda. *Mycologia,* 60 : 1140-1159.

Isaac I (1953). A further comparative study of pathogenic isolates of *Verticillium : V. nubilum* pethybr. and *V. tricopus* sp. nov. *Trans. Br. mycol. Soc.,* 36 : 180-195.

Jagapat AP (1973). Studies on entomogenous fungus, *Metarrhizium inisopliae* affecting *Pyrilla* sp. on sugarcane III. Pathological history. *Maharashtra Vigyan Mandir Patrika,* 8 : 25-30.

Jatala P, Kaltenbach R, Bocangel M (1979). Biological control of *Meloidogyne incognita* and *Globodera pallida* on potatoes. *J. Nematol.*, 11 : 303.

Jones FR (1964). *Nematoctonus robustus* sp. nov. *Trans. Br. Mycol. Soc.,* 47 : 57-60.

Kamat MK, Dhande GW (1952). Occurrence of the green muscardine fungus on *Pyrilla* sp. in Bombay, *Curr. Sci.,* 21 : 317.

Kapoor JN, Chowdhry PN (1976). Notes on Indian microfungi. *Indian Phytopath.,* 29 : 348-352.

Kerry BR (1988). Fungal parasites of cyst nematodes. *Agric. Ecosys. Environ.,* 24 : 293-305.

Kumar D, Singh KP (2006). Variability in Indian isolates of *Arthrobotrys dactyloides,* a nematode trapping fungus. *Current Microbiol.,* 52 : 293-299.

Linnemann G (1968). *Ampelomyces quisquilis* Ces. ein Parasit auf Mucorineen. Achiv Fur Microbiol., 60 : 59-75.

Mains EB (1951). Entomogenous species *Hirsutella, Tilachlidium* and *Synnematium. Mycologia,* 43 : 691-718.

Morqver R, Viala G, Rouch J, Fayret J, Berge G (1963). Contribution a l'etude morphogenique du genre *Gliocladium. Bull. Soc. Mycol. Fr,* 79 : 137-241.

Morris EE (1963). The synnematous genera of fungi Imperfecti. Series the Biological Sciences, No. 3, Western Illinois University, : 137 p.

Nagaich BB (1973). *Verticillium* sp. pathogenic on aphids. *Indian Phytopath.,* 26 : 163-165.

Narain U (2018). Fungal biocontrol agents : an introduction and taxonomy. In : *Microbial based interventions for sustainable pest management and improving soil health* (Eds. Krishna Kumar, Singh, B, Mishra, R.K., Bandi, SM, Singh, NP.) ICAR-Indian Institute of Pulses Research, Kanpur, pp. 3-13.

Narendra DA, Rao VG (1972). Some additions to fungi of India. *Sydowia,* 26 : 282-287.

Nirwan RS, Upadhyay J (1976). Some entomogenous fungi from North India. *Indian Phytopath.,* 29 : 308-310.

Onions AHS, Barron GL (1967). Monophialidic species of *Paeciolomyces. Mycol. Papers, C.M.I,* 107 : 1-25.

Patil MS (1974). Occurrence of hyperparasite, *Darluca* (Biv.) Cast. and *Ampelomyces* Ces. on rust and powdery mildew fungi, respectively from Maharashtra. *J. Shivaji Univ.,* 7 (14) : 233-236.

Petch T (1930). Notes on entomogenous fungi. *Trans. Br. mycol. Soc.,* 16 : 55-75.

Phadke CK, Rao VG, Pawar SK (1978). Natural outbreak of muscardine fungus, *Nomuraea rileji* (Farlow) Samson on leaf eating catterpillar, *Spodoptera exigua* Hb. in Maharashtra. *Curr. Sci.,* 47 : 476.

Prasad N (1961). The occurrence of two entomogenous fungi, *Metarrhizium anisopliae* and *Hirsutella* sp. on sugarcane leaf hopper (*Pyrilla perpusilla*) in Bihar. *Indian Sugarcane Res.* & Dev., 5 : 167.

Raghavendra Rao NN, Pavgi, MS (1977). Two mycoparasites on powder mildews. *Sydowia,* 30 : 145-147.

Rahalkar DW, Thirumalachar MJ (1974). Mass production of spores in two species of *Beauveria* for biological control of insect pests. *Maharashtra Vigyan Mandi Patrika,* 8 : 13-15.

Rama Raje Urs NV, Govindu HC (1971). *Metarrhizium anisopliae* (Metchiikoff) Sorokin and its host range. *Mycopath. et Mycol. Appl.*, 44 : 317-320.

Rama Raje Urs NV, Govindu H, Sastry KSS (1965). A preliminary study of white mucardine fungus on cabbage semilooper from Mysore. *Curr. Sci.*, 34 : 382-383.

Ramaseshaiah G (1967). The fungus, *Entomophthora coronata* parasite on three species of aphids infesting crucifers in India. *J. Invert. Path.*, 9 : 128-130.

Rao VC, Vijaylakshmi U (1959). A note on the occurrence of certain parasitic fungi on insect pests of sugarcane. *Curr. Sci.*, 28 : 295.

Rao VG, Phadke CK (1977). A muscardine disease of tobacco leaf eating catterpillar. *Curr. Sci.*, 46 : 648-649.

Rao VG, Vijaylakshmi U (1959). A note on the occurrence of certain parasitic fungi on insect pests of sugarcane. *Curr. Sci.*, 28 : 295.

Rifai M (1969). A revision of genus *Trichodera. Mycological papers*, 116 : 1-56.

Roy AK, Pujari KC (1979). Infection of banana leaf beetle by *Beauveria basiana. Curr. Sci.*, 48 : 115-116.

Sachidananda J, Swarup G (1966). *Nematophagous* fungi in Delhi soils. *Indian Phytopatto,* 19 : 279-285.

Sachidananda J, Swarup G (1967). Additional nematophagous fungi from Delhi soils. *Curr. Sci.*, 36 : 677-678.

Sachidananda J, Ramakrishnan K (1971). Nematophagous fungi of agricultural soil-I. *Mycopath. et Mycol. appl.*, 43 : 235-241.

Sawal P, Mishra PC, Nayak P (1978). *Entomophthora fumosa* Speare - an entomogenous fungus on rice brown plant hopper. *Curr. Sci.*, 47 : 241-242.

Sen Vineeta (1999). Kalisena on eco-friendly biopesticide-cum-biofestilizer from *Asperigillus niger* AN 27. Division of Plant Pathology, IARI, New Delhi, 10 pp..

Sharma A, Trivedi PC (1989). Influence of inoculum levels of the fungus, *Paecilomyces lilacinus* (Thom) Samson on the biocontrol of root knot nematode, *Meloidogyne incognita* (Chitwood). *Int. Nematol. Network Newsl.*, 6 : 27-29.

Singh HB, Sharma, BK, Keswani C (2016). *Agriculturally important microorganisms : Commercialization and regularly requirements in Asia.* Springer, Singapore, 336 pp.

Singh KP, Gupta P (1986). Observation on *Catenaria anguillulae* on *Stetarodera sorghi. Advances in Biol. Res.*, 4 : 240-250.

Singh KP, Stephan RA, Makesh Kumar T (1993). Development of *Catenaria anguillulae* in *Steterodera cajani. Mycological Research,* 97 : 100 : 1204-1206.

Singh VK (2012). Biological control of plant parasitic nematodes. In : *Ecofriendly innovative approaches in plant disease management* (Eds. Singh VK, Singh Y. Singh, A.). International Book Distributors, Dehradun, pp. 637-646.

Speare AT (1920). On certain entomogenous fungi. *Mycologia,* 12 : 62-76.

Subhedar AW, Rao VG (1975). Some interesting fungi from Western India. *Biovigyanam,* 1 : 191-196.

Subhedar AW, Rao VG (1979). Some noteworthy Coelomycetes. *J. Univ. Poona,* 52 : 317-322.

Subramaniam CV (1953). *Dactylella* (*Monacrosporium* and *Dactylaria*). *J. Indian Bot. Soc.* 52 : 291-299.

Thontadarya TS, Jayaramaiah M, Govindam R, Shishu Reddy KV (1973). Incidence of the entomogenous fungus, *Entomophthora* sp. on the Bihar hairy caterpillar, *Diacrisia obliqua. Curr. Sci.,* 42 : 106.

Tribe HT (1980). Prospects of the biological control of plant parasitic nematodes. *Parasitology,* 81 : 619-639.

16

Disease Management of Palms in Subtropical Zone of Gangetic Plains

Ruby Rani[1], AbhaKumari[1], Feza Ahmad[1], H.P. Maheshwarappa[2] Ankita Aman[1], Soni Kumari[1] and Neha Kumari[1]

[1]*Department of Horticulture (Fruit & Fruit Technology)*
Bihar Agricultural University, Sabour, Bhagalpur-813210, Bihar, India
[1]*ICAR-CPCRI, Kasaraggod, Kerela, India*

Abstract

Palms are generally grown commercially in tropical climate. But some of the palms like coconut, areca nut and palmyra palm are cultivated successfully in West Bengal, Orissa, Assam, and some pockets of Bihar that lies under sub tropics of India.Due to unsuitable climatic factor their production is more affected by abiotic and biotic stress including different kinds of diseases. The important disease are bud rot, basal stem end rot, nut shedding,stem bleeding in coconut, mahali disease, foot rot, stem breaking in arecanut and palmyra palm in the region have negligible incidence of diseases. These destructive diseases are the major constrain in production and causes severe yield loss in these palm fruits. Therefore effective management strategies are required by continuous monitoring the incidence and severity of these diseases caused by different pathogens.

Integrated disease management is the most accepted strategies for sustainable crop production that involves the holistic approach integrating cultural, physical, mechanical, chemical and biological means to control the disease. However, results of the disease management trials depend upon soil condition, age of the crop, stage of disease development and weather parameters of that particular area. Although it is impossible to manage a field free of pathogen but considerable reduction of the disease can be achieved through a proper integrated disease management system. Thus the causes and remedy of the diseases prevalent mainly in palms particularly in subtropical conditions has been reviewed for better management and sustainable production.

Keywords: Coconut, Areca nut, Palmyra palm, Disease, Symptoms, Management

Introduction

Palms such as coconut, areca nut, palmyra palm, date palms that belongs to family Palmeae are considered as palm crops. These crops usually require tropical climate having moderate climate with respect to temperature with high humidity for their successful cultivation and do not thrive well under extremes of climate.An average temperature of about 25-35^{0}C and humidity above 60 per cent and well distributed annual rainfall of 1200-1800 mm is considered ideal for most of the plantation crops. Thus they are mostly grown in coastal area of the world. In India it is mainly cultivated in the states like Tamil Nadu, Kerala, Karnataka, Andhra Pradesh, Orissa, Gujrat and Maharashtra, Goa, Andaman and Nicobar Islands etc. But crops like coconut, areca nuts and palmyra are grown in small area in the West Bengal, Assam, Bihar, Chhattisgarh, also, where the climate are subtropical.But climate in sub tropics like Bihar have distinct winter, summer and rainy season where average temperature is 35-40 ^{0}C throughout the summer months and the average minimum temperature during the coldest month of December and January goes down to 5 to 10 ^{0}C.Most of the annual rainfall received between the June and October with an average annual rainfall of 900-1500 mm.Thus the climate of subtropics is not much suited for cultivation of plantation crops. Coconut, arecanut and palmyra palm is the major palms of Bihar. The major coconut growing districts in the state are Supaul, Purnea, Madhepura, Katihar, Kishanganj, Madhubani and Bhagalpur. Coconut planted in these areas is mostly of tall type and most of the plantation is as stray, backyard or bund plantation. However few orchards in Katihar and Purnea districts have also been established. Due to unsuitable climatic factor their production is more affected by abiotic and biotic stress including different kinds of diseases.

The coconut palm (*Cocos nucifera* Linn.) is the most useful palm in the world. It is the versatile palm popularly known as 'King of Palms', 'Tree of Heaven', 'Tree of life', 'Tree of Abundance', as well as 'God's gift to mankind'. Every part of the tree is useful to human life for some purpose or the other. Hence, the coconut palm is endearingly called 'kalpavriksha' meaning the tree of heaven. India with about 2088 thousand hectares under coconut and an annual production of 15,256 thousand MT is the second largest coconut producing country in the world (NHB 2015-16). Bihar is one of the non-coconut growing state with an area 14.90 thousand hectares, production 97.30 thousand MT and productivity 6.53 MT/ha (NHB 2015-16). The successful cultivation of any crop depend on upon various factors, like yearly rainfall and climate,varieties, age of the plant, soil type and management systems pertaining to nutrient,moisture and pest management (Samarajeewa *et al*., 2001).The diseases like root (wilt), bud rot, basal stem rot (Ganoderma wilt or Thanjavur wilt), stem bleeding and leaf rot diseases causes heavy crop loss consequently lower productivity in coconut.

The arecanut commonly known as betel nut or Supari palm is the source of common chewing nut. In India it is extensively used by large sections of people as masticatory and is very much linked with religious practices also. India is the largest producer of areca nut with an area of 474 thousand hectares under, production 714 thousand MT and productivity 1.5 MT/ha and at the same time largest consumer of area not as well also. But, areca nut cultivation is also suffering a number of diseases and pest causing reduced productivity.Among the various factors causing considerable loss in production of arecanut in the state is basal stem rot, mahali disease, foot rot, stem breaking disease are the most common.

Palmyra palm (*Borassus flabellifer* L.), a multipurpose tree and it are referred to as tree of life with nearly 500 uses including food, beverage, fibre, medicinal and timber (Arulraj and Augustine 2008).

Proper disease management is very important for sustainable production of a crop in a particular region. A proper understanding of the factors associated with cessation and dissemination of any disease is very important to manage it. Also it is essential to know the basic principles of disease and growth habil of these palm. The broad principles of management of disease are to under following head: cause of Disease, mode of spread and effect of environment.

This topic is a general overview of some of the many methods, control measures and strategies to control or management of common diseases of palms in subtropical climate.The incidence of a disease are mainly depends on the status of the crop, its location, disease severity and management practices. To identfy the target pathogen of any disease, correct diagnosis is very essential.

Integrated approach is taken to manage the disease involving cultural, chemical and biological means. However age of the tree, soil and climatic conditions is also taken into consideration. The goal of plant disease management is to reduce the economic and aesthetic damage caused by plant diseases.

A. Coconut

1. Bud Rot

Bud rot disease was first noticed in Grand Cayman in 1834 (Tucker, 1926). In India, bud rot was first reported from the then Madras State in 1906 by Butler. Now it is reported from almost all coconut growing countries in the world.In India it was confined to west and east coasts in 1950, where coconuts were grown with rubber and palmyrah (Menon and Pandalai, 1958). And outbreaks of epidemics were also noticed (Radha and Joseph, 1974). Bud rot incidence is now prevalent in almost all growing state of like Karnataka, Maharashtra and Goa, particularly in the newly planted gardens. Bud rot was reported as a problem of serious concern in non-traditional coconut growing areas of Madhya Pradesh like Bastar, Raipur and Durg (Dantre *et al.*, 1997). India, According to Renard and Darwis (1992) there has been resurgence of symptoms in almost all the coconut growing zones. In certain regions of the Ivory Coast up to 50% of the coconut initially planted are killed by bud rot and up to 25% of the nut fall can be recorded each year. The extent of the damage depends upon climatic conditions and type of planting material (Quillec *et al.*, 1984). In Behar bud not is same problem in seedling slog as well as in beang palm as especially during winter.

Causal Organism: *Phytophthora palmivora*

Symptoms of damage

Palms of all age are liable to be attacked but normally young palms are more susceptible, particularly during monsoon and cloudy winter in subtropics when the temperature is low and humidity is comparatively high. In seedlings, the earlier symptom is the yellowing of one or two younger leaves. Black spots appear on spindle leaves the spear leaf turns pale and comes off with a gentle pull basal tissues of the leaf rot quickly and from the crown.In the later stages the spindle withers and drops down. In bearing palni the tender leaf base and soft tissues of the crown will rot into a slimy mass of decayed material emitting foul smell. Ultimately the entire crown falls down and the palm dies.In adult palms, the first visible symptom is the colour change of the spear, which becomes pale and breaks at the base and hangs down. The rotting slowly progresses downwards, finally affecting the meristem and killing the palms. This is accompanied by drooping of successive leaves. Even then, nuts that are retained on the palm may grow to maturity. Observational evidence indicates the wind principal agent.

Management: A number of factors are involved in bud rot incidence. Hence it is essential to take integrated approach to manage it like cultural, chemical and biological methods.

Cultural Method

Coconut gardens should have adequate drainage and aeration.Broadley (1992) suggested mounding near coconut basin to avoid water logging and to provide the soildrainage to a depth of 1.5 metres. Proper spacing should be adopted betwar the plant avoiding overcrowding in bud rot prone gardens. He also suggested plantation of cover crop in coconut garden in order to increase microbial population and to suppress Phytophthora population. Selection of varieties resistant to *P. palmivora* and *P. nicotianae* has been advocated by (Mangindaan *et al.*, 1992). The production of antifungal compounds like phytoalexins in plants in response to Phytophthora infection has been reported in a number of hosts (Erwin and Ribeiro 1996). The application of chemicals like salicylic acid analogue, Bion (acibenzolar-S-methyl) is known to activate systemic acquired resistance in plants that can increase resistance to Phytophthora (Ali *et al.*, 2000) in palms also.

Chemical Method

Variousstudies have been conducted to test the effectiveness of different fungicides to control bud rot disease in coconut in different coconut growing countries (Radha and Joseph, 1974 Chandra Mohanan and Babu, 2010). For young palm bud is readily accessible to diagnose the disease and to drench the affected region with fungicides. But disease management in mature palms is difficult due to tall trunk to diagnose the symptom in early stage. The affected palm can be saved only if they are treated properly in the very initial stage of the disease.

Removal of infected tissues of the crown region including those bordering the infected lesion and followed by crown drenching with a solution of any copper based fungicide at 0.25% has been recommended by Abad (1985). The primary reason for applying fungicide in nursery situation was to preventdisease development on remaining palms (Elliott, 2009). Placing of mancozeb (Dithane M-45) sachets of 2g in the leaf axils during the rainy season has been suggested by various workers in southern part of India (Nambiar and Rawther, 1993 and Jose, 2002). Injection of the coconut stems or with systemic fungicides like Ridomil(Metalaxyl) at 3g a.i./palm were found effective in protecting the palms from bud rot (Brahmana *et al.*, 1992). Removal of all the affected tissue of the crown region followed by crown drenching with Copper oxychloride 0.25% is the general recommendation.

Prophylactic Measures

Prophylactic spray of 1% Bordeaux mixture and application of Bordeaux paste as curative treatment were recommended as a general recommendation in

India for bud rot disease management. Pre and post monsoon spray with 0.25% Copper oxychloride on the crown of the neighboring palms is also recommended as a prophylactic measure. Are winter spray has also, found effective is subtropical zone. A Small, perforated sachets containing 2 g of mancozeb may be tied to the top of leaf axil. When it rains, a small quantity of the fungicide is released from the sachets to the leaf base, thus protecting the palm (Jose, 2002). However, Elliott (2009) reported drench with thiophanate-methyl was effective as a preventive measure to control it.But no fungicide has been recommended for the palms after the terminal bud is badly affected or dead. Elliott and Broschat (2012) demonstrated that the xylem mobile fungicides could move in to the palm canopy and persisted for at least 90 days. Therefore, they advocated trunk injection of the pesticides as the most effective method for managing Phytophthora bud rot of coconut.

Biological Method

This biological control is an important approach in this direction by use of micro-organism, gene or gene products to keep the inoculum density below the economic threshold level, to retard or exclude infection and to maximize the self-defense system of plantsystem (Cook, 977). Moosa (2002) identified 3 *Bacillus* spp. viz., *B. amylo* liquefaciens (endophyte), *B.subtilis* and *B.megatarium* and two fungi such as *Penicillim pinophilum* and Trichoderma virideas potential antagonists against *P. palmivora* causing bud rot disease of coconut in India based on *in vitro* interaction studies. Two species of the soild welling fungi like Trichoderma sp., Myrothecium roridum and Myrothecium verrucaria were found to reduce growth of *P. palmivora* and *P. katsurae* in coconut. This fungal genus is found in temperate, subtropical and tropical soils, and hence provides a possible option for biocontrol of bud rot in coconut (Tuset *et al.* 1992). However, the highest inhibition of *Phytophthora capsici* was recorded by *T. viride* (native isolate) Jahagirdar (1998). Trichoderma-based biocontrol agents exhibited better ability to promote plant growth and soil remediation activity compared to other microbes such as virus, bacteria, nematodes and protozoa (Esposito and Silva 1998; Gamal *et al.*, 2007). Thus in India application of talc powder formulation of *Pseudomonas fluorescence* or *Trichoderma viride* in crown region of coconut seedlings, is recommended at the rate of 150 g and 200 g for 6-10 years and above 20 years age of coconut seedlings respectively. 6 Spraying of 10 to 15 day old culture filtrate of *Pseudomonas fluorescens* at 100% concentration twice at 30 days interval on crown region and on nuts of coconut has been recommended (Rao *et al.*, 2012).

Integrated Management

Preventive measures such as sanitation (cutting and burning of affected palms) and fungicide application to neighboring palms in infected areas to prevent further spread should be under taken. Monocropping with highly susceptible cultivars should bed is couraged. Nursery stock should be closely monitored at all times for bud rot disease symptoms. The affected palm should be treated at the very initial stage of the disease. Thus orchard sanitation, proper drainage, use of healthy planting materials and biological method using recommended dose of *Pseudomonas fluorescence* or *Trichoderma viride* as per age of the palm is suggested as integrated approach to control it.

2. Thanjavur Wilt/ Basal Stem End Rot/ Anabe Roga/ Ganoderma Wilt

Among the several disease affecting coconut, Thanjavur wilt is the most serious and devastating disease. This disease first appeared in the coastal areas of Thanjavur district of Tamilnadu after cyclones of 1952 and 1955 and hence the names Thanjavur wilt, Bole rot or anaberoga (Karnataka) in different parts of India (Naik 2001).

Causal Organism: *Ganoderma lucidem* and *Ganoderma applanatum.*

In India, infector *Ganoderma lucidum* on coconut was first recorded in Karnataka state during the year 1913 by Butler (Petch 1916). Similar disease symptoms were reported to be caused by *Ganoderma applanatum* and *Ganoderma lucidum* in Andhra Pradesh by Papa Rao and Govinda Rao (1966) and Satyanarayana *et al.* (1985). Extent of incidence is as much as high up to 30 per cent and it is unattended entire coconut garden may damage within 6-7 years of span.

Symptoms of Damage

The disease is starts with the infection in roots without showing any external symptoms. Initially a few roots get infected and rot. In severely infected palms, extent of root rotting may be up to more than 70 % (Rethinam 1984, Srinivasulu and Rao 2007). The infection continuously goes to stems causing internal disintegration of cortical tissue. Initial visual symptoms of Thanjavur wilt (Ganoderma wilt) start with withering, yellowing and drooping of the outer whorl of leaves followed by exudation of reddish brown viscous fluid through cracks at the base of the trunk and oozing spread upward. In severe cases the bleeding patches begin from the base may extend up to 3 meters upwards with the progress of disease. The tissue on the bleeding spots are soft to touch and get rotten. The bark turns brittle and often gets peeled off in flakes, leaving open cracks and crevices. The internal tissues are discolored and disintegrated, emitting a bad smell. Reduction in nut size and nut yield is seen. Ganoderma appears at the base of the trunk. Ultimately causes complete collapse of tree. The disease is severe in hot and dry climate and more in sandy soil.

Management

Cultural Method

The pathogen can survive in soil for several years ,thus cultural operations are not much effective in controlling the disease(Soepena 1996). However it can be minimized to some extent by adopting proper cultural practices. Clean cultivation should be adopted by removing all source of ganoderma in the fieldand all affected palms should be removed immediately (Bhaskaran *et al.* 1990, Bhaskaran *et al.* 1994). Earlier Bhaskaran *et al* (1978) advocated irrigation along with farm yard manure + burying coconut husks in circular trenches around the palms + Bordeaux mixture drenching was the most effective in reducing the disease intensity. Karthikeyan and Bhaskaran (2001) reported that intercropping with green manuring crops like *Crotalaria juncea*, *Calopogonium mucunoides*, *Tephrosia purpurea*, *Curcuma domestica* and *Musa* sp. reduced disease incidence, increased soil antagonistic microorganisms and bio fertilizers, viz. PSB, Azotobacter and Azospirillum.

Chemical Method

Chemical method to control stem end rot is effective if the measure is taken at early stage of infection. Application of Bordeaux mixture (1%), Aureofungin-sol (0.2%) chemicals alone or in combination have been reported as effective chemicals by several workers (Bhaskaran and Ramanathan 1982, Bhaskaran *et al.* 1984). Sindha Mathur and *Balasubramaniam* (1987) reported that soil drenching with 0.1% IBP, carboxin, tridemorph or 0.05% carbendazim in combination with 5 kg neem cake per palm reduced disease intensity. Application of aureofungin-sol 2 g with 1 g Copper Sulphate in 100ml water or 2 ml of Tridemorph in 100 ml water applied as root feeding at quarterly intervals for a year effectively controlled the disease (Bhaskaran *et al.* 1994). Chemical control with trunk injection or root feeding with Calixin 3 ml/tree.Palanna *et al.* (2009) found that the disease spread was less (70.31% reduction over control) with root feeding of Hexaconazole (1%) at quarterly intervals along with soil application of 5 kg neem cake and 50 g of Trichoderma harzianum per palm at 6 month interval.

Biological Method

A number of micro-organisms antagonistic to *G.lucidum* havebeen reported by various workers. Organism like Bacillus coagulans, Streptomyces sp., Trichoderma viride, T. harzianum were found to inhibit the growth of G. lucidum (Menon 1963; Jollands,1983; Garrett, 1955; Bhaskaran *et al.*, 1988a). Neem cake application to diseased palms also enhanced the soil microflora especially Trichoderma in coconut basins and was found effective *in* the control of Thanjavur wilt (Gunasekaran *et al.*,1986). Significant reduction in pathogen has been found with application of banana rhizome extract and *Tephrosiapurpurea* root extract (Bhaskaran *et al.*, 1987; Bhaskaran*et al.*, 1988a; Bhaskaran *et al.*, 1988b). Antagonistic microorganisms: Trichoderma species (*T. harzianum, T. viride, T. hamatum, T. longibrachiatum, T. virens, T. polysporum*), *Pseudomonas fluorescens*, *Bacillus subtilus* are the antagonistic microorganisms reported against *Ganoderma spp.* in India.*Pseudomonas fluorescens* was reported to be having antagonistic activity against *Ganoderma spp.* under in vitro conditions and treatment ofganoderma with application of *Pseudomonas fluorescens* (Pf1) @ 200g/palm + *Trichoderma viride* @ 200g/palm/year effectively control the disease(Srinivasulu *et al.* 2004b, Karthikeyan *et al.* 2005, George *et al.* 2012).Rajendran *et al.* (2010) suggested endophytic Bacillus subtilis as effective bio control agent for management of BSR.Earlier application of FYM 50kg + neem cake 5 Kg once in 6 months along with fertilizers could effectively control the BSR in coconut (Prakasam *et al.* 1997).

Integrated management

The integrated approach to control BSR involves clean cultivation, adoption of cover crop, removal of infected plants, use of bio fertilizers , biocontrol agents and organic manures with recommended fertilizer dose has been found effective in controlling the disease.Soil drenching with 1% Bordeaux mixture (40 l/palm) around the trunk in a radius of 1.5m and application of neem cake (5 kg/palm) in basins followed by root feeding with Tridemorph (6 ml/palm) was found more effective in reducing the disease index of BSR in Andhra Pradesh (Srinivasulu *et al.* 2005).

3. Grey Leaf Spot/ Leaf Blight

Grey leaf spot diseases every year attacks the coconut gardens and decreases the growth and development of the palm and consequently yield .The disease has been reported from various coconut growing countries (Ghose ,2000). He also reported that grey leaf spot or blight caused by *Pestalotia palmarum* (Cooke.) had no immune or resistant sources against the disease.

Causal Organism: *Pestalosia palmivora*

Symptoms of Damage

The symptom is only developed in the mature leaves. Initially, minute yellow or grayish white spots surrounded by grayish bands appear on the surface of mature leaves of the outer whorl. Later they become grayish white and several such spots coalesce together and form irregular grey necrotic patches and show burnt or blighted appearances. The upper surface of the affected leaves reveals dark grey eruptions like pin heads.Fungal fruiting structures are visible as tiny black dots within the spots, especially on the upper surface of the leaves. Rain and wind spread the spores of both these leafspot fungi, so the diseases are more common during wet weather. In advanced stage, tip and margin or the whole leaflets dry and shrivel giving the leaf a burnt appearance. This condition is generally referred to as leaf blight (Karthikeyan *et al.*, 1994). In young plants bearing is delayed in affected palms.

Management

Cultural Method

The older 2-3 disease affected leaves should be removed. The disease infestation is more in the soil with low nutrient status especially during cold and humid condition, Thus proper nutrition should be given to palms.

Chemical Method

Spraying the foliage with 0.25% Copper oxychloride check the spread of the disease.The systemic fungicides thiophanate methyl and carbendazim at 0.05% were most effective, followed by the contact fungicides mancozeb (dithane M45) and copper oxychloride (COC) at 0.3% (Sanjay *et al.*, 2007). Spray with 1% Bordeaux mixture or propiconazole 0.3% also found to be effective. As and Mahata, (1985) reported that the growth of the fungus was also completely inhibited by brestan-60 at 300, 400 and 500 ppm as well as difolatan 80 w and Dithane M 45 at 500 ppm.

Biological Method

Biocontrol agents such as *Trichoderma*, *Gliocladium* and *Pseudomonas* gave satisfactory control when applied along with a food base as reported by Sanjay *et al.*, (2007). Application of 200g *Pseudomonas fluorescens* along with 50 kg of FYM+5 kg of Neem cake/palm/yr could effecting control the disease.

4. Stem Bleeding Disease

The disease is a mainly soil borne plant-pathogenic fungus that infects wounds and openings in the coconut stem. Severely affected or untreated palms may rot out completely inside and die, although it can takes years for a fatal rot to develop. But in severe infestation disease causes irreversible damage and becomes untreatable in its advanced stages. Thus it should be avoided by careful harvest, handling, and transport of palms.

Causal Organism: *Thielaviopsis paradoxa*

Symptoms of Damage

Exudation of a dark reddish brown liquid from the longitudinal cracks in the bark or wounds and seeping down the coconut stem.The liquid oozing out dries up and turns black. In initial stage of infestations the tissues below the lesions become rotten and turn yellow and become black at later stage. In advanced cases, the interior of affected trunks become hollow due to decay of interior tissues. The outer whorl of the leaves turn yellow, dry and shed prematurely.

Management

Cultural Method

Mechanical injury to trunk and contact of wounded palm stems with soil should be avoided (Scot Nelson, 2005). Adequate irrigation during summer and drainage during rainy season proper nutrient management should be done. Water should not be applied to trunk by installing sprinkler irrigation emitters but moisture and numerl shrubs shuuld be avoided (Scot Nelson, 2005).To control infection at early stage rotten portion should be scrapped and burnt off to avoid the spread of the disease.

Chemical Method

The affected tissues should be scraped out completely and the wounded area must be painted with tridemorph 5% or Bordeaux paste. Coal tar is applied after 1-2 days on the treated portion. Root feeding with tridemorph (5% Calixin) 5ml in 100 ml water should be done thrice a year during April-May, September-October and January-February to prevent further spread of lesions.

Biological Method

Along with 50 kg FYM, apply 5kg neem cake containing the antagonistic fungi, *Trichoderma* @ 200g/palm/year culture to the basin during September. Advanced symptoms may be virtually untreatable, requiring palm removal and destruction.

B. Arecanut

The areca nut palm (Areca catechu L.) is one of the important plantation crops in of India. It is commonly known as betel nut or supari and used in various religious and social ceremonies. Areca nut is infested by a number of insect pests and diseases. The major diseases of areca nut are fruit rot, leaf spot, bud rot , basal stem rot , nut cracking etc. Areca nut grown in subtropical climate also ... similar type of disease infestation.

1 Fruit Rot / Koleroga / Mahali Disease

Among the many diseases, fruit rot commonly called as *"Koleroga"* or *"Mahali"* is the most fatal disease that may cause fruit drop of 50 to 100 per cent in individual palms ,if proper control measures are not adopted. Fruit rot disease occurs in all the arecanut growing regions receiving heavy rainfall during southwest monsoon period (June- September) including Assam, Orissa, West Bengal and Bihar. Butler (1906) first recorded the disease in the Karnataka.

Causal Organism

Mainly caused by *Phytophthora meadii* but association of *P. palmivora , P. arecae* and *P. Heveae* are also been reported in rare occasions (Hegde and Chowdappa, 2015).

Symptom

Characteristic symptom is rotting and extensive shedding of the immature nuts which lie scattered near the base of the tree. Initial symptoms appear as dark green/ yellowish water-soaked lesions on the nut surface near the perianth (calyx). The infected nuts lose their natural green lustre, quality and hence have a low market value. The lesions on the fruits gradually spread covering the whole surface before or after shedding which consequently rot. With the advancement of the disease the fruit stalks and the axis of the inflorescence rot and dry and covered with white mycelial mats sometimes.

The severity, persistence and spread of fruit rot depends on the pattern of rain. The disease appears usually 15 to 20 days after the onset of regular monsoon rains and may continue up to the end of the rainy season. Continuous heavy rainfall with low temperature (20 to 23 °C), high relative humidity (>90%) and intermittent rain and sunshine hours favour the occurrence of fruit rot. Disease is spread through heavy wind and rain splashes.

Management

Cultural method

All dried and infected bunch of last season attached to the palm should be removed as phyto sanitary measures . Bunches of areca nut should be covered with polythene covers before the start of the heavy monsoon.

Prophylactic measures

The initial spray of one per cent Bordeaux mixture is to be done immediately after the onset of monsoon showers and the second spray after an interval of 40 to 45 days. If monsoon prolongs, third spray should also be given. A fine spray will be needed for effective spread of spray fluid over the surface of the nuts. Spraying operations are to be undertaken on clear sunny days.

Chemical control

Spray Bordeaux mixture 1% on all bunches twice in a year once before the onset of monsoon and another 40 days later could after control the disease. Remove and burn all fallen and infected nuts should be removed formt he field and burnt. Narayanaswamy *et al* (2017) recommended application of1 Bordeaux mixture at 1% before onset of monsoon that significantly reduced number of fallen nuts due to fruit rot of arecanut and increased the nut yield followed by one percent of stabilized Bordeaux mixture and Metalaxyl MZ.

Inetgrated Management: An integrated approach involving proper cultural practices, prophylactic measures application of bio control agents, fungicidal sprays and host plant resistance is need to be employed for effective control of the disease.

Basal Stem Rot / Foot Rot Or Anabe

Basal stem rot is one of the important diseases of arecanut accounting to severe yield loss in areca nut growing areas of India.

Causal Organism: *G. lucidum*

Management

Management of the disease is possible with continuous monitoring and implementing biocontrol based integrated management approaches. Narayanaswamy *et al.* (2018) reported that application of Tridemorph as root feeding at 2ml per 100ml water during January, April and September along with application of both Neem cake @ 2kg per palm and Trichoderma harzianum at 100g per palm performed better in controlling the disease.

An integrated method by applying both neem cake and Trichoderma harzianum, continuous monitoring and implementing biocontrol based management can effectively control it Root feeding with Tridemorph or Hexaconazole has also found very effective.

Affected palms have to be isolated by digging trenches all rounds. The severely affected palms should be cut and destroyed. The stumps should be pulled out by digging and the drainage improved.Soil application of neem cake @ 2 kg / palm / year followed by root feeding with 125 ml of 1.5 % (15 ml/litre of water) Tridemorph at 3 months interval or Soil drenching of Bordeaux mixture (1%).

The control measures of bud rot, leaf spot and root wilt disease are similar to that of in coconut.

References

Ali Z, Smith I, Guest DI (2000). Combinations of potassium phosphonate and Bion (acibenzolar-S-methyl) reduce root infection and dieback of Pinusradiata, Banksiaintegrifoliaand Isopogoncuneatus caused by Phytophthoracinnamomi. *Australasian Plant Pathology*. 29: 59-63.

Arulraj S, Augustine BJ (2008). Underutilized palms. In: Peter KV, editor. Underutilized and underexploited horticultural crops. New India Publishing Agency: New Delhi. 3:415–429.

Bhaskaran R, (1994). Perennial crop diseases caused by Ganoderma. Wallingford, UK: CAB International. Management of basal rot disease of coconut caused by Ganoderma lucidum. 102–108.

Bhaskaran R, Ramanathan T, (1982). Management of Thanjavur wilt of coconut. Proceeding PLACROSYM V. pp. 521-526.

Bhaskaran R, Chandrasekar G, Jaganathan T (1978). Control of Thanjavur wilt disease of coconut. *Food Farming and Agriculture*. 10(4): 115-116.

Bhaskaran R, Ramadoss N, Ramachandran TK (1988 a). Biological control of Thanjavur wilt disease of coconut. *Indian Coconut Journal*. 19(6): 3-8.

Bhaskaran R, Ramadoss N, Suriachandraselvan M, (1988 b). Effect of plant extracts on the growth of Ganoderma spp. associated with Thanjavur wilt of coconut. Proceeding of National Seminar on Management of Crop Diseases with Plant Products/ Biological Agents. Agricultural College and Research Institute., Madurai. p.24.

Bhaskaran R, Suriachandraselvan M, Ramachandran TK (1990). Ganoderma wilt disease of coconut – a threat to coconut cultivation in India. *Planter* 66(774): 467–71.

Bhaskaran R, Ramadoss N, Ramachandran TK (1987). Plant extracts on the growth of Ganoderma lucidum. *Newsletter* 17(7): 2.

Bhaskaran R, Ramanathan T, Ramiah M (1984 b). Chemical control of Thanjavur wilt of coconut. Proceeding of All India Symposium on Coconut Diseases. Coconut Reserch Station, lieppankulam. pp. 22-24.

Bhaskaran R, Ramanathan T, Ramieh M (1984 a). Thanjavur wilt of coconut, its occurrence, spread and management. Proceeding PLACROSVM. VI. pp.107-113.

Brahmana J, Lubis AU Lubis RA (1992). Resistance of coconuts to premature nutfall in relation to varieties and fruit age. Coconut *Phytophthora* workshop- Manado, Indonesia. 137-147.

Broadley RH (1992) Protect your avocados. Brisbane, Australia, Queensland Department of Primary Industries.

Butler EJ (1906). Some diseases of palms. *Agric J Ind* 1: 299-310

Butler EJ (1913). Rept. Imperial Mycologist Rept. Res. Inst. Colle., *Pusa* 60: 1911-12.

Cook RM, Hubbard S F (1977) Adaptive searching strategies in insect parasites. *J. Anim. Ecol.* 46, 115-125.

Dantre R K, Verma S S, Srivastava L K, Prakash R (1997). A survey on bud rot incidence in non – traditional coconut growing areas of Eastern Madhya Pradesh. *Indian Coconut.*27: 4 – 7

Elliott M L (2009). Emerging palm diseases in Florida. *Hort Technology*. 19: 717–718.

Elliott ML, Broschat TK (2012). Detection of Thiabendazole Fungicide in Coconut Palms Using a Bioassay. *Systemic Fungicide*. 56(1): 21-27.

Erwin DC, Ribeiro OK (1996). Phytophthora diseases world wide. St Paul, Minnesota, USA, APS Press.

Esposito E, da Silva M (1998). Systematics and environmental application of the genus *Trichoderma*. *Critical Reviews on Microbiology*. 24: 89-98.

Gamal M, Abdel-Fattah Shabana Y M, Ismail AE, Rashad YM (2007). Trichoderma harzianum: A biocontrol agent against bipolaris oryzae. *Mycopathology*, 164: 81-89.

Garrett SD (1955). A century of root disease investigations. *American Applied Biology*. 42: 211-219.

George P, Gupta A, Gopal M, Chandra MR, Thomas L, Thomas GV (2012). In vitro antagonism of rhizospheric fluorescent pseudomonads of coconut against Ganoderma applanatum and Thielaviopsis paradoxa, fungal pathogens of coconut. *Journal of Plantation Crops*. 40(2): 75-81.

Gunasekaran M, Ramadoss N, Ramiah M, Bhaskaran R, Ramanathan T (1986). Role of neem cake in the control of Thanjavur wilt of coconut. *Indian Coconut Journal*. 17(1): 7-12.

Jollands P (1983). Laboratory investigations on fungicides and biological agents to control three diseases of rubber and oil palm and their potential applications. *Tropical Pest Management* 29: 33-38.

Karthikeyan A, and Bhaskaran R. (2001). Effect of intercrops on the intensity of basal stem rot of coconut and soil microbial population. *Tropical Agricultural Research and Extension*. 4(2): 117-119.

Karthikeyan G, Karpagavalli S, Rabindran R, Natarajan C, (2005). Biological control of basal stem rot disease in coconut. *Planter* 81(957): 777-784.

Mangindaan HF, Thevenin JM, Kharie S, Motulo HF (1992) The susceptibility of coconut varieties to Phytophthorain Indonesia: the effect of environmental factors. Paper read at coconut Phytophthora workshop held at Manado, Indonesia.

Menon KPV, Pandalai, KM (1958). The coconut palm - A monograph. Indian Central Coconut Committee, Ernakulam. 384.

Menon R (1963). Transmission of yellow leaf disease *Phytopath. Z.* 48: 82-88.

Mohanan RC, Babu M (2011). Integrated management of diseases in arecanut based cropping systems. In: Arecanut based cropping/furming systems (eds. Thoma GV Krishnakumar V, Maheshwarappa HP, Bhat R and Balasimha D). Central Plantation Crops Research Institute, Kasaragod, Kerala. 83-103.

Moussa TAA (2002). Studies on biological control of sugarbeet pathogen *Rhizoctonia solani* Kuhn. *J. Biol. Sci. 2*(12): 800- 804.

Nambiar KK, Rawther TSS (1993). Fungal diseases of coconut in the world. In: Advances in Coconut Research and Development (Ed. M. K Nair, P.Gopalsundaram, H. H. Khan., and E.V.V.B.Rao), Oxford and IBH Publ.Co.Pvt.Ltd., New Delhi. 546-561.

Narayanaswamy H, Raju J, Jayalakshmi K, Syed Sannaulla, Shesragiri KS, Dinesh Kumar M (2018) Integrated management of basal stem rot disease of arecanut. *International Journal of Chemical Studies* 2018; 6(5): 530-531

Narayanaswamy H , Raju J, Jayalakshmi K (2017) Management of Fruit Rot Disease of Arecanut Incited by *Phytophthora meadii I nt.J.Curr.Microbiol.App.Sci* (2017) *6*(7): 2824-2828.

Palanna KB, Naik RG, Basavaraju TB, Boraiah B, Thyagaraj NE (2009). Etiology and management of coconut basal stem rot (Ganoderma wilt) in sandy soils of Karnataka. *Journal of Plantation Crops*. 37(1): 26–29.

Papa Rao A, Govinda Rao P (1966). A survey of coconut diseases in Andhra Pradesh. *Andhra Agricultural Journal*. 13: 208-217.

Petch T (1916). A preliminary list of Ceylon polypori. Ann. Roy. Bot. Gard. *Peradeniya* 6: 87-114.

Prakasam V, Valluvaparidasan V, Raguchander T, Prabakar K, Thiruvudainambi S (1997). Field crop disease. Coimbatore, *India: A. E. Publications*. 111–112.

Radha K, Joseph T (1974). Investigations on the bud rot disease (Phytophthora palmivora Bud.) of coconut. Final report, PL 480 scheme. 32.

Rajendran L, Karthikeyan G, Raguchander T, Samiyappan R (2010). Cloning and sequencing of novel endophytic Bacillus subtilis from coconut for the management of Basal Stem Rot disease. *Asian Journal of Plant Pathology*. 4(1): 20-33.

Rao MS, Sowmya DS, Chaya MK, Kumar M R, Rathnamma K, Gavaskar J, Priti K, Ramachandran N, (2012). Management of nematode induced wilt disease complex in capsicum using *Pseudomonas fluorescens* and *Paecilomyces lilacinus*. *Nematol. Medit*. 40: 101-105.

Renard J L, Darwis S N(1992). Report on coconut phytophthora disease seminar.Coconut Phytophthora Workshop Proceedings 26-30. October 1992.Monado, Indonesia 9-12

Rethinam P (1984). Thanjavur wilt disease of coconut in Tamil Nadu. Indian Coconut Journal. 15(2): 3 -11.

Retlllnam P, Roy, A.K., Baranwal, V.K., Chakraborthy, B.K. and Nambiar, K.K.N. (1990). Crown choke disease of coconut. *Indian Coconut* 1. 20: 3-6

Samarajeewa, S.R., Thanaweera arachchi PT, Fernando MTN, Rathnasiri NGSC (2001) Supply response analysis in coconut production. Sri Lanka Assoc. Adv. Sci., Proc. 57th Ann. Session, Part 1.

Sanjay R, Ponmurugan P, Baby UI (2007). Evaluation of fungicides and biocontrol agents against grey blight disease of tea in the field. *Crop protection*. 27(3-5): 689-694.

Satyanarayana Y, Ramapandu S, Rajamannar M, Chiranjeevi V (1985). Control of Ganoderma wilt disease of coconut. *Indian Coconut Journal*. 16(5): 3-5.

Scot Nelson (2005). Stem Bleeding of Coconut Palm. Cooperative Extension Service at Manoa. PD-30.

Sindha Mathar A, Balasubramaniam M (1987). Control of Thanjavur wilt disease of coconut. International Symposium on Ganoderma wilt diseases on palm and other Peremial Crops. Tamil Nadu Agricultural University, Coimbatore. (Abstract). pp.11-12.

Soepena H (1996). Seranganpenyakit Ganoderma padakelapasawit di kebunpadanghalaban. Pusat Penelitian Karet, Sungei Putih.

Srinivasulu B, Rao DVR (2007). Coconut Diseases, P 114. International Book Distributing Co., Lucknow, UP, India.

Srinivasulu B, Kumar KVK, Aruna K, Rao DVR (2005). Biocontrol of basal stem rot (Ganoderma wilt) disease of coconut. Technical Bulletin II, AICRP on Palms, ARS, Ambajipeta, ANGRAU.

Srinivasulu B, Vijay Krishna Kumar K, Aruna K, Lakshmi BKM, Rao DVR (2004b). An ecofriendly technology to manage basal stem rot (Ganoderma wilt) disease of coconut. *Andhra Agriculture Journal* 50: 264-267.

Tucker CM (1926). Phytophthora bud rot of coconut palms in Puerto Rico. *J Agric Res*. 32: 471-499.

Tuset JJ, Hinajeros C, Buj A, Molins A, Cebolla C (1992). Myrothecium roridumand M. verrucaria as potential antagonists of *Phytophthora* spp. of coconut. Paper read at coconut Phytophthora workshop held at Manado, Indonesia.

17

Genotypic Screening as a Tool for Developing Resistance to *Sclerotinia Sclerotiorum* in Vegetables

Shirin Akhtar[1*], Chanda Kushwaha[2] and Randhir Kumar[1]

[1]*Department of Horticulture, Vegetable and Floriculture, Bihar Agricultural University, Sabour, Bhagalpur Bihar – 813210, India*
[2]*Department of Plant Pathology, Bihar Agricultural University, Sabour Bhagalpur Bihar – 813210, India*

Abstract

Fungal rot and wilt caused by Sclerotinia sclerotiorum is a devastating disease of vegetables causing huge loss. The fungus has a broad host of more than 400 species including diverse vegetable crops, viz., *carrot, potato, tomato, green pepper, eggplant, lettuce, peas and beans, cole crops, bottle gourd, pointed gourd, etc. Being able to overwinter in the soil in form of sclerotia upto 5 years and having such a wide host range, management of the disease becomes very difficult. Thus development of resistant varieties can be the only long term strategy for control of the pathogen. The screening of the existing genotypes and identification of resistant genotypes forms the base of any resistant breeding programme. The widely available genotypes of different crops have been screened by several researchers and resistant genotypes have been identified in cauliflower, vegetable soybean, peas, tomato, etc. These genotypes are further used in breeding programmes for as donors for resistance to* Sclerotinia sclerotiorum.

***Keywords*:** Vegetables, *Sclerotinia*, Resistance breeding, Genotypic screening

Introduction

Vegetables comprise of the most important horticultural crops and also form the chief constituent of nutritional security. Added advantages of vegetables are that they are short duration crops, high yielding, nutritionally rich and generate on-farm and off-farm employment. The total area under vegetables crops is 10.29 million hectare with a total production of 175.01 million tonnes (Anonymous, 2017). India is the second largest producer of vegetables in the world after China. However, the productivity of major vegetables is quite low compared to the leading countries of the world and diseases causing a huge loss are a major reason for this. Of the various diseses affecting vegetable production, fungal rot and wilt caused by *Sclerotinia sclerotiorum* is widespread occurring extensively in various vegetable crops causing huge losses.

Sclerotinia sclerotiorum is a fungus belonging to the family Sclerotiniaceae, the order Helotiales, the phylum Ascomycota (Whetzel 1945). Like all other species in the Helotiales, *S. sclerotiorum* forms cup or disk-shaped apothecia from sclerotia; the apothecia produce inoperculate asci which contain ascospores (Bolton *et al.* 2006, Whetzel 1945). Under cool and humid weather very serious problem in vegetable crops occur's especially when they are cultivated in contaminated soils (Reis and Lopes 2007). The pathogen overwinters in the soil and remains viable for even upto 5 years without any host. Having a broad host range control of this fungus is very tough and development of resistant varieties seems to be a viable option. Resistant breeding is one of the most powerful means of management of plant diseases and play an effective role in disease management. Screening is the first step towards resistance breeding.

Disease development and symptoms

Sclerotinia rot and wilt is a very serious problem in vegetable crops, especially when they are cultivated in contaminated wet soils and the weather is cool and wet (Reis and Lopes 2007). The optimum temperature for disease development ranges from 15 to 21°C. The structure resistant to degradation - sclerotia serve as survival structures that can remain viable for 3-5 years in soil under natural conditions (Ayers and Adams 1979, Cook *et al.* 1975). The pathogen overwinters as sclerotia in soil (Cook *et al.* 1975, Merriman 1976), as mycelium in infected seeds (Cook *et al.* 1975, Nicholson *et al.* 1972) or as mycelia in dead or living hosts (Boland and Hall 1994). They require high soil and relative humidity and free water on the plants for germination and to infect its hosts (Lobo 999; Lobo and Abreu 2000). When environmental conditions are favourable, the sclerotia germinate carpogenically and produce apothecia. Over a period of 2-3 weeks, large numbers of ascospores are discharged from mature apothecia into the air (Clarkson *et al.* 2003).

Initial symptoms are recorded as yellowing of the foliar parts followed by wilting of lateral branches. If the main stem is attacked then the whole plant is affected leading to the death of plants. Lesions on infected stem are initially light brown, which later becomes dark brown. At advanced stages of infestation, lesions coalesce to girdle the lower stem, the sheathing mycelium produces round, light-brown to dark-brown sclerotia at the same place on the stem and adjoining soil surface of the infected plants. White cottony mycelial growth is observed between basal portion and sheaths of the stem. Later mustard seed like, dark black coloured sclerotia are observed on the basal portion of the stem, inside the leaf sheaths as well as the soil near to the collar region. The rot symptom accompanied by white mass of mycelia growth is referred to as white mould (e.g., in bean) and fruit, blossom or seedling rot as the case may be. If the infection is at the base of main stem, the entire plant wilts. Partial or total wilt is characteristic symptom of stem and branches in many crops. Such symptom is seen in tomato, eggplant, potato and chickpea. On opening the dry portion of stem, the pith can be seen full of dark brown to black fungal sclerotia.

Kulkarni *et al.* (1995) reported that *Sclerotinia sclerotiorum* damaged stem, root or tuber in potato, infected the stem and produced dark brown lesion at collar region causing wilt and ultimately plants became dry. Brownish sclerotia resembled mustard seed, developed at later stages on the root and collar region of the infected plants. Afterwards the tubers were infected and rotten in field. Prova *et al* (2014) first reported *Sclerotinia sclerotiorum* in hyacinth bean (*Lablab purpureus*) while surveying hyacinth bean fields in the Gazipur district of Bangladesh. Plants with light tan to brown blighted stems and pods were observed. Within the pod pith, large dark irregular sclerotia embedded in a white fluffy mycelium were found. Velastegui and Eall (1991) observed tree tomato (tamarillo) plants with stem lesions in an orchard in Tungurahua province, Ecuador. Dissection of the stems showed the presence of black sclerotia. Further laboratory analyses and pathogenicity tests revealed that *S. sclerotiorum* was the causal agent of the disease. Iqbal *et al* (1998) reported that symptoms of *Sclerotinia sclerotiorum* in pea included development of fluffy white mycelial mats on infected tissues of stems, leaves and pods along with prominent dark sclerotia of irregular shape and size, measuring from 2.0 to 8.0 mm in diameter. Sclerotia were also observed inside the infected stem and pods. Johnson *et al* (1998) reported that symptoms and signs on soyabean included stem bleaching, fluffy white mycelial growth on stems and foliage, and presence of sclerotia typical of white mould, and the mean incidence of white mould ranged from 0 to 6.8% in different varieties.

Host range and losses

Sclerotinia sclerotiorum is a necrotrophic pathogen that has a wide host range. It is one of the most non-specific and omnivorous plant pathogen that infects more than 400 species of plants (Gao *et al.*, 2015). It has a long list of hosts that includes many vegetable crops, *viz.*, carrot, potato, tomato, green pepper, eggplant, lettuce and cole crops (Mendes *et al.*, 1998). *Sclerotinia sclerotiorum* was recorded for the first time in England in 1837 on lettuce and thereafter it was reported on different hosts from all over the world, *viz.*, cabbage seed crop in Washington (Mclean 1949), peas in Kincardineshire in Britain (Gray and Findlater 1957), cabbage and cauliflower in Denmark during 1953-1958 (Neergaard 1958), groundnut in USA (Porter and Beute 1974), cauliflower and tomato in New South Wales in 1971 (Letham *et al.* 1976), beans in north central region of the United States during 1992-1994 (Yang *et al.* 1997), grapes in Chile (Latorre and Guerrero 2001), carrot in northeastern Scotland (Couper *et al.* 2001) and Canada (Kora *et al.* 2003), potato plants in Iran (Ojaghian 2009), pyrethrum flowers in Australia (Pethybridge *et al.* 2010), blueberry in Argentina in 2007 (Perez *et al.*, 2011) and Mexican sunflower in California (Koike 2013). Brinjal was first listed as one of the many hosts of *Sclerotinia sclerotiorum* in New Zealand in 1932 and the same was later reported from Morocco, Netherlands, Bermuda, Brazil, Argentina and Scotland, and from the United States (Gray and Findlater, 1960). Other hosts include cultivated plants such as canola (oilseed rape, *Brassica napus* L.) (Morrall and Dueck 1982), soybean (*Glycine max* L. Merr.) (Boland and Hall 1988), bean (*Phaseolus vulgaris* L.) (Abawi and Grogen 1975), and sunflower (*Helianthus annuus* L.) (Hiang and Hoes 1976). Wild plants species are also reported as *S. sclerotiorum* host and this is considered to be an important factor in *Sclerotinia* stem rot epidemiology (Boland and Hall 1994). This pathogen was also recorded on different hosts all over India such as cauliflower (Sharma *et al.*, 1983; Sandhu 1986), brinjal (Singh 1985), radish (Kapoor *et al.* 1987), potatoes (Singh and Agrawal 1989; Dutta *et al.* 2009), rosemary (Mohan 1994), gram (Sharma 1995), soybean (Pant and Mukhopadhyay 2001), Indian mustard (Chattopadhyay *et al.* 2004), pea (Kapil and Kapoor 2005), carrot (Bharat *et al.*, 2012) and lettuce (Bharat *et al.*, 2014). Scannavini *et al.* (1993) reported that *Sclerotinia minor* and *S. sclerotiorum* are the principal agents of collar rot of lettuce, endive and chicory.

Bag (2000) studied the status of vegetable diseases caused by *Sclerotinia sclerotiorum* under jhum (shifting cultivation) land and regularly cultivated agricultural land in the West Siang district (at 660-880m MSL) of Arunachal Pradesh. The disease incidence was highest in French bean (22.5%) followed by sponge gourd, chilli, brinjal, ridge gourd order under jhum cultivation. However, percent occurrence of the disease in regularly cultivated agricultural land was maximum in pea (56.0 %), followed by French bean, cabbage, cauliflower, brinjal, broad bean, ridge gourd and so on. Under both conditions, yam, cowpea, taro, sweet gourd, bottle gourd, okra, squash, cucumber, bitter gourd were free from infection.

Solanaceous crops grown in greenhouses and fields in Korea were surveyed from 1994 to 2000 by Kim and Cho (2003). *Sclerotinia* rot was most severe in potato (up to 60%), followed by tomato (20%), brinjal (5%) and less than 1% in red pepper. Kumar *et al.* (2003) conducted a study with 24 plant species from 9 families (Chenopodiaceae, Compositae, Cruciferae, Cucurbitaceae, Euphorbiaceae, Leguminosae, Malvaceae, Solanaceae and Umbelliferae), including field crops and weed species, by inoculating with mycelial suspension of *S. sclerotiorum*. The pathogen successfully infected 21 plants of 18 species from 8 families, suggesting that *S. sclerotiorum* was not host-specific but had a wide host range. The infected plants belonging to Cruciferae, Leguminosae and Umbelliferae developed the inoculum fast, thus facilitating secondary infection. Dutta *et al.* (2009) reported severe symptoms of *Sclerotinia sclerotiorum* on the lower parts of potato plants, which was the first report of the pathogen on potato in West Bengal, India. Hansda *et al.* (2014) observed that brinjal isolate of *S. sclerotiorium* is not host specific and bottle gourd, cabbage, cauliflower, carrot, French bean, pea, mustard and parthenium showed highly susceptible reaction along with pointed gourd, which was believed to be new addition to the host range of *S. sclerotiorum.*

S. sclerotiorum is a widespread plant pathogen affecting many economically important vegetables and cause huge losses from time to time in different crops. It caused 50-80 per cent losses of celery in Florida (Tisdale and Kelbert 1936), 25 per cent of potato in Ireland (Eddins 1937), 100 per cent of beans in South Florida (Moore 1948), 100 per cent in experimental fields in Washington (McLean 1949), over 50 per cent of peanuts in North Carolina and Virginia in U.S.A. (Beute *et al.* 1975; Woodward *et al.* 2008), 30 to 50 per cent of carrot in Canada (Finlayson *et al.*, 1989) and up to 50 per cent reduction in seed yield in cauliflower (Sharma and Sharma 1984). Stem rot (*S. sclerotiorum*) on brinjal with 26.7 to 47.3% disease incidence has been reported by Iqbal *et al.* (2003).

Singh *et al.* (1988) observed the pathogen on *Brassica oleracea* var. *gongylodes* (kohlrabi) for the first time in Nagaland and the disease incidence ranged from 1 to 50%. Chaudhury *et al* (1993) studied grain yield, plant height, number of siliqua/plant and 1000 grain weight in rape and mustard plants infected by *S. sclerotiorum* in Nepal and reported that yield was reduced by 75% in infected plants. Iqbal *et al.* (1998) reported an epidemic of Sclerotinia rot of peas during March 1996 for the first time in seed production plots of varieties

Meteor (local) and Green Feasts (exotic) at the National Agricultural Research Centre, Islamabad, Pakistan and disease incidence was 80-90%. Anahosur *et al.* (1998) reported that the losses on different potato varieties in North Karnataka due to the pathogen ranged between of 25-90 per cent wilting of potato plant and upto 25 per cent tuber infection in storage. Dhaliwal *et al.* (2004) reported 6.5 and 8% incidence of white mould caused by *Sclerotinia sclerotiorum* in on potato cv. Kufri Badshah during 2002-03 in Khanaura and Nakodar, Punjab, India when potato was sown after bitter gourd and sunflower, respectively. Schwartz and Singh (2013) reported that under favorable weather conditions white mould causes 100% crop and yield loss in common bean.

Peltier *et al.* (2002) observed that this disease, caused by the fungus *Sclerotinia sclerotiorum* (Lib.) De Bary, varies in incidence and severity from year to year because of its sensitivity to weather conditions. Losses due to *Sclerotinia* stem rot can be substantial when environmental conditions and management practices favour high yield potential. Employing a disease management plan based on knowledge of field history and best disease management practices can help reduce losses from *Sclerotinia* stem rot.

Survival of the Pathogen

Long term survival of this pathogen in soil is attribuited to formation of hard resting structure called sclerotia. Many aspects of the development and structure of sclerotia have been reviewed by several workers and methods of sclerotia formation have already been studied. Usually three developmental stages or phases can be distinguished during sclerotia formation – initiation, development and maturation in *S. sclerotiorum* (Willets and Wong, 1980; Chet and Henis, 1975). Initiation and formation of sclerotia in *S. sclerotiorum* is a programmed and controlled process. Under stalling conditions, nutritient deficiency and poor aeration the fungus forms small hyphal aggregates, which indicate unsuccessful attempts to produce sclerotia. Long term survival of this pathogen makes it a pathogen of concern in crops owing to its extensive host range and use of host resistance is often deployed to manage this pathogen in host crops.

Genotypic screening against *Sclerotinia* rot

The long term strategy against prevention of any disease is to develop resistant varieties. The first step towards any resistance breeding programme is genotypic screening of the existing germplasm for resistance. The resistance source may thereafter be directly used as variety or as the donor parent in breeding programmes.

Singh and Kalda (1995) screened 69 cauliflower lines for resistance to *Sclerotinia* rot caused by *Sclerotinia sclerotiorum* under artificial inoculation of the leaf tissue and reported that only four winter cultivars i.e. Janovan, EC 103576, EWAWH and EC 177283 were resistant.

Thakur *et al.* (2001) carried out crosses between susceptible parents and resistant genotypes (Janavon and RSK 1301) of cauliflower. The disease reaction recorded in the F_1 and segregating generations revealed that resistance was recessive to susceptibility. The intermediate disease reaction in F_2 and low in the back cross generations indicated the polygenic control of the resistance.

Kim *et al* (1999) evaluated 18 soyabean genotypes for resistance of 18 soyabean genotypes to *Sclerotinia* stem rot over several field locations and compared these disease ratings with seed yields, other agronomic traits, and parentage. The average disease severity index (DSI) of the 18 genotypes at a single environment ranged from 2.1 to 49.9. Mean DSI values over locations differed ($P < 0.05$) among the genotypes. The genotypes NKS1990, Asgrow A2506, Colfax and Corsoy 79 showed the greatest resistance to *Sclerotinia* stem rot.

Sharma and Kapoor (1999) conducted a study where twenty-day-old seedlings of 97 pea lines/cultivars inoculated with *S. sclerotiorum* were kept in humidity chambers for 7-8 days before being transferred to a cage house. The same genotypes were evaluated under field conditions in Himachal Pradesh, India. Under caged conditions, resistant genotypes (with <50% of the disease severity of the control cultivar Lincoln) were Dark Skin Perfection, DPH-64, HPPC-75, HPPC-77, HPPC-95, HPPC-96, 7104 and PI 189171. Under field conditions, resistant genotypes were Dark Skin Perfection, DPP-19, DPP-54, DPP-58, DPP-71, DPH-9, DPH-86, HPPC-95, P-3471, P-3496, P-3549, P-3611, P-3641 and P-3673.

Ghasolia and Shivpuri (2004) reported that four genotypes of tomato, *viz.*, PCR-10, RW-8410, RW-8006 and RGH-8006 had resistance against *S. sclerotiorum* as compared to susceptible check. Prajapati *et al.* (2005) screened 96 dolichos bean (*Lablab purpureus*) cultivars to stem and pod rot caused by *S. sclerotiorum* in a field experiment conducted in Kanpur, Uttar Pradesh, India during the *kharif* seasons under natural conditions and found that 18 cultivars were resistant, whereas 16 were moderately resistant to the pathogen. Under artificial conditions, 10 (Arka Vijay, 6009, 6022, 6802, 7011, 7020B, 7101, 7202, 8101 and Rajani) were resistant and 18 were moderately resistant to the pathogen.

Conclusion

Sclerotinia rot in vegetables cause a huge loss and is a production constraint for vegetable production throughout the world. While management strategies for the fungus control may not be very effective for this pathogen due to its broad host range and capacity to remain viable in soil without host plant for many years, screening out resistant genotypes in different crops for cultivation and use of these in further breeding programmes as donors for resistance is a long term strategy to control it.

References

Abawi GS, Grogen RG (1975) Source of primary inoculum and effect of temperature and moisture on infection of beans by Whetzeliniasclerotiorum. *Phytopathology*, 65: 300-309.

Anahosur Kh, Gaddanakeri MA, Sataraddi A, Kulkarni S (1998) Biological control of potato Sclerotium wilt. Paper presented at Indian Phytopathology Society Symposium (SC), University of Agricultural Sciences, Bangalore, 10-12, Dec. 1998, p 45.

Anonymous (2017) Horticultural statistics at a glance, National Horticultural Board, Gurgaon.

Ayers WA, Adams PB (1979) Ecology of Sclerotinia species. *Phytopathology*, 69(8): 896-899.

Bag TK (2000) Status of vegetable diseases caused by *Sclerotinia sclerotiorum* in differen land use systems of Arunachal Pradesh. *Environment and Ecology*, 18(1): 88-91 .

Beute MK, Porter DM , Hadley BA (1975) Sclerotinia blight of peanut in North Carolina and Virginia and its chemical control. *Plant Disease Reporter*,59(9): 697-701.

Bharat NK, Kumar R, Gupta P (2012) Two new diseases on carrot seed crop in dry temperate zone of Himachal Pradesh. *International Journal of Farm Sciences*, 2(2): 44-47.

Bharat NK, Thakur M, Bhardwaj RK, Kumar S (2014) Occurrence of Sclerotinia rot and Botrytis gray mould on lettuce under protected conditions in Himachal Pradesh. *International Journal of Farm Sciences*,4(2): 86-91.

Boland GJ, Hall R (1988) Epidemiology of *Sclerotinia* stem rot of soybean in Ontario. *Phytopathology*, 78:1241-1245

Boland GJ, Hall R (1994) Index of plant hosts of *Sclerotinia sclerotiorum*. *Canadian Journal of Plant Pathology*, 16: 93–100.

Bolton MD, Thomma BPHJ, Nelson BD (2006) *Sclerotinia sclerotiorum* (Lib.) DBary: Biology and Molecular Traits of a Cosmopolitan Pathogen. *Molecular Plant Pathology*, 7(1): 1-16.

Chaudhury BN (1993) Yield loss estimation by (*Sclerotinia sclerotiorum*) (LIB.) de Bary. *Journal of the Institute of Agriculture and Animal Science*, 14: 113.

Chet I, Henis Y (1975). Sclerotial morphogenesis in fungi. *Annual Review of Phytopathology*. 13: 169-192.

Clarkson JP, Staveley J, Phelps K, Young CS, Whipps JM, 2003. Ascospore release and survival in *Sclerotinia sclerotiorum*. *Mycological Research*, 107: 213-222.

Cook GE, Steadman JR, Boosalis MG (1975) Survival of *Whetzelinia sclerotiorum* and initial infection of dry beans in western Nebraska. *Phytopathology*,65: 250-255.

Couper G, Litterick A and Leifert C (2001) Control of Sclerotinia within carrot crops in NE Scotland: the effect of irrigation and compost application on sclerotia germination. Presented at the 11th International Workshop, 12-18th July 2001, Central Scientific Laboratory, York, UK 79-82.

Dhaliwal HJS, Thind TS, Mohan C (2004) White mold, a new disease of potato in Punjab. Plant Disease Research Ludhiana, 19(2): 192 .

Dutta S, Ghosh PP, Kuiry SP (2009) Stem rot, a new disease of potato in West Bengal, India. *Australasian Plant Disease Notes*, 4(1): 80-81.

Eddins AH (1937) Sclerotinia rot of Irish potatoes. *Phytopathology*,37(1): 100-103.

Finlayson JE, Rimmer SR, Prichard M K (1989) Infection of carrot by *Sclerotinia sclerotiorum*. *Canadian Journal of Plant Pathology*, 11: 313-316 .

Gray EG, Findlater WT (1960) *Sclerotinia sclerotiorum* in Kincardineshire. *Plant Pathology*, 9(4): 130-132.

Ghasolia RP, Shivpuri A (2004) Screening of rapeseed-mustard genotypes for resistance against Sclerotinia rot. *Indian Phytopathology*, 58(2): 242 .

Hansda S, Nanda RK, Dutta S, Ray SK (2014) Sclerotinia rot of brinjal and its host range in West Bengal, *The Journal of Plant Protection Sciences*, 6(1): 27-30.

Iqbal SM, Mirza MS, Bakhsh A, Tariq M (1998) Sclerotinia rot of peas (*Pisum sativum* L.) in Pakistan. *Sarhad Journal of Agriculture*, 14(2): 157-159 .

Iqbal SM, Ghafoor A, Ahmad Z, Haqqani AM (2003) Pathogenicity and fungicidal efficacy for Sclerotinia rot of brinjal. *International Journal of Agriculture and Biology*, 5(4) 618-620 .

Johnson SB, Kleinhenz MD, Dwyer JD, Griffin T, Olanya OM, Lambert DH, Porter GA (1998). First report of white mold (*Sclerotinia sclerotiorum*) on soybean in Maine. *Plant Disease*, 82(7): 832

Kapil R, Kapoor AS (2005) Management of white rot of pea incited by *Sclerotinia sclerotiorum* using *Trichoderma* spp. and biopesticides. *Indian Phytopathology* 58(1): 10-16.

Kapoor KS, Gill HS, Sharma SR (1987) Sclerotinia root rot of radish. *Indian Phytopathology*, 40: 118-120.

Kim WG, Cho WD (2003) Occurrence of Sclerotinia Rot in Solanaceous Crops Caused by *Sclerotinia* spp. *Mycobiology*, 31(2): 113-118

Kim HS, Sneller CH, Diers BW (1999) Evaluation of soybean cultivars for resistance to *Sclerotinia* stem rot in field environments. *Crop Science*, 39(1): 64-68 .

Koike ST (2013) First report of white mold caused by Sclerotinia minor on Mexican sunflower in California. *Plant Disease*, 97(9): 1250.

Kora C, McDonald MR, Boland GJ (2003). Sclerotinia rot of carrot: an example ofphonological adaption and bycyclic development by *Sclerotinia sclerotiorum. Plant Disease*, 87(5): 456-470.

Kulkarni S, Hiremath RV, Padaganur GM (1995) Diseases of potato and their management. Research Highlights on Potato, University of Agricultural Sciences, Dharwad, pp. 22-30.

Kumar B, Pandey P, Verma AK (2003) Studies on host range of *Sclerotinia sclerotiorum* of broccoli. *Progressive Agriculture*, 3(1/2): 131-132 .

Latorre BA, Guerrero MJ (2001) First report on shoot blight of grapevine caused by *Sclerotinia sclerotiorum* in Chile. *Plant Disease*, 85: 1122.

Letham DB, Huett DO, Trimboli DS (1976) Biology and control of Sclerotinia sclerotiorum in cauliflower and tomato crops in coastal New South Wales. *Plant Disease Reporter*, 60(4): 286-289.

Lobo JM (1999) Epidemiologia da podridão de esclerotínia em tomateiro para processamento industrial. Brasília: Universidade de Brasília. 117 p (Tese doutorado).

Lobo JM, Abreu MS (2000) Inhibition of *Sclerotinia sclerotiorum* mycelial growth by non-volatile metabolites produced by some antagonists under different temperatures and pHs. Ciênciae*Agrotecnologia* 24:521-526.

Mclean DM (1949) Occurrence of Sclerotinia stalk rot in cabbage seed plants in Skagit County, Washington in 1948. *Plant Disease Reporter*,33(5): 222-223.

Mendes MAS, Silva VL, Dianese JC,Ferreira MASV, Santos CEN, Gomes NE, Urben AF, Castro C (1998) Fungos em Plantas no Brasil. Brasília: Embrapa Cenargen. 569p.

Merriman PR (1976) Survival of sclerotia of *Sclerotinia sclerotiorum* in soil. *Soil Biology and Biochemistry*, 8: 385–389.

Mohan L (1994) Sclerotinia rot in rosemary. *Indian Phytopathology*, 47(4):443.

Moore WD (1948) Weather and the incidence of *Sclerotinia sclerotiorum* on vegetables in South Florida during the years 1944-1948. *Plant Disease Reporter*,39(6): 470-472.

Morrall RAA, Dueck J (1982) Epidemiology of sclerotinia stem rot of rapeseed in Saskatchewan. *Canadian Journal of Plant Pathology*, 4:161-168.

Neergaard P (1958) Mycelial seed infection of certain crucifers by Sclerotinia sclerotiorum (Lib.) de Bary. *Plant Disease Reporter*, 42(10): 1105-1106.

Nicholson JF, Dhingra OD, Sinclair JB (1972). Internal seed-borne nature of Sclerotinia sclerotiorum and Phomopsis sp. and their effects on soybean seed quality. *Phytopathology*, 62:1261-1263.

Ojaghian MR (2009) First report of *Sclerotinia sclerotiorum* on potato plants in Iran.Australasian *Plant Disease Notes*,4(1): 39-41.

Pant R, Mukhopadhyay AN (2001) Integrated management of seed and seedling rot complex of soybean. *Indian Phytopathology*, 54(3): 346-350.

Peltier AJ, Bradley CA, Chilvers MI, Malvick DK, Mueller DS, Wise KA,Esker PD (2002) Biology, yield loss and control of Sclerotinia stem rot of soybean. *Journal of Integrated Pest Management* 3: 1-7.

Perez BA, Farinon OM, Berretta MF (2011) First report of Sclerotinia rot on blueberry caused by *Sclerotinia sclerotiorum* in Argentina. *Plant Disease*, 95(6): 774.

Pethybridge SJ, Hay FS, Gent DH (2010) Characterization of the spatiotemporal attributes of *Sclerotinia* flower blight epidemics in a perennial pyrethrum pathosystem. *Plant Disease*, 94: 1305–1313.

Porter DM, Beute MK (1974) Sclerotinia blight of peanut. *Phytopathology*,64(2): 263-264.

Prajapati, CR, Shukla HP, Pandey R (2005) Screening of Dolichos bean cultivars/germplasms against *Sclerotinia sclerotiorum*. *Annals of Plant Protection Sciences*, 13(1): 259-261

Prova A, Akanda MAM , Islam S, SultanaF , Islam MT, Hossain MM (2014) First report of stem and pod blight of hyacinth bean caused by *Sclerotinia sclerotiorum* in Bangladesh. *Journal of Plant Pathology*, 96(3): 607.

Reis A, Lopes CA (2007) Principais fungos de solo em Hortaliças: Epidemiologia e manejo. In: Zambolim L,Lopes Ca, Picanço Mc, Costa H (orgs). Manejo integrado de doenças e pragas: Hortaliças. Viçosa: UFV. p. 189-224.

Sandhu KS (1986) Sclerotinia sclerotiorum: history, disease and symptomatology, host range, geographical distribution, and impact. *Phytopathology*, 69(8): 875-880.

Scannavini M, Antoniacci L, Cobelli L, Brunelli A (1993) Experiments in soil solarization in Emilia Romagna for the control of lettuce drop. *Informatore Fitopatologico*, 43(10): 30-35.

Schwartz HF, Singh SP (2013) Breeding common bean for resistance to diseases: a review. *Crop Science* 53: 1832-1844.

Sharma RC, Sharma SL (1984) Evaluation and economies of fungicidal sprays against *Sclerotinia* rot of cauliflower seed crop. *Seed Research*, 12: 95-97.

Sharma SK (1999) Management of the stem rot of gram caused by *Sclerotinia* sclerotiorum (Lib.) De Bary. M.Sc. Thesis, Himachal Pradesh Kirshi Vishvavidhyalaya, Palampur, India p 67.

Sharma SL, Kaith DS, Khan MA (1983) Cultural control of Sclerotinia stalk rot of Cauliflower. *Indian Phytopathology*, 36(4): 601-603.

Singh H, Kalda TS (1995) Screening of cauliflower germplasm against *Sclerotinia* rot. *Indian Journal of Genetics and Plant Breeding*, 55(1): 98-102 .

Singh HB (1988) Sclerotinia rot of knol khol. *Indian Journal of Plant Pathology*, 6(1): 81.

Singh RB , Agrawal JM (1989) Outbreaks of *Sclerotinia* white mould disease in India. *Current Science* 58(8): 456.

Singh RS (1985) Diseases of Vegetable Crops. Oxford and IBH Publishing Coperator, New Delhi pp 112-136.

Thakur BS, Korla N, Dohroom NP (2001) Resistance to stalk rot and its inheritance in cauliflower. *Crop-Improvement*, 28(1): 109-114.

Tisdale WB, Kelbert GA (1936) Pink rot of celery in Floida. *Plant Disease Reporter* ,20(8): 134-135.

Velastegui JR, Ball SFL (1991) First record of *Sclerotinia sclerotiorum* on tree tomato in Ecuador. *Plant Pathology*, 40(3):476-477.

Whetzel HH (1945) A synopsis of the genera and species of the Sclerotiniaceae, a family of stromaticinoperculatedi scomycetes. *Mycologia*, 37:648–714.

Woodward JE, Batla MA, Dotray PA , Wheeler TA (2008) First report of Sclerotinia Minor infecting Ipomoea hederacea and I. Coccinea in Texas. *Disease Notes*, 92(3): 482.

Willets HJ, Wong JAL (1980). The biology of *Sclerotinia Sclerotiorum, S. trifolionum and S. minor* with emphasis on specific nomenclature. *The Botanical Review* 46:101-165.

Yang B, Workneh F, Lundeen P (1997) First report of Sclerotium production of *Sclerotinia sclerotiorum* in soil on infected soybean seeds. *Plant Disease*, 82(2):26.

18

Emerging Threat to Mango Production

Chanda Kushwaha[1], Sanjay Sahay[3], Munishwar Prasad[3], Samik Sengupta[3], S N Ray[2], Ravindra Kumar[3], Amit Kumar[3] and Girija Shankar Yadav[3]

[1]Department of Plant Pathology, Bihar Agriculture University Sabour Bhagalpur, Bihar, India
[2]Department of Entomology, Bihar Agriculture University Sabour Bhagalpur, Bihar, India
[3]Department of Fruits and Fruit Technology, Bihar Agriculture University Sabour, Bhagalpur, Bihar, India

Abstract

India ranks first among world's mango producing countries accounting for about 50 % of the world's total mango production. In Bihar it is the most important fruit crop as well as occupies a large area affecting socio economic conditions of the region. The crop suffers from over 140 diseases all over the world. From young seedlings to mature trees and fruits in their all stages from start to storage may suffer from a number of biotic and abiotic stresses. All parts of the plant namely, trunk, branch, twigs, leaf, petiole, flower and fruits are prone to attack by a number of pathogens The changes in climatic patterns and shifting towards commercial cultivation of this crop has seen the emergence of some diseases which can cause huge losses to the production of mango over the years. One such problem, decline in mango is reported to be a complex problem involving multitude of factors. Decline disorders are recognized in virtually all mango-producing regions of the world. In most cases, the disease has been characterized by leaf drooping and drying; bark splitting, gum secretion from branches and main trunk, bud necrosis, dieback, vascular discoloration and death of the whole tree. The bark beetle Hypocryphalus mangiferae *is closely associated with trees affected by mango sudden decline disease. Report suggests the causal agent to be* Botryodiplodia theobromae, Ceratocystis manginecans, Fusarium spp, Colletotrichum sp, Pestalosiopsis maniferae. *In most of the cases* Botryodiplodia theobromae, Ceratocystis spp *are associated with it. Although, none of the pathogens isolated could singly incite the complete decline symptoms under artificial inoculation on mango seedlings indicating towards complex etiology of the disease. Since pathogens are endophytic in nature; mangement of the pathogen after infection is difficult and relies more upon prohytalctic measures. Over all plant health, its nutritional status and abiotic conditions of flood and drought are also the pre disposing factors to decline in Mango. Effective management of decline in mango needs holistic approaches using optimum nutrition, general sanitation, routine crop protection schedule, weed management and appropriate intercropping practices.*

Keywords: *Ceratocystis* spp, decline, *Hypocryphalus mangiferae*, Mango

Introduction

India ranks first among world's mango producing countries accounting for about 50% of the world's mango production. Other major mango producing countries include China, Thailand, Mexico, Pakistan, Philippines, Indonesia, Brazil, Nigeria and Egypt. India's share is around 52% of world production. Bihar ranks fifth in total mango production in the country after Uttar Pradesh, Andhra Pradesh, Karnataka and Telangana. Mango is susceptible to many diseases as many as over 140 all over the world (Ploetz, 1997). From young seedlings to mature trees and fruits in their all stages from start to storage may suffer from a number of biotic and abiotic stresses. All parts of the plant namely, trunk, branch, twigs, leaf, petiole, flower and fruits are prone to attack by a number of pathogens particularly fungi. Besides the perennial nature of biennial bearings, important diseases include anthracnose, malformation, die-back, powdery mildew, decline, stem end rot and decline have become some constraints in production of Mango.

With the intensification of mango cultivation in Bihar various newer concerns with regards to pests have come up. One such concerns being Decline in Mango. Periodic surveys in major mango growing regions of Zone III B of agro ecological zone of Bihar showed very low but increasing trends in incidence of Mango decline over the past five years. Usually the tree starts showing symptoms after the monsoon season and in next 2-3 months have resulted in the complete drying of the trees. Often at the farmers level the symptoms are confused with those of attack by stem borer. Therefore, critical evaluations are necessary to diagnose the incidence of wilting/ decline in mango after a farmer's perception.

Although, the nature of the disease is complex. Many pathogens like *Botryodiplodia theobromae*, *Fusarium* spp, *Colletotrichum* sp, *Pestalosiopsis manifera* were isolated from the bark and roots of the declining trees. Under artificial inoculated conditions known of the pathogens completely induced declining symptoms in the seedilings. However, *Botryodiplodia theobromae* induced characteristic browning at the point of inoculation initially at 20 days of inoculation. Therefore, for timely intervention awareness and proper diagnosis of this complex problem is essential for its effective management.

Mango Decline: Symptoms, etiology and its management

This problem is reported to be a complex problem involving multitude of factors. It is reported from all most all mango-producing regions of the world *ie* India, Pakistan, Australia, and Oman (Al-Adawi *et al.*, 2006). Decline disorders are recognized in virtually all mango-producing regions of the world. In most cases, the disease has been characterized by leaf drooping and drying; bark splitting, gum secretion from branches and main trunk, bud necrosis, dieback, vascular discoloration and death of the whole tree. The conducting tissues are damaged, blocking the food supply to roots and other parts, resulting in partial to full drying of the plant. As a preliminary symptom, drying of tip, discoloration and darkening of the bark from the tip becomes visible. It progresses downward involving bigger branches. As a result, the leaves shed. Sometimes, gum oozes from the diseased portions. Bark splitting or cracking may also be noticed in severe cases. These symptoms are found alone or in combination with other symptoms in different mango orchards. On removal of the affected bark, a thick liquid with foul smell ooze out. As the infection progresses, tree death occurs, perhaps 6 months from first appearance of symptoms. Initially, a portion of the bark is affected and gradually the whole tree trunk rots causing collapse of the tree. The wood is stained dark brown, spreading from a point of infection; under acute conditions, form in the decline syndrome. The tree appears normal but suddenly starts to wilt. Within a couple of days the affected portions of the tree (twigs or branches) completely wilts and dies. Usually begin on one side and later spreads to the entire tree. Amber-colored gum from the bark of their trunks or branches. Vascular tissues are discolored. Xylem tissue appears as striated brownish streaks. In most cases, the disease has been characterized by leaf drooping and drying; bark splitting, gum secretion from branches and main trunk, bud necrosis, dieback, vascular discoloration and death of the whole tree. Sometimes, gum oozes from the diseased portions. Bark splitting or cracking may also be noticed in severe cases.

Damage caused by a bark beetle (*Cryphalus scabrecollis*) was also reported to be associated with the disease. A close inspection of dried plants often reveals tiny holes, numerous small beetles running under the bark, probably acting as carriers of this disease. In Oman, the bark beetle *Hypocryphalus mangiferae* is closely associated with trees affected by mango sudden decline disease caused by *Ceratocystis manginecans*. Report suggests the causal agent to be *Botryodiplodia theobromae, Ceratocystis manginecans*. and *Fusarium* spp. In most of the cases *Botryodiplodia theobromae, Ceratocystis spp* are associated with it (Van Wyk *et al*, 2007). *Botryodiplodia theobromae* is a well known opportunistic tree pathogen in the tropics and sub-tropics.

The fungus *Ceratocystis fimbriata, Lasiodiplodia theobromae (syn. Botryodiplodia theobromae)*. *Ceratocystis moniliformis* is a colonist of fresh wounds on trees, mainly in the tropics. *Ceratocystis moniliformis* has been reported on many taxonomically different plants and in many different climatic zones. It is thought to represent a complex of morphologically similar but physiologically and phylogenetically different species, some of which have recently been described. The phylogenetic relationship of *C. moniliformis* isolates from various hosts and origins, based on comparisons of DNA sequences of the Internal Transcribed Spacer (ITS) regions including the 5.8S gene of rDNA, β-tubulin and EF1-α genes war studied. Four distinct clades were discernable in the phylogenetic tree. Two recently described species, *C. bhutanensis* and *C. moniliformopsis*, were confirmed to be phylogenetically distinct. *Ceratocystis moniliformis sensu stricto* isolated from Bhutan, Costa Rica, Ecuador and South Africa represented a well-resolved monophyletic group. A collection of isolates initially identified as *C. moniliformis*, from *Pinus merkusii* in Sumatra, Indonesia was found to reside in a distinct clade. *Ceratocystis tribiliformis* sp. nov. is described here to accommodate this group of isolates. Morphologically, *C. tribiliformis* differs from *C. moniliformis* in having obpyriform to globose ascomata and both smooth and granular hyphae. *Ceratocystis tribiliformis* also has distinct optimal growth at 20-25°C on malt extract agar (Al-Sabhi *et al*, 2006). Bark beetles (*Hypocryphalus mangiferae*) are shown to carry *C. fimbriata* and *L. theobromae* and are presumably responsible for transmitting both pathogens to healthy mango trees.(Masood *et al.*, 2012 a; Masood *et al.*, 2012 b) In Pakistan, the Asian Ambrosia beetle (*Xylosandrus crassiusculus)* (Motschulsky) is associated with the disease complex (Masood *et al.*, 2011). The beetle is known to spread the fungus to healthy trees. As the fungus grows, the beetle feeds on them.

Some reports also suggest association of Plant parasitic nematodes with declining trees that include *Criconemella sphaerocephala, Helicotylenchus dihystera, Hemicriconemoides mangiferae, Hoplolaimus indicus, Meloidogyne* spp., *Pratylenchus brachyurus, Rotylenchulus reniformis, Trichodorus* spp., *Tylenchorhynchus claytoni, Tylenchus filiformis* and *Xiphinema* spp. Populations of *H. mangiferae, Macroposthonia* spp. and *Rotylenchulus reniformis* were very high in the roots of trees showing decline. Such factor may likely cause mango decline including *H. mangiferae and R. reniformis* (Anwer *et al*, 2012).

Role of nutrition was also studied by some workers and nutrient application was found to be correlated with vigor of trees and in disease management results indicated application of zinc sulphate along with copper sulphate, nitrogen phosphorous and humic acid improved the overall health of mango trees and reduced the incidence of decline in chousa variety of mango (Masood *et al*, 2012)

Various strategies have been put forward for management of this complex problem in Mango essentially relying upon management of fungi and its vector both by various workers some of them being as follows.

- Alternate host trees such as sheeshum, gular, golmohar, sareenh etc., should not be planted in and around mango orchards.
- Soil solarization by polyethylene mulching has proved to be an effective and environmentally safe alternateive to chemicals for controlling various soil-borne pests, weeds and phytopathogens including *L. theobromae* by increasing the soil temperatures. It should be practiced in mango orchards in order to minimize the primary inoculums of soil-borne casual pathogen (*L. theobromae*) especially in the nursery beds and pits in orchards before transplanting.
- The disease-free trees should be selected for propagation and planting. Suitable fungicide or bio-agent may be applied at the nursery level.
- The best managed gardens are free from the decline disease. Regular monitoring of orchards is most essential to identify the problem at an early stage.
- Painting the tree trunks with the Bordeaux mixture twice a year and spraying with systemic fungicides help in reducing the fungal inoculums on the tree.
- The diseased branches should be pruned and the cut portions painted with the Bordeaux mixture. Any injury to the plants should be avoided to minimize the chances of microorganism infection.
- The diseased trees should be removed and burnt at the earliest to reduce the inoculums of pathogen.
- Two foliar sprays with (Thiophanate-methyl) @1 g L^{-1} or foliar spray with Carbendazim @ 0.1%, or Chlorothalonil @ 0.2% at fortnightly interval helps in reducing the fungal infection in mango plants, suppressing the

gum exudation, dieback and wilting resulting in significant enhancement in vegetative growth of plants.

- The bark beetles or caterpillar borers are the carriers of this fungus for which trunk spray may be done at regular intervals with long residual pyrethroids besides application of systemic fungicides.
- The orchard was also found to be free from termite attack after planting turmeric as intercrop in mango. Turmeric comes up well in partial shade and hence can be grown as an intercrop in several fruit orchards. Its plantation as intercrop can find application in organic farming systems, to control various soil borne pests and diseases in several fruit orchards.

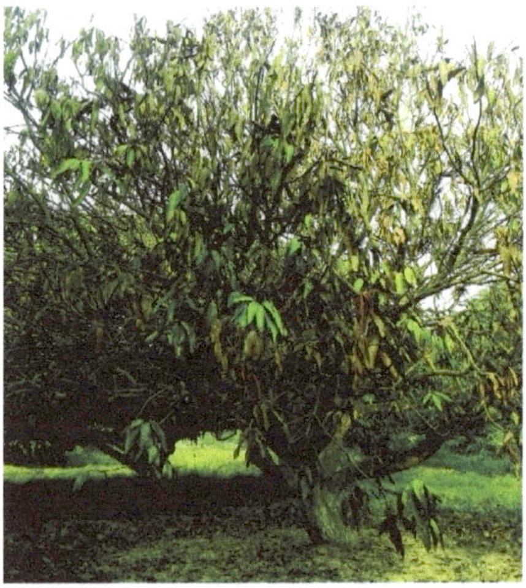

(a) Mango trees affected with sudden decline in Mango.

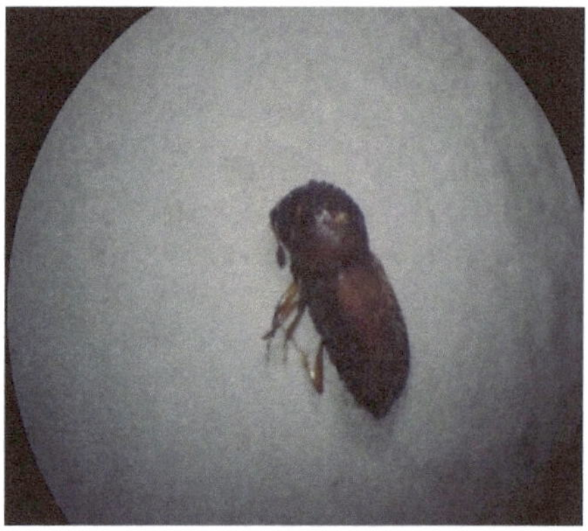

(b) Bark beetle associated with the trees affected by sudden decline in Mango.

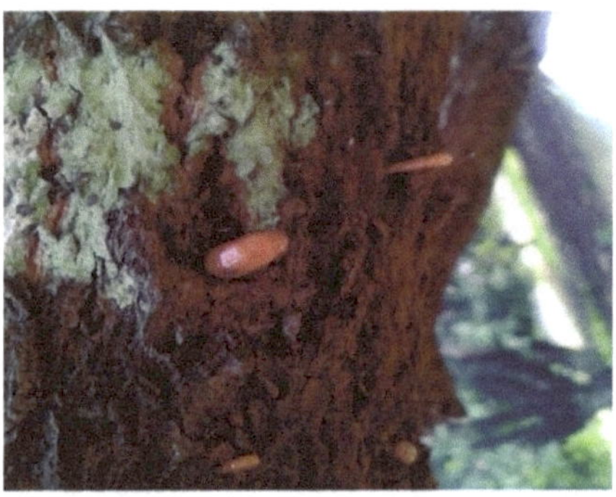

(c) Exudation of gum from the bark of affected trees

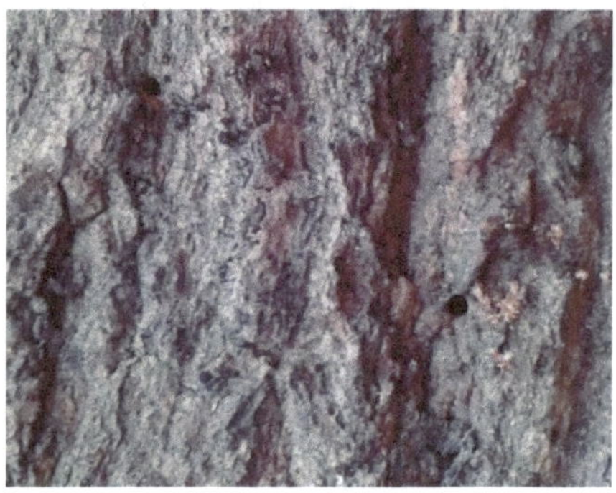

(d) Presence of minute holes on the bark of affected trees.

Fig. 1: Symptoms of Mango sudden decline, associated bark beetle (adult and grub)

References

Al-Subhi, AM, Al-Adawr, AO, Van Wyk, M, Deadman, Michal L and Wingfield, MJ (2006). Ceratocystis Omanensis, a new species from diseased mango trees in Oman. *Mycologcal Research* 110:237-245.

Al-Adawi AO, Deadman ML, Al Rawahi AK, Al Maqbali YM, Al Jahwari AA, Al Saadi BA, Al Amrapaliri IS, Wingfield MJ (2006) Aetiology and causal agents of mango sudden decline disease in the Sultanate of Oman. *Eur J Plant Pathol* 116:247–254

Anwar S A, McKenry M V, Ahmad H A (2012) Nematode and Fungal Communities Associated With Mango Decline of Southern Punjab. *Pakistan J. Zool.* 44: 915-922.

Fateh FS, Kazmi MR, Ahmad I, Ashraf M (2006) *Ceratocystis fimbriata* isolated from vascular bundles of declining mango trees in Sindh, Pakistan. *Pak. J. Bot* 38:1257–1259

Masood A, Saeed S, Silveira SFD, Akem CN, Hussain N, Farooq M. (2011) Quick decline of mango in Pakistan: Survey and pathogenicity of fungi isolated from mango tree and bark beetle. *Pakistan J Bot.* 43:1793-1798.

Masood A, Saeed S, Mahmood A, Malik SA (2012) Husain N. Role of nutrients in management of mango sudden death disease. *Pakistan Journal of Zoology* 44: 20-21

Masood A, Saeed S. Bark Beetle (2012) *Hypocryphalus mangiferae* Stebbing (Coleoptera: Curculionidae: Scolytinae) is a vector of Mango Sudden Death Disease in Pakistan. *Pak. J Bot.* 44:813-820.

Ploetz RC, Prakash O (1997) Foliar, floral and soil borne diseases. In: Litz RE (ed) The mango: botany, production and uses. CABI Publishing, UK, pp 281–326.

Shukla P K, Varma S, Fatima T, Bajpai A, Mishra R, Mishra AK, Gundappa, Muthukumar, M (2018) First report on wilt disease of mango caused by Ceratocystis fimbriata in Uttar Pradesh, India, Indian Phytopathology 71: 135. https://doi.org/10.1007/s42360-018-0021-3

Van Wyk M, Al Adawi AO, Khan I A, Deadman M.L, Al Jahwari AA, Wingfield BD, Ploetz R and Wingfield MJ (2007). *Ceratocystis manginecans* sp. nov., causal agent of a destructive mango wilt disease in Oman and Pakistan. *Fungal Diversity* 27: 213-230.

19

Stemphylium Leaf Blight of Onion and Garlic

Sangeeta Shree[1*], Mohammad Ansar[2], A. P. Bhagat[3], Bahadur S. Bamaniya[4] and Chandan Kumar Bagchi[5]

[1&5]Department of Horticulture (Veg. and Flori.), BAC, Sabour, Bihar, India
[4]Department of Horticulture, Sikkim University,Gangtok, Sikkim, India
[2&3]Department of Plant Pathology, BAC, Sabour, Bihar, India
Bihar Agricultural University, Sabour - 813 210, Bhagalpur, Bihar, India

Abstract

Onion (Allium cepa L.) and garlic (Allium sativum L.) are important members of the family Amaryllidaceae. Bulbs, which are the edible component in both onion and garlic grow underground and are of nutritional and medicinal importance. These underground bulb vegetables are affected by many diseases caused by different microorganisms like fungi, bacteria, nematode and viruses causing huge economic loss. Stemphylium leaf blight caused by Stemphylium vesicarium, is the major fungal disease affecting their productivity of the edible bulbs adversely.The fungus primarily attacks the leaves but can affect bulbs in storage. Initial infection is characterised by appearance of small greyish white oval spots on the leaves. These spots are often surrounded by a yellowish halo with irregular margins. Fungal pseudothecia may over-winter in contaminated plant material or may survive in the soil having plant debris and ascospores are the primary inoculums in the following season. Spores require rain or persistent dew to cause infection. This disease can spread rapidly when environmental conditions are favourable for spore development. Suitable integration of more efficient treatments like fungicides, bio agents in combination with appropriate cultural control provide better management of the Stemphylium blight disease

Introduction

Onion and garlic is the important bulb vegetables which are produced underground. They have vertical shoots and underground modified leaves which are used as food storage organs by the dormant plants. Onion and garlic are believed to have originated from Central Asia (Vavilov 1951) and Southern Europe. However, the highest onion diversity is observed in the eastern Mediterranean region and through Afghanistan, Tajikstan, Pakistan and India (Brewster, 2008 and Kik, 2008).These vegetables belong to the genus *Allium*. Among vegetables, *Alliums* are perhaps the most important genus and are consumed throughout the world. In genus *Allium*, onion (*A. cepa*) and garlic (*A. sativum*) are mostly consumed throughout the globe. Apart from being used as a prime vegetable, garlic also has numerous medicinal properties. In India, references about cultivation of onion and garlic are found from ancient times onwards as is evidenced by Charaka-Samhita, a famous early medical treatise of India. The varied medicinal uses and pharmacological actions like the anti-inflammatory, antihelmintic, and heart friendly nature of garlic were known many centuries ago (Kirtikar and Basu, 1975).Onion and garlic are the most important commercial crops grown all over the world and consumed in various forms. In India, onion and garlic have been under cultivation for the last 5000 years.

Onion (*Allium cepa*) is a popular vegetable and is the most widely cultivated species of the *Allium* (Bock, 2010).The bulb group is generally commercially propagated from seed and the aggregate group of onion is propagated vegetatively (Hanelt 1990; Rabinowitch and Currah 2002). The onion is normally a biennial or a perennial plant, but for commercial purposes it is taken usually as an annual crop.The onion plant has bluish-green leaves which are tubular and hollow and the underground bulb is primarily used for vegetable and salad purposes.The crop accumulates and stores food in the underground bulb as it approaches maturity by forming several bladeless scales at the base of the plant (Heath and Hollies 1965; Fritschand Friesen 2002). Leaves are also consumed for culinary purposes. Green bunch onions are harvested when they are of pencil thickness with a small bulb. The flowering shoot known as scape is also used as vegetable. The typical flavour of onion is due to presence of a volatile compound known as allyl propyl disulphide and the red colour is due to the presence of another pigment quercetin. Bulb formation starts when a certain day length is reached.

Garlic also enjoys almost universal cultivation for its valuable bulb. It is grown throughout the world and used as spices and flavouring agent for many foods (Velisek*et al.,* 1997). Other parts of the garlic plant are also edible. Garlic, produces narrow flat leaves. The leaves and flowers (bulbils) on the head are sometimes eaten. They are milder in flavour than the bulbs, and are most often consumed while immature and still tender. Immature garlic is sometimes pulled, rather like a scallion, and sold as "green garlic". Immature scapes are tender and edible. They are also known as "garlic spears", "stems" or "tops". Scapes generally have a milder taste than the cloves. They are often used in stir frying or braised like asparagus. Garlic leaves are a popular vegetable in many parts of Asia.The leaves are cleaned, cut and then stir-fried with eggs, meat or vegetables. Therefore healthy and disease free leaves are desirable. Garlic contains allicin, which imparts it garlicky flavour.

The area under onion cultivation in India is 1320.13 thousands hectares producing 20931.25 thousands metric tonnes with an average national productivity of 15.86 tonnes/ha. In Bihar the area, production and productivity under onion are 54.03 thousands ha,1247.34 thousands metric tonnes and 23.09 t/ha (DOGR, 2015-16). The area under garlic cultivation in India is 280.95 thousands hectares producing 1617.34 thousands metric tonnes with an average national productivity of 5.76 tonnes/ha. In Bihar the area, production and productivity under garlic are 4.25 thousands ha, 4.00 thousands metric tonnes and 0.94 t/ha (DOGR, 2015-16). Both onion and garlic can be cultivated on a range of soil types, but the ideal is sandy loam with a pH of 6 – 7 (Currah and Proctor 1990) and grown in almost all parts of India except higher altitudes. The major onion and garlic producing states are Madhya Pradesh, Gujarat, Maharashtra, Karnataka, Rajasthan, Uttar Pradesh, Bihar and Andhra Pradesh. Onion and garlic can be grown a under wide range of climatic condition. It, however cannot withstand too hot or too cold temperature. It requires cool and moist period during growth and relatively dry period during maturity of bulb. Bulb development takes place during longer days and at higher temperature. In general, cool growing period gives more yield than warm. These crops form important foreign exchange earner of India.Major onion importing countries are Sri Lanka, Malaysia, Maldives, Nepal, Dubai, Kuwait, Indonesia, UAE, Singapore, Seychelles, Pakistan, Saudi Arabia,Qatar, Bangladesh while Bangladesh, Philippines, Singapore, UK and USA are the major garlic importing countries. In the year 2017-18 India exported 26527.72 MT of garlic worth Rs.11858.11 lakhs. (DOGR, 2018-19).

Losses and Distribution

Onion as well as garlic is affected by many diseases caused by different microorganisms like fungi, bacteria, nematode and viruses but fungi are the most important pathogens causing huge economic loss. Stemphylium leaf blight is an important fungal disease of onion in both tropical and temperate countries (FAO/IPGRI 1997). Stemphylium leaf blight of onion is caused by *Stemphylium vesicarium* Wallr (Simmons). It is an Ascomycete belonging to the family Pleosporaceae. The pathogen is very much related to *A.* porri, (Simmons 1967; Bessey 1968). Diseases that occur due to these fungi are very often misdiagnosed because the early symptoms are more or less alike (Simmons 1967; Jakhar *et al.* 1996; Suheri and Price 2001). In Ontario, *S. Vesicarium* was reported on onion in 2008 (Roddy 2011). The disease led to 90% yield losses on onion inTexas and New York State in 1978 (Miller *et al.*, 1978 and Lorbeer, 1993), 80 85% yield loss in Portugal (Tomaz and Lima, 1988), and huge losses in Egypt (Hassan *et al.*, 2007), India (Rao and Pavgi 1975), Japan (Misawa and Yasuoka, 2012), New Zealand (Suheri and Price, 2001), South Africa (Aveling, 1992) and Spain (Basallote, 1993).

In garlic *fungal strains like Sclerotium cepivorum, Fusarium spp.* and *Penicillium spp. cause diseases* of the root system (Dugan *et al.*, 2007 and Schwartz and Mohan, 2008). As for the, shoot system, Stemphylium leaf blight, caused by *Stemphylium* spp (Basallote *et al.*, 1993), is the major fungal diseases that cause serious infestation in the field affecting the productivity adversely and the same has been described in many countries worldwide, including India (Raghayendra and Pavgi, 1975), South Africa (Aveling and Naude, 1992), Spain (Basallote *et al.*, 1993), Australia (Suheri and Price, 2000), China (Zheng *et al.*,2008), and Turkey (Polat *et al.*, 2012).

Different species of Stemphylium have been reported to be responsible in different localities as reported by Gálvez *et al.*, 2016 in his review study on Stemphylium Leaf Blight of Garlic (*Allium sativum).* The most widespread species in China is *S. solani* as reported by (Zheng *et al.*, 2008). Not only in garlic, it has also been reported that *Stemphylium spp* cause serious disease and affect yield and quality in other crops such as onion, asparagus, lentil, alfalfa, pear, parsley and also several horticultural crops (Falloon *et al.*, 1987; Koike *et al.*,2013; Lamprecht *et al.*, 1984; Llorente and Montesinos, 2006; Mentha, 1998; Miller *et al.*, 1978; Nasehi *et al.*, 2013a, 2013b; Reis *et al.*, 2011; and Vakalounakis and Markakis, 2013). Rao and Pavgi, 1975 also have reported pathogen from India on several hosts including onion. On asparagus, 100% loss of spears can occur (Falloon, 1987 and Hausbeck, 2009). Zheng *et al.*, 2010 reported the decreases in yield of garlic up to 70% each year in a number of fields and in onion loss from 40 to 75% in the absence of fungicides.

In India, Stemphylium blight (*Stemphylium vesicarium*) was first reported in Kullu, Himanchal Pradesh during 1973 (Singh and Sharma, 1977). Katoch and Kumar, 2016 also reported that garlic is prone to several fungal diseases and that Stemphylium leaf blight (*Stemphylium vesicarium*) is the most important disease in lower and mid hill areas of the State, Himachal Pradesh, India.The disease in this region was observed to occur in low profile (PDI <5%) till 2000-

01 but emerged in an epidemic form during 2003 and was very devastating, causing huge damage to the crop in some pockets (Sugha and Kumar, 2005). The disease severity was assessed using 0–9 disease scale (Zheng *et al.* 2010). A foliar infection up to 90% has been reported by Bisht and Agrwal, 1993 in susceptible cultivars of garlic. Stemphylium leaf blight appears every year in a moderate to severe form in garlic growing areas of Bihar. Severe outbreak of leaf blight of garlic was reported from Bihar during 1995 on varieties Vanarshi and P-49 (Patna selection), ranging the disease severity from 25.6 to 76% and 20.16 to 75% respectively (Anon., 2013). Molecular procedures can be used to precisely categorize *Stemphylium* species, based on specific primers in polymerase chain reaction of the internal transcribe spacer (ITS) region or DNA sequencing of the glyceraldehyde-3-phosphate dehydrogenase (*gpd*)gene sequence (Câmara *et al.*, 2002 and Köhl *et al.*, 2009).

Symptomatology

The early symptoms of Stemphylium leaf blight on onion comprise of small, yellowish brown to tan, water-soaked patches (Rao and Pavgi, 1975). Aveling and Snyman, 1993 have observed that in onion leaves and inflorescences are normally infested by Stemphylium leaf blight pathogens. Stemphylium leaf blight first affects crop when it is at the 3-4-leaf stage, reaching maximum severity when leaves begin to senescence. As Stemphylium leaf blight advances, widespread necrosis of infected leaves build up back from the tip which is related with host-specific toxins produced by *S. Vesicarium* after infection (Singh *et al.*, 2000 and Wolpert *et al.*, 2002). The disease also causes parchedness and premature lodging of onion, which can lead to a drastic reduction in bulb yield and bulb size. Severely infected plants produce small bulbs that fetches only low price (Rao and Pavgi, 1975; Miller *et al.*, 1978 and Lorbeer, 1993). In garlic the fungus primarily attacks the leaves but can affect bulbs in storage. Mature leaves and plants are more susceptible than young and juvenile plants. In the beginning symptoms of leaf blight disease caused by *Stemphylium spp*. infection in garlic are characterised by appearanceof small greyish white oval spots measuring about 1-3mm in length on the leaves. These spots are often surrounded by a yellowish halo with irregular margins. Centres of spots are more or less tan, and it is difficult to differentiate between leaf blight and damage from insect feeding, mechanical damage or herbicide injury. Lesions enlarge with age and when abundant, may cause leaftips to dieback. Ultimately, leaf dies and severely affected garlic fields develop a blighted look. Bulbs from infected plants have smaller size because growth is reduced by leaf loss. Secondary infection often follows as injury caused either by other fungi, bacteria, viruses, insects, or by sand or dust particles on windy days.

Fungal pseudothecia may over-winter in contaminated plant material or may survive in the soil and ascospores are the primary inoculum in the following season (Basallote *et al.*, 1998, 1999). Once the disease is established, conidia form in primary lesions and quickly spread to infect healthy plants, and as a result there is decline in photosynthesis and consequently there is reduction in bulb yield (Zheng *et al.*, 2010). Prados-Ligero *et al.*, 1998 have observed that both pseudothecia maturation and ascospore release are very much related with high relative humidity and mild temperature. During moist periods with moderate temperatures, fungal spores are dispersed from infected leaves and debris to initiate infection. Spores require rain or persistent dew to cause infection.This disease can spread rapidly when environmental conditions are favourable for development.

Management/ Control of Stemphylium leaf Blight of Garlic

Stemphylium leaf blight in garlic and onion has emerged as a major disease in recent years. The disease causes premature senescence of crops leading to substantial reduction in yield and the control of leaf blight of onion and garlic is not well established. Although chemical control of Stemphylium leaf blight had been practiced, its success depends largely on high number of spraying. Today there are strict regulations on chemical fungicide use, due to residual toxicity problems and environmental pollution. Further, use of synthetic fungicides can cause development of fungicide-resistant strains of the pathogen. This implies that management of Stemphylium leaf blight by the use of fungicides alone may be unsustainable. Therefore, a large number of studies have been devoted to searching for alternative control strategies to plant pathogens. As such integrated management strategy for control of Stemphylium leaf blight of onion and garlic would prove quite beneficial.

Bio Agents

Trichoderma species are regarded as largely accepted and environment friendly bio-control agents against various phytopathogenic fungi. They successfully suppress leaf fungal pathogens and many other soil-borne pathogens . Hussein *et al.,* 2007 have reported that application of bioagents, *Bacillus subtilis*, *Pseudomonas fluorescens* and *Trichoderma harzianum* exhibited highest reduction in disease severity in onion, caused by fungal pathogen, *Stemphylium vesicarium*. Kamal *et al.,* 2017 in their study in onion have observed that application of *Trichoderma harzianum* and *Stachybotrys chartarum has* resulted in reduction in disease incidence by 67.9 and 71.3%, respectively. Plant extracts of *Azadirachta indica* and *Datura stramonium* showed reduction in the growth of fungal pathogen, *Alternaria porri* and *Stemphylium vesicarium* under green house conditions (Abdel-Hafez *et al.,* 2014). The effectiveness of

Pseudomonas fluorescens and hexaconazole against onion leaf blight pathogen was found out by seed treatment, root dip as well as foliar spraying, alone or in combination. Treatment with *P. Fluorescens* exhibited lower disease severity and higher yield of onion bulbs as concluded by Barnwal *et al.,* 2003. *Azadirachta indica* (66.5%) and *Datura metel* (64.5%) showed check in the growth of pathogen over control against leaf blight pathogen. In the evaluation of bioagents, *T.harizianum* and *T. Viride* were found to be significantly effective in restricting the growth of leaf blight pathogen (Kumar *et al.*, 2012). Prasad and Barnwal (2004) also reported antifungal activity of 20%leaf extract of *Azadirachta indica* and *Datura metel* against *Stemphylum vesicarium* and improved bulb yield in onion. Work done on garlic in this regard is rather scanty. However, similar line of treatment can be followed in garlic to check Stemphylium leaf blight pathogen in garlic and augment the yield. Biological control agents such as *Bacillus subtilis, Saccharomyces cerevisiae,Pseudomonas fluorescens* and *Trichoderma* species reduced the severity of Stemphylium leaf blight in onion under controlled conditions (Kamal *et al.* 2008). However, these products do not provide effective management of Stemphylium leaf blight when used as the sole management strategy under field conditions (Wright *et al.*, 2005).

Cultural Control

It is a well established fact that debris of onion and garlic plays a vital role in overwintering of the fungus. *Stemphylium vesicarium* overwinters in leaf debris and provide a source of inoculums for succeeding crops i.e. the debris left in the field from the previous year serve as a source of inoculums into new season crop. Therefore clean culture should be practiced .The debris of garlic should be buried deep down the ground to check the release and spread of ascospores (Johnson, 1990). Cultural control like crop rotations, lesser hours of leaf wetness, wider plant spacing, good drainage facility and other good cultural control should be practiced to avoid and evade such fungal infections. Old onion culls should be destroyed and debris must be buried or burnt. Care should be taken so as to avoid injuring bulbs during harvest. As has been reported, infections may be carried onto bulbs also; therefore wounded, bruised, and damaged bulbs should be removed before storage. Proper curing of bulbs in the field is recommended. Optimum drying of bulbs before is advised. Sundaram and Kalb, 2001 also have supported cultural strategies like sanitation, crop rotation, reduced plant densities, and removal or burying of crop residue for managing Stemphylium leaf blight on onion while, Pathak *et al.*, 2001 and Mishra *et al.*, 2009 recommends the use of host resistance as the most efficient way to manage Stemphylium leaf blight on Allium crops. Therefore tolerant or resistant varieties must be planted. Usually, white cultivars have been reported to be more prone to infection *of Stemphylium* spp. as compared to the purple cultivars (Gálvez *et al*, 2016). Excess doses of nitrogenous fertilizers must be avoided. (Mishra *et al*, 2014). Too much and too heavy irrigation is often the culprit.

Chemical control

Various management strategies like cultural practices, field sanitation, and biological control have been suggested for the management and control of Stemphylium leaf blight. All these methods are effective only when employed well in advance as defensive measure (Kata, 2000). But once the disease has appeared, these methods become less effective. Under such circumstances, chemical control offers a good choice to grower for managing the disease. Chemical fungicides have been used since long and have the advantage of providing quick, effective and economic management of plant diseases. Regular calendar-based application of precautionary dose of fungicides has been suggested as an efficient way of managing Stemphylium leaf blight on onion, garlic, asparagus and pear (Basallote *et al.*, 1993; Meyer *et al.*, 2000; Gupta *et al.*, 2010 and Llorente *et al.*, 2012). On the other hand, Alberoni *et al.*, 2010 and Hoepting, 2015 have reported that the pathogens are insensitive to a number of fungicides, which suggests that this approach may not be sustainable.

From a range of *in vitro* experiments it is evident that tebuconazole, procymidone and chlorothalonil are ineffective in controlling growth of *S. Vesicarium* isolated from onion and asparagus (Aveling *et al.*, 1993 and Grinstein *et al.*, 1988). As opposed to this field trials indicate that chlorothalonil and procymidone reduce to some extent the occurrence of Stemphylium leaf spot of onion and asparagus, respectively (Grinstein *et al.*, 1988). At high concentrations, some chemicals such as mancozeb, azoxystrobin, propiconazole and propineb inhibit *in vitro* fungal growth of *S. Vesicarium* isolated from onion (Mishra and Gupta, 2012).The propiconazole has been proved effective against *S. vesicarium*in asparagus (Hausbeck &Bousds, 2005), lentil (Huq & Khan, 2007) and onion (Vyas, 2000; Gupta & Gupta, 2014), whereas the effectiveness of mancozeb has been reported on onion (Srivastava *et al.,* 1992 and Vyas, 2000) and garlic (Kumar *et al.*, 2011). However, there is only limited number of literature available on the effectiveness of chemical treatments to control *Stemphylium* spp. on garlic. Regular spray of tebuconazole or procymidone during vegetative phase of growth of garlic inhibited the incidence of leaf spots caused by *S. Vesicarium* in Europe (Basallote*et al.*1998). Furthermore, mancozeb and flusilazole were suggested to be the most effective fungicides for the control of *S. Solani* in Chinese garlic fields by Zheng *et al.*, 2008. Thus it is obvious that judicious application of fungicides can effectively reduce the incidence of Stemphylium leaf blight and consequently augment the overall bulb yield.

Suitable integration of more than one efficient treatments like fungicides, bioagents in combination with appropriate cultural control may provide a better management of the Stemphylium blight disease in onion and garlic. However, in integrated approach of diseases management under organic crop production, bio-insecticide (neembicidine) and bio-control agent (*T. harzianum*) may be looked upon as promising alternative for the management of purple blotch and Stemphylium blight of onion and garlic.

Refrences

Abdel-Hafez,S.I.J, Abo-Elyousr, K.A.M and Abdel-Rahim, I.R. (2013). Effect of certain plant extracts to control purple blotch disease of onion plants (*Allium cepa*). *J. Phytopathol.* 162:567-574

Alberoni, G., Cavallini, D., Collina, M., and Brunelli, A. (2010). Characterisation of the first *Stemphylium vesicarium* isolates resistant to strobilurins in Italian pear orchards. *European Journal of Plant Pathology* 126 (4): 453–457.

Anonymous. (2013). A new disease of garlic Stemphylium blight discovered. http://aripatna.com.> accessed 1 May, 2013.

Aveling, .T.A.S. and Naude, S.P.(1992). First report of Alternaria porri on garlic in South Africa. *Plant Dis.*76:643.

Aveling, T.A.S., Synman, H.G. and Naude, S.P. (1993). Evaluation of seed treatments for reducing *Alternaria porri* and *Stemphylium vesicarum* on onion seed. *Plant Dis.* 77:1009–1011.

Barnwal, M.K., Prasad, S.M. and Maiti, D. (2003). Efficacy of fungicides and bioagents against *Stemphylium*blight of onion. *Indian Phytopathology,* 56(3): 291-292.

Basallote- Ureba, M. J., Prados Ligero, A.M. and Melero Vara, J.M. (1999). Aetiology of leaf spot of garlic and onion caused by *Stemphylium vesicarium* in Spain. *Plant Pathology* 48:139–145.

Basallote, M.J., Prados, A.M., Pégrez, de., Algaba, A. and Melero, J.M.(1993). First report in spain of two leaf spots of garlic caused by Stemphylium vesicarium. *Plant Dis.*77:952.

Basallote-Ureba, M.J., Prados, A.M., Melero-Vara JM. (1998). Effectiveness of tebuconazole and procymidone in the control of Stemphylium leaf spots in garlic. *Crop Prot.* 17:491–495.

Bessey, E.A. (1968). Fungi imperfecti: The imperfect fungi. In: Morphology and Taxonomy of Fungi. New York: Hafner Publishing Company pp. 572–627.

Bisht, I.S. and Agrawal, R. C. (1993) Susceptibility to purple blotch (*Alternaria porri*) in garlic (*Allium sativum*).*The Annals of Applied Biology* 122: 31-38.

Bock, C.H., Poole, G.H., Parker, P.E., and Gottwald, T.R. (2010). Plant disease severity estimated visually, by digital photography and image analysis, and by hyperspectral imaging.

Brewster, J.L. (2008). Onions and Other Vegetable Alliums. 2nd ed. Cambridge, MA: CAB International.

Câmara, M.P.S., O'Neill, N.R., and van Berkum, P. (2002). Phylogeny of *Stemphylium* spp. based on ITS and glyceraldehyde-3-phosphate dehydrogenase gene sequences. *Mycologia* 94 (4): 660–672.

Conn, K.E., Lutton, J. S. and Rosenberger, S. A.(2012). Onion disease Guide, A practical guide for seedsmen, growers and agricultural advisors. Seminis Vegetable Seeds, Inc.

Critical Reviews in Plant Sciences 29 (2): 59–107.

Currah, L. and Proctor, F.J. (1990). Onions in Tropical Regions. *Natural Resource Institute Bulletin* 35, Chatham, UK.

Davis, R.M., Hao, J.J., Romberg, M.K., Nunez, J.J., and Smith, R.F. (2007). Efficacy of germination stimulants of sclerotia of Sclerotium cepivorum for management of white rot of garlic. *Plant Disease* 91(2), 204-208.

DOGR (2015-16) http://dogr.res.in/index.php/en/download/20-downloads/69-statistic

DOGR(2018-19) http://dogr.res.in/index.php/en/download/20-downloads/69-statistic

Dugan, F.M., Hellier, B.C. and Lupien, S.L. (2007). Pathogenic fungi in garlic seed cloves from the United States and China, and efficacy of fungicides against pathogens in garlic germplasm in Washington state. *J. Phytopathol.* 155:437–445.

Etoh, T. and Simon, P.W. (2002). Diversity, fertility and seed production of garlic. *Allicrop science Evolution* 11: 130-162.

Falloon, P.G., 1987. Etiology and epidemiology of stemphylium leaf spot and purple spot of asparagus in California. *Phytopathology* 77 (3): 407-413.

Falloon, P.G, Falloon, L.M. and Grogan, R.G.(1987). Etiology and epidemiology of Stemphylium leaf spot and purple spot of asparagus in California. *Phytopathology.*77:407–413.

Figliuolo, G.C., Logozzo, V., Miccolis, G.V. and Spagnoletti, Z.P.L. (2001). Genetic evaluation of cultivated garlic germplasm (*Allium sativum* L. and *Allium ampeloprasum* L.). *Euphytica* 3: 325-334.

Fritsch, R.M. and Friesen, N. (2002). Evolution, domestication and taxonomy.*In*: H.

Gálvez,L., Gil-Serna, J., García, M., Iglesias,C. and Palmero, D. (2016). *Stemphylium* Leaf Blight of Garlic (*Allium sativum*) in Spain: Taxonomy and *In Vitro* Fungicide Response. *Plant Pathol J.* 32(5): 388–395.

Grinstein, A., Frankel, H., Austerweil, M. and Kritzman, G. (1988). Air-assisted placement spraying for *Stemphylium* control in seed onions. *Crop Prot.* 7:356-360.

Gupta, R. C. and Gupta, R. P. (2014). Epidemiological studies on *Stemphylium vesicarium* causing Stemphylium blight disease of onion (*Allium cepa* L.). *The Indian Journal of Agricultural Sciences*. 84: 9.

Gupta, R.P., Srivastava, P.., and Sharma, R. (2010). Plant health management. In: National Horticultural Research and Development FoundationNashik Report FoundationNashik Report. Maharashtra, India: The Directorate: National Horticultural Research and Development Foundation, pp. 13–15.

Hanelt, P. (1990). Taxonomy, evolution and history. In: H..Rabinowitch and J.L. Brewster, eds. *Allium* and allied crops Vol. I. Botany, Physiology and Genetics. Florida: CRC Press, pp. 1–26.

Hassan, M.H.A., Allam, A.D.A., Abo-Elyousr, K.A. M., and Hussein, M.A.M. (2007). First report of stemphylium leaf blight of onion caused by *Stemphylium vesicarium* in Egypt. *Plant Pathology* 56 (4): 724–724.

Hausbeck, M. and Bousds. R. (2005). New products for onion disease management. *Vegetable Production and Marketing News*. 15: 5.

Hausbeck, M.K. (2005). Pest management in the future, a strategic plan for the Michigan onion industry Workshop Summary Michigan State University East Lansing, MI. Available from: http://www.ipmcenters.org/pmsp/pdf/MIonion.pdf [Accessed 8 May 2015]

Heath, O.V. and Hollies, M. (1965). Studies in the physiology of the onion plant. *Journal of Experimental Botany* 16 (46): 128–144.

Hoepting, C. (2015). Managing Stemphylium leaf blight - Spray by number to prevent fungicide resistance. Cornell Cooperative Extension Vegetable Program. *Onion World* pp. 6-8.

Huq, M. I. and Khan, A. Z. M. N. A. (2007). Efficacy *in vivo* of different fungicides in controlling Stemphylium blight of lentil during 1998-2001. *Bangladesh Journal of Scientific and Industrial Research*. 42 (1): 89-96.

Hussein, M.A.M., Hassan, M.H.A., Allam, A.D.A. and Abo-Elyousr, K.A.M. (2007). Management of stemphylium blight of onion by using biological agents and resistance inducers. *Journal of Phytopathology*, 35(1), 49-60.

Ipek, M., Ipek, A. and Simon, P.W. (2003).Comparison of AFLPs, RAPD markers, and isozymes for diversity assessment of garlic and detection of putative duplicates in germplasm collections. *J. Amer. Soc., Hort. Sci.* 128: 246-252.

Ipek, M., Ipek, A., Almquist, S.G. and Simon, P.W. (2005). Demonstration of linkage and development of the first low-density genetic map of garlic, based on AFLP markers. Theor. *Appl.Genet.*110:228-236.

Jakhar, S.S., Duhan, J.C., and Suhag, L.S. (1996). Studies on conidial germination and factors affecting disease development of stemphylium blight of onion. Indian Phytopathology 49 (4): 362–365.

Johnson, D.A. (1990). Effect of crop debris management on severity of Stemphylium purple spot of asparagus. *Plant Dis*., 74: 413–415

Kamal, A.E. M., Mohamed, H.M., Aly, A. D., and Mohamed, H. H. (2008). Enhanced onion resistance against Stemphylium leaf blight disease, caused by *Stemphylium vesicarium*, by di-potassium phosphate and benzothiadiazole treatments. *Plant Pathology Journal* 24 (2): 171–177.

Kamal, A.M., Abo-Elyousr, Sobhy, I.I., Abdel-Hafez and Ismail, R. A. (2017). Control of stemphylium leaf blight disease of onion and elevation of seed production using certain bioagents. *International Journal of Plant Pathology,* 8:1-7.

Katoch, S. and Kumar,S. (2016). Status, distribution and symptomatology of Stemphylium blight of garlic in Himachal Pradesh *Himachal Journal of Agricultural Research* 42(2): *184-186*

Kik, C. (2008). Allium genetic resources with particular reference to onion. In: O. Dae- Geun and K. Chieri, (eds.). Proc. XXVII IHC - Cultivation and Utilization. Asian, Sub-Tropic, Underutilized Horticultural Crops. Wageningen: Acta Horticulture, pp. 135–138.

Kirtikar, K.R., Basu, B.D. (1975). International Book Distributors, Dehradun, *Indian Medicinal Plants*, Vol II, 4th ed., 1325-27.

Köhl, J., Groenenboom-De Haas, B., Goossen-Van De Geijn, H., Speksnijder, A., Kastelein, P., De Hoog, S., and Gerrits van Den Ende, B. (2009). Pathogenicity of *Stemphylium vesicarium* from different hosts causing brown spot in pear. *European Journal of Plant Pathology* 124: 151–162.

Koike, S.T., O'Neill, N., Wolf, J., Van Berkum, P. and Daugovish, O. (2013).Stemphylium leaf spot of parsley in California caused by Stemphylium vesicarium. *Plant Dis.* 97:315–322.

Kumar, U., Naresh, P. and Biswas, S.K. (2012). Ecofriendly management of stemphylium blight (*Stemphylium botryosum*) of garlic by plant extract and bioagents. *HortFlora Research Spectrum*, 1(1): 42-45.

Kumar, U., Singh, J., Prem, N. and Singh, R.(2011). Management of Stemphylium blight of garlic through chemicals. *Ann Pl Prot Sci.* 19 (1):126-128.

Lamprecht, S.C., Baxter, A. and Thompson, A.H. (1984).Stemphylium vesicarium on Medicago spp. in South Africa. *Phytophylactica.*16:73–75.

Llorente, I. and Montesinos, E. (2006). Brown spot of pear: an emerging disease of economic importance in Europe. *Plant Dis.* 1368–1375.

Llorente, I., Moragrega, C., Ruz, L., and Montesinos, E. (2012). An update on control of brown spot of pear. *Trees - Structure and Function* 26: 239–245.

Lorbeer, J.W. (1993). A serious outbreak of Stemphylium leaf blight of onion in New York. in: Proceedings of the 1993 National Onion Research Conference. Ithaca, NY, USA.: Cornell University, pp. 32–37.

Lorbeer, J.W. (1993). A serious outbreak of Stemphylium leaf blight of onion in New York. In: Proceedings of the 1993 National Onion Research Conference. Ithaca, NY, USA.: Cornell University, pp. 32–37.

McCollum, G.D. (1987). Onion and allies Evolution of crop plants in N.W. Simmonds (ed.) Longman S. & T. *London, England* 186-190.

Mentha, Y.R. (1998). Severe outbreak of Stemphylium leaf blight, a new disease of cotton in Brazil. *Plant Dis.* 82:333–336.

Meyer, M.P., Hausbeck, M.K., and Podolsky, R. (2000). Optimal fungicide management of purple spot of asparagus and impact on yield. *Plant Disease* 84 (13): 525–530.

Miller, M.E., Taber, R.A. and Amador, J.M. (1978) Stemphylium blight of onion in South Texas. *Plant Dis Rep.*62:851–853.

Miller, M.E., Taber, R.A., and Amador, J.M. (1978). Stemphylium blight of onion in South Texas. *Plant Disease Reporter* 62 (10): 851–853.b 2016].

Misawa, T. and Yasuoka, S. (2012). The life cycle of *Stemphylium vesicarium,* the causal agent of Welsh onion leaf blight. *Journal of General Plant Pathology* 78: 18–29.

Mishra, R. K., Jaiswal, R. K., Kumar, D., Saabale, P. R. and Singh, A. (2014). Management of major diseases and insect pests of onion and garlic: A comprehensive review. *Journal of Plant Breeding and Crop Science.* 6(11): 160-170.

Mishra, R.K. and Gupta, R.P. (2012). In vitro evaluation of plant extracts, bio-agents and fungicides against Purple blotch and Stemphylium blight of onion. *Journal of Medicinal Plants Research,* 6(48): 5840-5843.

Mishra, R.K., Verma, A., Singh, S., and Gupta, R.P. (2009). Screening of garlic lines against purple blotch and stemphylium blight. *Pest Management in Horticultural Ecosystems* 15 (2): 138–140.

Nasehi, A., Kadir, J.B., Esfahani, M.N., Mahmodi, F., Ghadirian, H., Ashtiani, F.A and Golkhandan, E. (2013). An outbreak of leaf spot caused by Stemphylium solani on eggplant in Malaysia. *Plant Dis.* 97(689):2.

Nasehi, A., Kadir, J.B., Esfahani, M.N., Mahmodi, F., Ghadirian, H., Ashtiani, F.A. and Soleimani, N.(2013). Leaf spot on lettuce (Lactuca sativa) caused by Stemphylium solani, a new disease in Malaysia. *Plant Dis.* 97(689):3.

Pathak, S.S., Black, S.J., Cherng, T.C., and Ko, S.S. (2001).Breeding onions for stemphylium leaf blight resistance. Proc. II IS Edible Alliaceae Acta Horticulturae 555: 77–81.

Polat, Z., Besirli, G., Sönmez, I. and Yavuz, B. (2012). First report of Stemphylium leaf blight of garlic (Allium sativum) caused by Stemphylium vesicarium in Turkey. *New Dis Rep.* 25:29.

Prados-Ligero, A.M., González-Andújar, J.M., Melero-Vara ,J.M. and Basallote-Ureba, M.J. (1998). Development of Pleospora allii on garlic debris infected by Stemphylium vesicarium. *Eur J Plant Pathol.* 104:861–870.

Prasad, S.M. and Barnwal, M.K. (2004). Evaluation of plant extracts in management of Stemphylium blight of onion. *Indian Phytopathology*, 57(1): 110-111.

Rabinowitch and L. Currah (eds.). *Allium Crop Science: Recent Advances .New York: CAB International,* 5–30.

Raghayendra, N.N. and Pavgi, M.S. (1975). Stemphylium leaf blight of onion. *Mycopathologia* 56:113–118.

Rao, R.N.N. and Pavgi, M. (1975). Stemphylium leaf blight in onion. *Mycopathologia* 56 (1): 1–6.

Reis, A., Boiteux, L.S., Fonseca, M.N.(2011). Identification of solanaceous and non-solanaceous species as hosts of Stemphylium solani isolates in Brazil. *Phytopathology* 101:152.

Roddy, E. (2011). Asparagus diseases - Purple spot (*Stemphylium*) [online]. Available from: http://www.omafra.gov.on.ca/english/crops/hort/asparagus-diseases-purplespot. htm Accessed 11 Fe

Schwartz, H.F. and Mohan, S.K. (2008).Compendium of onion and garlic diseases and pests. APS Press; St. Paul, MN, USA. 127.

Shanmugasundaram, S., Kalb, T. (2001). Suggested cultural practices for onion. AVRDC training guide. Shanhua, Taiwan. www.http://www.avrdc.org.

Simmons, E.G. (1967).Typification of *Alternaria*, *Stemphylium*, and *Ulocladium*. Mycologia, 59 (1): 67.

Singh, B.M. and Sharma, Y.R. (1997).Occurrence of leaf blight of garlic caused by *Stemphylium botryosum* in India. *Indian phytopathology* 30: 272-273.

Singh, P., Park, P., Bugiani, R., Cavanni, P., Nakajima, H., Kodama, M., Otani, H., and Kohmoto, K. (2000). Effects of host-selective SV-toxin from *Stemphylium vesicarium*, the cause of brown spot of European pear plants, on ultrastructure of leaf cells. *Journal of Phytopathology* 148 (2): 87–93.

Srivastava, K. J., Srivastava, P. K. and Gupta, R. P. 1992. Management of garlic disease in India. *News letter AADF*. 12: 4.

Sugha, S. K. and Kumar, S. (2005). Outbreak of Stemphylium blight of garlic in Himachal Pradesh. *J. Plant Disease Research (Ludhiana)* 20(2): 190-191

Suheri, H. and Price, T. V. (2000). Infection of onion leaves by *Alternaria porri* and *Stemphylium vesicarium* and disease development in controlled environments. *Plant Pathology* 49 (3): 375–382.

Suheri, H. and Price, T. V. (2001). The epidemiology of purple leaf blotch on leeks in Victoria, Australia. *European Journal of Plant Pathology* 107 (5): 503–510.

Suheri, H., and Price, T.V.(2000). Stemphylium leaf blight of garlic (Allium sativum) in Australia. *Australas Plant Pathol.*29:192–199.

Tomaz, I..and Lima, A. (1988). An important disease of onion caused by *Stemphylium vesicarium* (Wallr.) Simmons in Portugal. *Horticultural Abstracts* 68: 618.

Tsiaganis, M.C., Laskari, K. and Melissari, E. (2006). Fatty acid composition of Allium species 40 lipids. *J. of Food Composition and Analysis* 19: 620-627.

Vakalounakis, D.J., Markakis, E.A.(2013). First report of Stemphylium solani as the causal agent of a leaf spot on greenhouse cucumber. *Plant Dis.*97:287–288.

Vavilov, N.I. (1951). The origin, variation, and immunity and breeding of cultivated plants. *Economic Botany.* 13: 1–6.

Velisek, J., Kubec, R. and Davidek, J. (1997). Chemical composition and classification of culinary and pharmaceutical garlic-based products. *Z Lebensem Unters Forsch*. 204: 161–164.

Vyas, U. M. (2000). Investigation on Stemphylium blight of onion (*Allium cepa* L.) caused by *Stemphylium vesicarium* (Wallr.) Simmons. Comb. nov. M.Sc. (Agri.) Thesis (Unpublished) Gujarat Agricultural University, Sardarkrushinagar, Gujarat.

Wolpert, T.J., Dunkle, L.D., and Ciuffetti, L.M. (2002). Host-selective toxins and a virulence determinants: what's in a name? *Annual Review of Phytopathology* 40: 251–285.

Wright, M.G., Hoffmann, M.P., Kuhar, T.P., Gardner, J., and Pitcher, S. A. (2005). Evaluating risks of biological control introductions: A probabilistic risk-assessment approach. *Biological Control* 35: 338–347.

Zheng, L., Huang, J. and Hsiang, T. (2008). First report of leaf blight of garlic (Allium sativum) caused by Stemphylium solani in China. *Plant Pathol.* 57:380.

Zheng, L., Lv, R., Huang, J., Jiang, D., Liu, X. and Hsiang, T. (2010). Integrated control of garlic leaf blight caused by Stemphylium solani in China. *Can J Plant Pathol.* 32:135–145.

20

Diagnosis of Bacterial Diseases of Solanaceous Vegetable Crops

Dinesh Singh[1] and Amit K Kesharwani[1,2]

[1]*Division of Plant Pathology, ICAR- Indian Agricultural Research Institute New Delhi -110 012, India*
[2]*Amity Institute of Biotechnology, Amity University Campus, Noida-201303 India*

Abstract

Bacterial diseases of solanaceous crops like tomato, brinjal, chilli, capsicum and potato are the most serious and destructive diseases affecting both under field and greenhouse conditions. Under moist field conditions they can cause epidemics to affect total crop loss, quality of the produce and reduce market value. These diseases can be distinguished from each other on the basis of their symptoms appearance of the various parts of the plant as well as by using advanced techniques of diagnosis. Diagnosis of the disease is important step to detect pathogen at early stage of disease and subsequently manage it effectively in efficient manner.

Keywords: Bacterial diseases, solanaceous crops, symptoms, diagnosis.

Introduction

Bacterial diseases of solanaceous crops like tomato, brinjal, chilli, capsicum and potato are the most serious and destructive diseases affecting both under field and greenhouse conditions. Under moist field conditions they can cause epidemics to affect total crop loss, quality of the produce and reduce market value. These diseases can be distinguished from each other on the basis of their symptoms appearanceofthe various parts of the plant as well as by using advanced techniques of diagnosis. Diagnosis of the disease is important step to detect pathogen at early stage of disease and subsequently manage it effectively in efficient manner. Therefore, the early detection of the bacterium from asymptomatic plants, soil, and water and plant residues could facilitate elimination and certainly reduce the risk of crop loss. Powerful tools for the identification and detection of the bacterium in diverse substrates (plant, seed, water and soil) are available for diagnosis of the bacterial diseases. DNA amplification of pathogen offers many advantages over classical techniques; neither purification nor cultivation of the pathogen is required and the specificity, sensitivity and response time of tests are improved. Nevertheless, the PCR method has not yet become a routine diagnostic tool for many laboratories, mainly because of the inhibition of the amplification reaction by compounds contained in crude bacterial extracts, which give false negative results or low detection sensitivity.

Materials and Methods

Population of plant pathogenic bacteria on/ in the seeds, soil and crop residues are declined in the absence of host and survive comparatively for lesser period than the wilted plants. Sometimes the bacteria could not be detected even through common PCR method. Therefore, to improve the sensitivity of PCR primer, enrichment of targeted bacteria is done by incubating samples on general or selective media followed by PCR with specific primers has been used earlier to detect bacteria from samples. A list of bacterial diseases of solanaceous crops is given Table 1. Most common diseases of solanaceous crops such as bacterial leaf spot, canker, wilt, soft rot and common scab are discussed in detail particularly diagnosis of diseases.

Table 1: List of bacterial diseases of solanaceous crops.

Sr. No.	Name of disease	Causal organism	Host	Mode of survival
1.	Bacterial Canker	Clavibacter michiganensis subsp. michiganensis	Tomato, capsicum, chili	Seed borne, transplant
2.	Bacterial speck	Pseudomonas syringae pv. tomato	Tomato	Seed borne, field as long as there is infected crop debris
3.	Bacterial spot	Xanthomonas spp.	Tomato, capsicum, chili	Seed borne, crop residues and soil
4.	Bacterial stem rot and fruit rot	Pectobacterium carotovorum subsp. carotovorum, P. atrosepticum and Dickeya spp. (Formely Erwinia carotovora subsp. carotovora)	Tomato, potato	Seed tuber, crop residues and soil
5.	Syringae leaf spot		Tomato, capsicum, chili	Seed borne, crop residues and soil
6.	Pith necrosis	Pseudomonas corrugata	Tomato	infected plant debris and soil, seed
7.	Bacterial wilt	Ralstonia solanacearum	Tomato, capsicum, chili eggplant, potato	Soil borne, seed
8	Crown gall	Rhizobium radiobacter (previously Agrobacterium tumefaciens)	Tomato, capsicum, chili	Soil
9.	Common scab	Streptomyces scabies	Potato	Tuber and soil
10.	Ring rot	Clavibacter michiganensis subsp. sepedonicus	Potato	Seed potato, plant and soil debris, potato bags, machinery and other equipment

Results and Discussion

1. Bacterial spot of tomato and capsicum

The disease symptoms appear all the aerial parts of the plant. Spots are generally brown, circular and up to 3 mm in diameter both on leaves and stems. In the presence of dew during rainy season, these spots become dark colour water soaked and with and without any halo yellow around it. Later the spots coalesce together and lightening of foliage takes place by giving scorchy appearance. On young fruits, lesions appear as small, dark slightly raised dots, sometimes with a narrow water soaked borders. On mature green fruits, the spots appear as brownish-black elevated scab like areas 2 to 6 mm in diameter with feathered or irregular margins.

The disease is caused by a relatively diverse set of bacterial strains within the genus *Xanthomonas*; strain nomenclature and classification for the strains that infect pepper and tomato plants have gone through considerable taxonomic revision in recent years. For a long time, it was described as *X. vesicatoria* (Doidge) Dawson as a causal organism of bacterial leaf spot. After a number of earlier revisions, (Dye 1978) proposed the name *X. campestris* pv. *vesicatoria*. Phenotypically and phylogenetically, this pathovar was shown to be composed of at least four different populations, all of which are pathogenic on tomato; those groups are named groups A, B, C and D (Vauterin *et al.,* 1995; Jones *et al.,* 2004). Based on DNA± DNA hybridization studies and accordingly bacteriological code, species level elevation of all four groups are name group A as *Xanthomonas euvesicatoria,* group B as *X. vesicatoria,* group C *X. perforans* and group Das *X. gardneri*. Presently, bacterial leaf spot causing xanthomonands are placed in four different species, viz.*Xanthomonas euvesicatoria*, *X. vesicatoria, X. perforans*and *X. gardneri*(Jones *et al.,* 2004).The main host plants of *X. vesicatoria*, *X. euvesicatoria* and *X. gardneri* are tomato and pepper, *X. perforans* affects mainly tomato but there is one report on affecting the pepper. Some races infect both pepper and tomato (P/T strains), whereas other races are specific for tomato (T races) or pepper (P races). On pepper 11 races have been reported based on the pathogenicity reaction on pepper differentials having five resistance genes in peppers *Bs1*, *Bs2*, *Bs3*, *Bs4*(Stall *et al.*, 2009).

The pathogen is rod shaped, gram negative, strictly aerobic, motile by with a single polar flagellum, forms colonies yellow in colour, liquefies gelatine, attacks, starch and digests protein and measures 0.7-1.0 x 2.0-2.4 µm. However, on nutrient agar, it grows relatively slowly and is smooth, flat glistening, convex, circular with fringed margins, measuring 1 cm after 4 days. An EPPO quarantine procedure has recently been developed (OEPP/EPPO, 1992) involving a preliminary screen of seed extract by immunofluorescence (IF), followed by isolation, serological testing (slide agglutination, IF or dot-ELISA; Lazarovits *et al.*, 1987) and, if necessary, confirmatory pathogenicity tests on leaves. EPPO diagnostic protocols PM 7/97(1) and PM 7/101(1) describe indirect immunofluorescence tests and ELISA tests for use with validated antibodies (EPPO, 2009, 2010). Tests are performed on seed or plant extracts and their 10-fold dilutions.

Koenraadt *et al.* (2007) have developed four species specific primers for identification of all four species of xanthomonads associated with bacterial spot of pepper and tomato species based AFLP based approach. For *X. vesicatoria*, Bs-XvF and Bs-XvR primers; for*X. euvesicatoria*, Bs-XeF and Bs-XeR primers; for *X. Perforanse*, Bs-XpF and Bs-XpR primers and for*X. gardeneri*, Bs-XgF and Bs-XgR amplifying fragment of 138 bp, 154 bp, 173 bp and 197 bp respectively. Moretti*et al.* (2009) developed the *X. euvesicatoria* specific primer set Xeu2.4 and Xeu2.5 which amplifies 208 bp specific regions from repetitive extra genic palindromic sequence of *X. euvesicatoria*. They reported that primer set developed by specific and consistence result with high sensitivity. Araujo*et al.* (2013) further validated the species specific primers developed by Koenraadt *et al.* (2007) developed a multiplex- PCR assay for simultaneous detection of all four species associated with bacterial leaf spot of pepper and tomato. Beran and Mraz (2013) developed *X. vesicatoria* specific primer that amplify *atp* D at 104 bp and proposed use of primer set for detection and identification this bacterium. Araujo*et al.* (2013) has also developed *X. vesicatoria* specific primer that amplify *gyr*B gene at 104 bp and proposed for further validation for using in identification and detection.

2. Bacterial canker of tomato

Plants at all stage of growth are susceptible to the disease. Infected seedlings may be quickly killed, or they may produce weak, stunted plants. The early symptoms of the disease are wilting, curling of leaflets, and browning of leaves, often only on one side of the plant. As the leaves die, the petioles remain green and firmly attached to the stem. On the fruit, the spots have a dark brown center, which becomes raised, and are surrounded by a distinct white halo; they have been termed "bird's-eye spots." Wilting progresses until the entire leaflet dies. Splitting of the stem lengthwise reveals reddish brown discoloration follows the phloem.

The disease is caused by *Clavibactermichiganensis* subsp. *michiganensis.* The bacterium is an aerobic, non-spore forming and Gram- positive. This pathogen can be isolated on Yeast peptone glucose agar (YPGA). It produces yellow colonies on nutrient agar. The colonies reach 3-4 mm in diameter after 5 days of incubation. The bacteria can also be isolated on specific medium SCM medium. Bacterial cells can be pleomorphic in nature, but rod shaped when isolated from plants. Optimum growth can occur at 24 -27^{0}C. Bacteria can occur on the seed coat as well as within the embryo. Seed borneinoculums may serve as one source of the bacterium. Immunofluorescence is the labeling of antibodies or antigens with fluorescentdyes, which is often used to visualize the subcellular distribution of biomolecules of interest. IF has been used in France for at least 20 years to assay tomato seeds for IF has been used in France for at least 20 years to assay tomato seeds for *C.michiganensis* subsp. *michiganensis*. In immunofluorescence colony-staining(IFC) method to assay seed health incorporates seed extract with an equal volume of agar medium. The mixture is incubated, dried, and exposed to target bacterium-specific antibodies conjugated with a fluorescent dye. Colonies stained with the antibody-dye conjugate can be visualized with fluorescent microscopy, and bacteria inside the colonies can be isolated with a glass capillary tube and transferred to a suitable growth medium. IFC was optimized for detecting *Xanthomonas campestris* pv. *vesicatoria (Xcv*) and *C.michiganensis*subsp. *michiganensis* (Nemeth *et al.*, 2006).

Molecular detection of *C. michiganensis* subsp. *Michiganensis* from seedlings and grafted plants, ISSR marker was used by Baysal*et al.*(2011). The PCR protocol suggested in EPPO standards PM 7/42 was used to confirm the pathogen by PCR. The primers were used as Forward primer PSA-4: (50-TCA TTG GTC AAT TCT GTCTCC C-30) and Reverse primer PSA-R: (50-TAC TGA GAT GTT TCA CTT CCC C-30)as developed by Pastrik and Rainey (1999). Improved the recommended detection protocol of EPPO (Anonymous, 2005), *i.e.* development of a new semi-selective medium (Ftayeh *et al.*, 2008) in combination with highly specific PCR primers (Bio-PCR) (Ftayeh *et al.*, 2009).

3. Bacterial wilt of solanaceous crops

Characteristic symptoms of bacterial wilt on most of the hosts are rapid and resulting in complete wilting of normal grown up plants. During wet and warm climatic conditions, the most conspicuous symptom seen on tomato plants is sudden drooping of leaves, without yellowing often accompanied by rotting of the stem. The roots appear healthy and often are well developed. Pathogen is mostly confined to vascular region. In advance cases, it may invade the cortex and pith and cause yellow brown discolouration of tissues. In potato, initial symptoms of the disease are slight wilting or drooping of foliage especially at end of branches during hot period of the day which recover at sunset. Later the leaves become yellow, the wilting become permanent and the plant collapse. Cross section of the stem reveals browning of vascular bundles and bacterial slime ooze out of vascular region. Bacterial mass emerges through the affected eyes of the tubers to which soil adheres at harvest. Freshly cut tubers show glistening droplets of bacterial ooze emerging from the vascular ring.

The disease in causal by *Ralstonia solanacearum* (Yabbuuchi *et al.,* 1995). The bacterium is gram negative, rod shaped, frequently occurs in pairs, motile with 1 to 4 polar flagella and measures 0.5-0.7 x 1.5-2.5 µm. It is aerobic and catalase and oxidase-positive and forms nitrites from nitrates. It, like some other non-fluorescent pseudomonads, produces intracellular, refractile, sudanophilic inclusions consisting of polyhydroxy-butyric acid. Some strains produce a brown diffusible pigment on complex media and a black pigment on autoclaved potato slants. The pathogen is negative for levan production and starch hydrolysis. Virulent isolates on tetrazolium chloride medium develop fluidial irregular shaped colonies with white to pinkish centre (Kelman, 1954) whereas avirulent types produce small round, dark red dry colonies.

Chakravarti *et al.* (1993) standardized the protocol of alkaline phosphatase based DAS-ELISA to detect *P. solanacearum* either from infected stems or tubers using antiserum produced against formalin killed bacteria (race 1). Robinson-Smith *et al.* (1995) developed both polyclonal and monoclonal antibodies to detect *R. solanacearum.* The polyclonal antibodies, when used with an indirect enzyme-linked immunosorbent assay detected *R. solanacearum* from infected plant or soil samples, but they were not able to distinguish between *R. solanacearum, P. celebensis, P. syzygii* and *P. picketti.* Further serological tests on *R. solanacearum* were carried out by Baharuddin *et al.* (1994) and since then there have been many serological kits developed to detect *R. solanacearum* from water, plant tissue and soil.

Rapid methods to detect pathogen in potato have been developed by Weller *et al.*(2000), Singh *et al.* (2014). Standardization of PCR and real time PCR analysis for the detection of latent infection by *R. solanacearum* where the organism survives in low number could play an important role in detection of the disease in the seed. The disease can be detected in conventional PCR assay ranging from 10^4 CFU ml^{-1} (Khakvar *et al.,* 2008) to 10^5 CFU ml^{-1}. PCR based methods for the detection of *R. solanacearum* are usually based on the amplification of ribosomal sequences (16S RNA or ITS region). Molecular based detection of *R. solanacearum* causing bacterial wilt of tomato, chilli, brinjal and potato done by using specific primers Y2 and OLII amplified at 288bp. The primer was also able to distinguish the *R. solanacearum* from other saprophytic bacteria through colony PCR within 2 days (Singh *et al.,* 2010). Because of high degree of conservation bacteria cannot be differentiated at species level, which can lead to positive signal to related species. To improve the sensitivity of a single round PCR, various modifications have been employed viz., enrichment in semi-selective SMSA broth prior to PCR, real time BIO-PCR (Ozakman and Schaad, 2003;Singh *et al.,* 2014; Ranjan *et al.,* 2016) and nested PCR (Khakvar *et al.,* 2008). DNA detection tools for reliable detection of latent infection by *R. solanacearum*, therefore, need to be standardized further to detect minimal amount of disease in large seed lots.For detection of *R. solanacearum* from asymptomatic tomato plants, *hrp* B-based sequence primers (Hrp_rs2F and Hrp_rs2R) amplified at 323 bp was used in bio-PCR to detect *R. solanacerarum* from crown, mid part of stem and upper parts of the plant (Singh *et al.,* 2014). Multiplex polymerase chain reaction (PCR)protocol was developed for simultaneous detection of *R. solanacearum* and *E. carotovora*subsp. *carotovora* frompotato tubers. A set of oligos targeting the pectatelyase (pel) gene of *E. carotovora* subsp. *Carotovora* and theuniversal primers based on 16S rRNA gene of*R. solanacearum* were used. The standardized multiplex PCR protocol could detect *R. solanacearum* and *E. carotovora*subsp. *Carotovora* up to 0.01 and 1.0 ng of genomic DNA, respectively (Ranjan *et al.,* 2016). Sebastien *et al.* (2014) developed a multiplex real-time PCR method to detect simultaneously *Clavibactermichiganensis* subsp. *sepedonicus* and *R. solanacearum,* causing ring rot and brown rot disease in potato respectively. The detection limit of developed duplex was at least 100 cfu/ml of potato macerate for each pathogen.

The LAMP technique utilizes a strand displacement strategy and is one of the most prominent of these methods explored to date. LAMPassays have been developed for *R. solanacearum*. The method as first described by Notomi et al. 2000 makesuse of four specially designed primers, a pair of outer primers and a pair of inner primers, which together recognize six distinct sites flanking the amplified DNA sequence. In place of heat denaturation of double-stranded DNA as in PCR, the LAMP reaction relieson a DNA polymerase with particularly highstrand displacement activity to remove newly amplified strands. Because of the hybrid design of the inner primers, amplified DNA structures take on a loop configuration at one or bothends of the elongated strands, which in turnserve as stem-loop structured templates forfurther displacement DNA synthesis. The final amplified product consists of a mixture of stem loop DNA strands with various stem lengths and structures with multiple loops. The rateof DNA amplification can be accelerated, and specificity increased, by additional loop primers designed to hybridize to the loop structure and uniquely amplify the stem-loop strands. The LAMP assay has captured the imagination of many in the world of diagnostics because its specific advantages make it suitable for adoption in on-the-spot testing devices. It canbe done in an essentially equipment-free environment. Only a water bath or heating block is needed to maintain temperature in the range of 60–68°C. LAMP assays are particularly specific because hybridization to at least six sites is required for the reaction to proceed and, as with other DNA amplification methods, the LAMP assay has exquisite sensitivity. Adetection level as low as 2 pg µl"1 of template DNA was achieved to detect latent stage wheat stripe rust infections. Methods for end-product analysis include direct visualization under ultraviolet light by addition of DNA-intercalating fluorescent dyes and, invisible light using other colorimetric procedures, measurement of turbidity caused by accumulation of insoluble salts from reactionof metal ions with the pyrophosphate ion, hybridization of single-stranded amplicons to DNA microarrays and detection with electrochemical sensors. LAMP assays can also be configured in real-time quantitative formats. Another attractive feature of the LAMP method for on-site testing is its tolerance to template contaminants (Peng *et al.,* 2013).

4. Bacterial soft rot and black leg of potato

On tubers, the disease appears as small soft water soaked spots around lenticels which enlarge under high humidity. The pith of infected tuber decay beyond the boundary of external lesion, turn cream to tan brown in colour and the tissues becomes soft and granular. A brown to black pigment may develop around the lesion. Immature, large tubers damaged by bruises at harvest, tubers infected with late blight and those grown with high nitrogen fertilizer especially ammonium chloride are more prone to soft. The soft rot affected tubers become slimy and foul smelling and brown liquid oozes out from the affected tubers. Blackleg symptoms appear on foliage at any stage of potato plant but are more frequent in dense canopies under warm and wet weather. The disease develops from soft rot affected tubers. A soft black lesion appears at base of stem which extend from the decaying mother seed tuber in soil to a little above ground level. The affected plants become stunted, exhibit yellow chlorotic foliage, wilt and die without producing fresh tubers.

The pathogen such as *Pectobacteriumatrosepticum* (van Hall) Gardan *et al.*(2003) (syn. *Erwiniacarotovora* subsp. *atroseptica*), *Pectobacteriumcarotovorum* subsp. *carotovorum* (Jones) Hauben *et al.*(1998) (syn. *Erwiniacarotovora* subsp. *carotovora*), *Dickeya* spp. (including *D. dianthicola, D. dadantii, D. zeae*) (syn. *Erwiniachrysanthemi*), *Bacillus polymyxa,B. subtilis,B. mesentericus,B. megaterium* de Bary, *Pseudomonas marginalis* (Brown) Stevens, *P. viridiflava* (Burkholder) Dowson, *Clostridium* spp., *Micrococcus* spp., and *Flavobacterium* have been reported to cause soft rot. *Pectobacteriumatrosepticum* the primary enterobacteria causing soft rots are gram negative bacteria, rod shaped with peritrichus flagella which can grow both under aerobic and anaerobic conditions, produce pectolytic enzymes and degrade pectin in middle lamella of host cells, breakdown tissues and cause soft rot and the decay. Czajkowski*et al.* (2015) studied on detection, identification and differentiation of soft rot causing pathogen *Pectobacterium* and *Dickeya* sp. using biochemical characters, serology, molecular techniques, which rely on DNA sequence amplification as well as several less investigated one. Multiplex polymerase chain reaction (PCR) assay was developed by Potrykus*et al.* (2014) for simultaneous detection of the main soft rot and blackleg potato pathogens in Europe. It utilized three pairs of primers and enables detection of three groups of pectinolytic bacteria frequently found in potato, *viz.,P. atrosepticum*, *P. carotovorum* subsp. *carotovorum* together with *Pectobacteriumwasabiae* and *Dickeya* spp. in a multiplex PCR assay. The developed assay was able to detect minimum of 0.01 ng of genomic DNA of *Dickeya* sp., and down to 0.1 ng of *P. atrosepticum* and *P. carotovorum* subsp. *carotovorum* genomic DNA *in vitro*.

5. Common scab of potato

Scab lesions on tubers may be shallow, raised or sunken. Symptoms on young tubers begin as inconspicuous round minute brown specks, less than 1mm in diameter under stomata or young lenticels. The lesions are initially shallow and typically circular with definite margin. As the lesion increase in size the periderm crack due to formation of cork layer around lesions and assume various shapes such as reticulate, shallow or deep pitted. The lesions may coalesce to affect large area on tuber surface. The lesions on mature tubers may be mere abrasions; star shaped with corky depositions; concentric wrinkled layers of cork around a central black core; raised and rough corky pustules or 3 to 4 mm deep pits surrounded by hard corky tissue. Tubers which protrude above ground are not invaded and tubers which grow faster than other develop higher infection. Quick bulking varieties in general suffer more than slow bulking varieties. The tuber lesions being corky and hard are generally not affected by secondary organisms and do not affect storage life of the produce. Russet scab of potato is a major problem in North- western plains especially in early crop (Arora *et al.*, 2006). The disease appears on potato tuber surface as brown netted or irregular superficial abrasions. Lesions of russet scab can also appear on emerging sprouts, stolon's, stem base besides potato tubers (Aroraand Jyotsana, 2007).

At least 13 different *Streptomyces* spp. have been found to cause common scab on potato worldwide. The prominent among them are *Streptomyces scabies* (Thaxter) Lambert and Loria, *S. acidiscabies* Bambert and Loria, *S. turgidscabis* Takeunchi, *S. collinus* Lindenbein; *S. griseus* (Krainsky) Waksman & Henria, *S. Longisporoflavus*, *S. cinereus*, *S.violanceoruber*, *S.alborgriseolus*, *S. griseoflavus*, *S. catenulae* and others. *Streptomces* are bacteria which resemble fungi due to formation of vegetative substrate mycelium that develop aerial filaments. However, the filaments are of smaller dimensions than the true fungi. These filaments produce spores through fragmentation. The pathogenic species produce thaxtomins which are phytotoxins and cause hypertrophy and cell death. *S. scabies* form grey, spiral spore chains on several media and produce brown pigment whereas *S. acidiscabis* produce peach coloured wavy chains of spores and brown pigment in medium.The identification and taxonomy of *Streptomyces* spp. has been based on morphological and physiological characteristics combined with thaxtomin production and pathogenicity tests *in vitro* and *in vivo*. Ability to produce thaxtomin toxin is strongly correlated with the pathogen's pathogenicity.

Diagnostic assays based on PCR have been developed to detect the pathogen (Cullen *et al.*, 2000). Recently, molecular techniques have become more important. DNA-based methods enable fast and accurate detection of thaxtomin and identification of various *Streptomyces* spp. Although *Streptomyces* taxonomy is complex, phylogenetic analysis using 16S ribosomal (r)RNA gene sequencing and DNA-DNA hybridization have been used successfully for species-level identification. The highly conserved genes responsible for pathogenicity among genetically diverse *Streptomyces* isolates are ideal molecular markers for determination of pathogenicity. The *nec1* gene, for example, is thought to be highly conserved in both structure and function among unrelated pathogenic *Streptomyces* spp., and is not known to be present in non-pathogenic species.

6. Bacterial speck of tomato and pepper

Bacterial speck is a common disease of tomato that occurs worldwide wherever tomatoes are grown. The disease can substantially reduce yield when it severely affects leaves early in the growing season. The disease can have an even greater impact on quality (and marketability for commercial tomato producers) when symptoms occur on tomato fruit. The disease can be diagnosed by appearance of the symptoms on leaf as speck consist of small black spots (approximately [! - ¼ inch in dia.) that often are more prominent on the undersides of leaves and as disease progress, a yellow halo may develop around the edge. Spots on fruit are very small (almost pinpoint-like) and do not penetrate very deeply into the tissue. The spots can be raised, flat or sunken, and range in color from brown to black. On unripe, green fruits, the spots often have darker green haloes, while on ripe fruits, the spots can have subtle, yellow haloes.

Bacterial speck of tomato is caused by the bacterium *Pseudomonas syringae* pv. *tomato*. Another diagnostic tool that has been reported to be reliable and fast is Biolog (Biolog Inc., Hayward, CA, USA) metabolic profiling. The Biolog system has been efficiently used in the identification of the isolates to the species level, as 53 of the 56 (94.6%) isolates of*P. syringae* pv. *Tomato* was identified as *P. syringae*. However, only 23 isolates out of the 56 (41.1%) were identified as *P. syringae* pv. *tomato*. The results of this work indicate the existence of *P. syringae* pv. *tomato* isolates that differ significantly from those used to create the Biolog database (Shenge *et al.,* 2008).

Antibodies were developed to the somatic, flagellar, cytoplasmic, and titers to the somatic and extracellular antigens of *P.syringae* pv. *tomato*. Precipitin tests have a little diagnostic value since antibodies to the cytoplasmic extracellular antigens cross-reacted with antigens of other bacteria and plant extracts. Conversely, agglutination tests are stable, sensitive, and differential. Long-term immunization increased titers to the somatic and flagellar antigens to 16,000 and reduced cross-reactivity. Elimination of polysaccharides from the immunogen and from the test antigen further reduced cross-reactivity (Fackrell and Sinha, 1983). Serological techniques such as indirect fluorescent antibody staining (IFAS) and enzyme-linked immunosorbent assay (ELISA) are also commonly used in some laboratory. All these approaches are laborious and time-consuming, not well suited for the high throughput screenings required for seed and plant certification programmes.

The molecular identification of *P. syringae* pv. *tomato* is often based on the isolation of bacteria in semi-selective media (VBTar) coupled to DNA hybridization using coronatine synthesis genes as probes (Cuppels *et al.,* 1990). RFLP analysis showed that the isolates were highly conserved in their *hrpZ* gene. The low level of genomic diversity within the pathogen shows that there is a possibility to use resistant tomato varieties as part of an effective integrated bacterial speck management plan (Shenge *et al.,* 2008).

PCR amplification of the *cfl* gene was reported by Bereswill *et al.* (1994) for the identification and genetic diversity analysis of coronatine-producing *P. syringae* pathovars. To approach the problem of developing a rapid and sensitive diagnostic tool for high-throughput screenings of infected tomato plants, a PCR method for the amplification of an internal fragment of hrpZPst. P. *syringae* pv. *tomato* hrpZ is a chromosomal gene located in the hrp/hrc pathogenicity island, which is essential for symptom production in host plants and hypersensitive response in non-hosts (Alfano and Collmer, 1997). Nevertheless, pathovar-specific sequences with appropriate (G+C)% content and potential for primer design was designed. The two oligonucleotide primers chosen for further analyses were MM5F (5¢- GAACGAGCTGAAGGAAGACA-3¢) and MM5R (5¢-CAGCCTGGTTAGTCTGGTTA-3¢), which amplify a 532-bp fragment from hrpZPst. The reaction mixture (50 µl) contained 0.4 lM of each primer, 200 lM of dNTPs, 2.5 mM of $MgCl_2$ and 1 U of Taq-DNA polymerase. The amplification programme consisted of a denaturation at 94°C for 5 min followed by 36 cycles of denaturation at 94 C for 1 min, annealing at 57°C for 1 min and extension at 72°C for 1 min, with a final extension at 72°C for 10 min and soak at 4°C. The amplicons are visualized by standard agarose gel electrophoresis and ethidium bromide staining. The expected pathovar-specific 532 bp amplification product is produced from all the *P. syringae* pv. *tomato* isolates, including the three coronatine-deficient isolates, but not from the other pathogenic and symbiotic bacterial isolates belonging to the genera *Pseudomonas, Xanthomonas, Erwinia, Rhizobium and Mesorhizobium*. Adetection threshold of 200 cells (determined as CFU on KB-agar) per PCR reaction tube when suspensions from pure cultures are used. When asymptomatic tomato plant materials which had been experimentally contaminated were used, detection threshold was 2.5×10^5 and 2.5×10^6 cells (CFU) per gram of leaves and seeds respectively. The detection threshold obtained with asymptomatic leaf tissue is comparable with or lower than that obtained using a nonradioactive DNA hybridization probe from the coronatine gene (Cuppels *et al.,* 1990). This PCR protocol is suitable for specific detection of *P. syringae* pv. *tomato* in pure culture and in symptomatic and asymptomatic tomato plant materials (Zaccardelli *et al.,* 2005).

7. Pith necrosis of tomato

Initial symptoms often appear just as the first fruit clusters reach the mature green stage and consist of yellowing and wilting of young leaves. Serious infections can result in chlorosis and wilting of upper portions of plants with brown to black lesions on infected stems and petioles. When stems are cut longitudinally, the center of the stem (pith) may be extensively discolored, hollow, and/or degraded. Stems may be swollen, numerous adventitious roots can form, and infected stems may shrink, crack, or collapse. The disease is caused by *Pseudomonas corrugate* (ex. Scarlett *et al.,* 1978). The strains in six different *Pseudomonas* species including *P. viridiflava*, *P. cichorii*, *P. corrugata*, *P. mediterraneae*, *P. fluorescens*, and unidentified *Pseudomonas* sp. were proven to be the causal agents of pith necrosis. Based on FAME analysis, *Pseudomonas* strains had 35 different fatty acids, respectively. For isolation of pathogen, diseased stem tissue is homogenized with a mortar and pestle in sterile water and extract is streaked onto King's B medium agar. Initially, colonies appear on the medium as white and smooth and after 5 days had irregular surface and margin and produced a tan diffuse pigment. The bacterium isnon-fluorescent *Pseudomonas* species. Gram-negative, rod-shaped, aerobic with multitrichous polar flagella, oxidase-positive, non-spore forming, grew at 37°C on nutrient broth yeast agar and was arginine dihydrolase positive (Powell *et al.,* 2013). *P. corrugata* produces wrinkled and, rarely, smooth colonies on yeast peptone glucose agar or nutrient dextrose agar; yellow to brown diffusible pigments are frequently produced. The *P. corrugata* species epithet "corrugata" refers to the typical morphology of bacterial colonies on NDA; slightly raised, with a wrinkled-rough surface and undulate margins that produce a yellow diffusible pigment (Scarlett *et al.,* 1978). It builds up medium sized chains of poly (hydroxyl alkanoates), and is incapable of producing levan (Catara *et al.,* 2002).

The available information about serological characterization of *P. corrugata* is limited to the serological variability among *P. corrugata* isolates observed on tube agglutination and detection of some isolates by enzyme-linked immunosorbent assay (ELISA) (Fiori *et al.,* 1983; Naumann *et al.,* 1990). *P. corrugata* lies in the possibility of developing specific methods for detection and identification and contributing to knowledge of the phenotypical heterogeneity of this species. The variation in biochemical and serological features of 128 isolates of *P. corrugata* has been studied with 56 isolates from Spain and 72 isolates from other countries. Isolates were analyzed with common diagnostic tests and with the API50CHE system. Variability among isolates for some standard tests usually listed as positive or negative for this species, such as arginine dihydrolase and gelatin hydrolysis, lipase and lecithinase activities, pigment production, and wrinkled colony morphology, was observed. Three antisera were raised against the type strain and two Spanish isolates from tomato and pepper plants. Serological reactions were studied by indirect immunofluorescence and indirect enzyme-linked immunosorbent assay. Eighty-three isolates reacted with a single antiserum, 6 reacted with two antisera, and none reacted with three antisera. Thirty-nine isolates did not react with any of the three antisera. These results suggest that serology will not be a useful method for routine diagnosis of *P. corrugata* unless common antigens can be identified. Electrophoresis and immune electrotransfer were used to study the antigens involved. Each antiserum reacted with whole-cell lysates, giving two common bands for *P. corrugata* isolates and other *Pseudomonas* species and a ladder-like pattern characteristic of lipopolysaccharides (LPS). Common bands were not observed after proteinase K treatment. More than 10 LPS patterns were distinguished in 98 isolates after silver staining of polyacrylamide gels. There was no correlation between the geographical origin or host of the isolates and the LPS patterns. A correlation between LPS groups and serological reaction was observed (Siverio *et al.,* 1993).

Catara *et al.* (2000) observed unique DNA bands from strains representative of two groups of *P. corrugata*, as shown by amplification of their genomic DNA by polymerase chain reaction using short random sequence oligonucleotide primers (RAPD-PCR), were isolated, cloned and sequenced. RAPD-PCR was performed using the above reaction mix with 10 pmol of the single OPA primer.

Two pairs of specific primer sequences, based on the ends of the cloned unique DNA bands from strains IPVCT10.3 and IPVCT8.1, were used in multiplex PCR with a range of *P. corrugata* strains. All strains produced one of the two specific bands, 1100 bp (from the IPVCT10.3-based primers) and 600 bp (from the IPVCT8.1-based primers), representing groups designated I and II, respectively. The primers were also tested on a wider range of *Pseudomonas* species, including the closely-related fluorescent *Pseudomonas* genomospecies FP1, FP2 and FP3: none of these bacteria produced any bands following amplification by PCR with these primers. The primer sets detected *P. corrugata* in tomato pith necrosis-infected plants providing a useful tool for rapid identification and epidemiological studies.Identification of *P. corrugata* and *P. mediterraneae* strains were confirmed by amplification of 1100 and 600 bp DNA fragment in PCR studies, respectively (Saygili *et al.,* 2008). Licciardello *et al.* (2011) developed a quantitative real-time PCR assay to screen tomato planting material reliably and to detect and/or discriminate both bacterial pathogens in a single tube. They designed two species-specific primer/probe sets on the sequences of two DNA fragments amplified. New real-time PCR primers were: PcoFw (5'-GGTGGTATCGGTTGCGTAGCG-3') and PcoRew (5'-GTGGGAACGTTTGGGCCTGG-3') for *P. corrugata* detection, amplifying a 149 bp DNA fragment, and PmeFor (5'-CTGTCCGAGACGATGGCGAC-3') and PmeRew (5'-CAGACGTGGCCTCAAGCAGAT-3') for *P. mediterranea* detection, amplifying a 85 bp DNA fragment. The corresponding probes were designed within the DNA segments to allow fluorescent detection of amplification and labelled with different reporter molecules: Pco (5'FAM-CCGCCCCATCTGCCCACCCTGC-3'BHQ-1) and Pme (5'TXR-CCCGCTCATCCGCTGGACCGGC-3'BHQ2) for *P. corrugata* and *P. mediterranea*, respectively. TaqMan real-time PCR assays were developed for individual (simplex PCR) and simultaneous (duplex PCR) amplifications. The assays were performed with the SmartCycler TD II System (Cepheid) and the fluorescence from both FAM and Texas Red channels were recorded at the annealing step. Specificity was tested with an extended range of *P. corrugata* and *P. mediterranea* strains, with other *Pseudomonas* spp. and with a number of tomato bacterial pathogens. The detection limit was approximately 10 cells per reaction for both bacteria, and quantification was linear over a six-log range. The duplex real-time PCR assay was validated on tomato plants artificially inoculated by pricking the stem with a strain of each species either separately or together.

8. Syringae leaf spot of tomato and pepper

The syringae leaf spot in tomato and pepper may be diagnosed based on symptomology as brown spots that lack a halo, to dark brown or black spots with bright yellow halos appear on leaves and they look very similar to those of bacterial speck. However, the leaf spots from syringae leaf spot can be larger than those of bacterial speck. Initial symptoms that developed 2-10 days after transplanting consisted of water soaked circular lesions (2-3 mm in dia.) on stem and petioles. These lesions eventually coalesced into brown to black areas as much as 1 cm in dia. In some cases, necrotic areas progressed from stem to petioles to leaf tissues. Thereafter plants wilted and died within a few days (Garibaldi *et al.,* 2007). The disease is caused by *P. syringae* pv. *syringae*. On nutrient yeast dextrose agar medium, light yellow colonies typical of *Pseudomonas* spp. are appear after 48h at 22±1°C. All colonies are levan production andtobacco positive and oxidase, potato soft rot and arginine dihydrase negative (LOPAT test group Ia), The colonies fluoresced under UV light when grown on King's B medium. Further all, isolates are positive for arbutin and aesculin hydrolysis and utilized erythitol but not adanitol, 1 (+)- tartrate or dl-homoserine as carbon source (Scortichini *et al.,* 2003). Most isolates were similar to pv. *syringae* in producing syringomycin, in using erythritol and DL-lactate as substrates, and in forming ice nuclei. The isolates typically caused necrotic leaf spots with halos on the cowpea cv. California Blackeye and necrotic reactions on the peach cv. Lovell, both known hosts of *P. syringae* pv. *syringae*, whereas pv. *tomato* usually caused no necrotic symptoms. The new bacterium also caused brown necrotic lesions without halos on leaves of the tomato cv. Chico III after infiltration with inoculum or when wound-inoculated. Evidently a fluorescent pseudomonad other than *P. syringae* pv. *tomato* can cause necrotic lesions on tomato transplants and additional testing is needed to differentiate these bacteria during certification procedures (Jones *et al.,* 1981). The pathogen also cause disease on pepper seedlings (*Capsicum annuum* cv. *Kurtovska kapija* (Mitrev *et al.,* 2000).

9. Crown gall

Crown gall disease is diagnosed as round, wart-like growths-2 inches or larger in diameter that appears at or just above the soil line, or on lower branches and stems. Plants with several galls may be unable to move water and nutrients up the trunk and become weakened, stunted and unproductive. Young plants can be killed by developing gall tissue. Crown gall is caused by *Agrobacterium* strains harbouring a Ti-plasmid (pTi)a Gram-negative, strictly aerobic, bacilliform rods measuring 1 x 3 µm, and whose nutritional requirements are non-fastidious. On solidified agar such as Yeast Mannitol (YM) medium, colonies of agrobacteria are white to cream colored, smooth, convex, glistening circular with entire edges and mucoid (Shams*et al.,* 2012). When *Agrobacterium* spp. is allowed to growth on carbohydrate containing media, considerable extracellular polysaccharide slime layers are often secreted, leave colonies a voluminous and slimy appearance (Murugesan, 2010). The rods bear flagella that are arranged subpolarly around the cylindrical circumference of the cell, referred as circumthecal flagellation that is normally associated with the roots of many different plants in the field. Disease symptoms are initiated by the transfer of a DNA fragment (T-DNA) located on pTi into the genome of recipient plant cells. In transformed plant tissues the T-DNA encodes genes that induce gall formation at the infection site. *Agrobacterium* strains were isolated from galls using semi-selective Schroth's medium and identified by fatty acid profiling (Stead *et al.,* 1992) as *Agrobacterium* biovar 1 strains (*A. radiobacter*). Based on some distinct phenotypic differences, *A. tumefaciens* isolates were originally classified into three biotypes or biovars (biotype I, II and III; biovar 1, 2, and 3). Biotype I or biovar 1 strains produce 3-ketosugars and usually have wide host ranges. Biotype II or biovar 2 strains mainly classify as the hairy root-forming organism, *A. rhizogenes*. Biotype III or biovar 3 isolates are mainly confined to grapevines, prefer L-tartaric acid over glucose and produce polygalacturonase. his system, basedon biochemical features encoded by chromosomal genes disagreed with the traditional species classification. However, the results of various taxonomic studies based on conventional, chemotaxonomic, numericaland DNA-based methods such asDNA: DNAhybridization, sequence analysis of16SrDNAand 23S rDNA indicate that biovaridentity of *Agrobacterium* is a reliable taxonomic trait.

A PCR assay (Pulawska and Sobiczewski, 2005) showed these strains possessed pTi. On the basis of 23S rRNA gene sequences, 1 universal forward and 4 taxon(species/biovar)-specific reverse primers were designed for multiplex PCR to aid in identification and differentiation of *Agrobacterium rubi*, *A. vitis* and *Agrobacterium* biovars 1 and 2. The primers developed for identification of *A. vitis*, *A. rubi* or *Agrobacterium*biovar 1 amplified only DNA of strains belonging to these taxa, producing fragments of the expected sizes Biovar 1(184 bp), Biovar 2 (1066 bp), *A. vitis* (478 bp) and *A. rubi* (1006 bp) with primers UFf (GTAAGAAGCGAACGCAGGGAACT), B1R r (GACAATGACTGTTCTACGCGTAA) B2Rr (TCCGATACCTCCA GGGCCCCTCACAA), vRr (AACTAACTCAATCGCGCTATTAACA), rRr (AAAACAGCCACTACGACTGTCTT). However, in the case of the primer developed for identification of *Agrobacterium* biovar 2, the characteristic 1066 bp PCR product was obtained not only with DNA of this biovar, but also with DNA of 3 atypical biovar 1 strains and some rhizobial strains. Differentiation between *Agrobacterium* biovar 2 and the other strains was possible using the restriction analysis of this product with endonuclease *Alw*26I. The method developed is an excellent tool for rapid classification of these 4 taxa of *Agrobacterium*. The affected tomato plants were located in a glasshouse previously affected with another *Agrobacterium*-induced disease, known as root mat and caused by strains harbouring a root-inducing Ri-plasmid (Weller *et al.*, 2000). Between-season amendment of soil with composted green waste eradicated root mat in this glasshouse. Ri-plasmid harbouring strains were not detected in the crown gall affected crop (Weller *et al.,* 2006).

10. Ring rot of potato

The symptoms shown by infected plants are variable and can sometimes be mistaken for potato blight, wilt or stem canker. The first symptoms are wilting in the lower leaves, either all around the plant or on one side of the plant. The margins of the leaves roll inwards and upwards and the leaf surface lose its light shiny appearance. Leaves become progressively dull light green, then grey-green with occasional mottling, then yellow and finally brown and necrotic. Symptoms are enhanced by hot, dry weather conditions. Tuber infection occurs through the stolon. The initial symptom is a soft cheese-like rotting of the vascular ring (hence the name "ring rot"). In severe cases the vascular ring rots completely and the skin of the potato may crack. External symptoms may consist of reddish brown blotches around the eyes, or irregular shaped cracks on the skin.

The disease is caused by *Clavibacter michiganensis* subsp. *sepedonicus* (Spickermann and Kotthoff, 1914) Davis *et al.,* 1984. The bacterium is Gram positive, non-motile, non-spore-forming and approximately 0.4-0.6 ìm x 0.8- 1.2 ìm. Cells are coryneform rods, slightly curved and club shaped, arranged singly or in pairs in L or V formations). It is strictly aerobic and nutritionally fastidious, requiring a specialized media such as NCP-88. When plated on to NCP-88, colonies of *C. michiganensis* subsp. *sepedonicus*are visible within 5 days at 25°C, and measure 0.5-1.5 mm in diameter after 7-10 days. The colonies are round to irregular with entire margins, white to cream in colour, raised, and usually mucoid and glistening. After 10-12 days of incubation, colonies become pale yellow (de la Cruz *et al.,* 1992). The bacterium can hydrolyse soluble starch, and utilize acetate, citrate and succinate. It can produce acid from the oxidation of mannitol and sorbitol. It cannot produce H_2S from the decomposition of organic sulphur compounds or from the reduction of sulphate under anaerobic conditions. It is unable to produce and maintain stable acid end products from glucose fermentation. The majority of *C. michiganensis* subsp. *Sepedonicus* bacterial cultures on agar medium are of the mucoid colony type, although intermediate- and nonmucoid-type strains are also found. Acidic bacterial exopolysaccharides (EPSs), which are produced in *C. michiganensis* subsp. *sepedonicus*, are also found in other subspecies of *C. michiganensis*. Bacterial EPSs protect the bacterial cells against moisture loss, whereas they inhibit transpiration and cause wilting in the plant through the physical occlusion of vascular bundle walls. Earlier attempts involved immunodiffusion, latex agglutination, and indirect fluorescent antibody staining. However, the sensitivity and specificity of these methods are unsatisfactory. Although *C. michiganensis* subsp. *sepedonicus*is a bacterial subspecies characterized by a relatively high phenotypic homogeneity, it exhibits diverse EPS levels, which makes immunological diagnosis difficult. Owing to numerous problems in the development of highly specific, sensitive polyclonal antibodies, most studies have been directed toward the production of monoclonal antibodies. The use of monoclonal antibodies has significantly improved the specificity of immunofluorescence assay-type serological tests (IFAS).However, it has also led to reduced sensitivity of detection and increased costs. Moreover, 9AI monoclonal antibodies, which are used in IFAS directed against an antigen from the bacterial cell walls, are not suitable for enzyme linked immunosorbent assay (ELISA). By contrast, monoclonal antibodies directed against polysaccharide components are highly sensitive in ELISAs. However, such antibodies are useful only for strains with high EPS levels, and they produce false positive results due to cross-reactivity with *C. michiganensis* subsp. *michiganensis* and *C. michiganensis* subsp. *insidiosus*. Using monoclonal antibodies, this assay enables the detection of 1×10^5 to 5×10^6 bacterial cells/ml of suspension. With current polyclonal antibodies, *C. michiganensis* subsp. *Sepedonicus* bacterial cells do not act as detectable antigens in ELISA. Instead, detection is mainly based on the free polysaccharides from mucus New Antibody for *C. michiganensis* subsp. *sepedonicus*. All currently available polyclonal and monoclonal antibodies are characterized by high levels of nonspecific reactions giving false-positive results, which precludes a definitive diagnosis. Bacteria are detected using a triple antibody sandwich (TAS-ELISA), in which the 1H3 monoclonal antibody constituted the primary antibody. However, the results were still unsatisfactory: nearly 20% of the samples giving positive PCR results were identified as negative in ELISA tests (Przewodowski and Przewodowska, 2017).

Polymerase chain reaction (PCR) based detection of *C. michiganensis* subsp. *sepedonicus* appears to have the potential to circumvent many of the problems currently associated with detection of this phytopathogen. PCR reactions using primers specific to *C.michiganensis* subsp. *sepedonicus* was detectable strains, including phytopathogens, did not produce any amplification products. *C. michiganensis* subsp. *sepedonicus* was detectable from a mixture of potato and bacterial DNA by amplification of a DNA sequence specific to *C. michiganensis*subsp. *sepedonicus*. Detection by DNA amplification allowed direct processing of plant tissue samples, and circumvented the need for prior isolation of the suspected phytopathogen (Schneider *et al.,* 1993).

Oligonucleotide primers derived from sequences of the 16S rRNA gene (CMR16F1, CMR16R1, CMR16F2, and CMR16R2) and insertion element IS1121 of *C. michiganensis* subsp. *Sepedonicus* (CMSIF1, CMSIR1, CMSIF2, and CMISR2) were used in nested PCR to detect the potato ring rot bacterium *C. michiganensis* subsp. *sepedonicus*. Nested PCR with primer pair CMSIF1-CMSIR1 followed by primer pair CMSIF2- CMSIR2 specifically detected *C. michiganensis* subsp. *sepedonicus*, while nested PCR with CMR16F1-CMR16R1 followed by CMR16F2-CMR16R2 detected *C. michiganensis* subsp. *sepedonicus* and the other *C. michiganensis* subspecies. In the latter case, *C. michiganensis* subsp. *sepedonicus* can be differentiated from the other subspecies by restriction fragment length polymorphism (RFLP) analyses of the nested PCR products (16S rDNA sequences). The nested PCR assays developed in this work allow ultrasensitive detection of very low titers of *C. michiganensis* subsp. *sepedonicus* which may be present in symptomless potato plants or tubers and which cannot be readily detected by direct PCR (single PCR amplification). RFLP analysis of PCR products provides for an unambiguous confirmation of the identity of *C. michiganensis* subsp. *sepedonicus* (Lee *et al.,* 1997)

A new multiplex PCR assay has been developed for the detection of *C. michiganensis* subsp. *sepedonicus* in potato tubers. The assay combines two different tests in one reaction mixture. First, a highly specific and sensitive detection of the pathogen and second, an indicator test for successful amplification (internal PCR control), which monitors potentially false-negative PCR results, caused by inhibition of the PCR. For the simultaneous amplification of two different targets in one reaction mixture, a mix of two different primer sets was used. For the detection of *C. michiganensis* subsp. *sepedonicus*, a pathogen-specific primer set PSA-1/PSA-R was used, based on the intergenic spacer region of the 16S–23S rRNA genes of *C. michiganensis* subsp. *sepedonicus*. For the simultaneous amplification of the internal PCR control, the plant-specific primer set NS-7-F/NS-8-R was employed, permitting amplification of target sequence from plant DNA present in DNA extractions from potato core fluid. The applicability of the multiplex PCR was verified in 3500 composite samples of 200 seed potato tubers from 143 different cultivars in a survey for *C. michiganensis* subsp. *sepedonicus* by parallel testing using immunofluorescence, a bioassay in eggplant seedlings and multiplex PCR.

Real-time PCR, with TaqMan probes that utilize the 52 exonuclease activity of Taq polymerase to separate quencher and fluorophore moieties on labeled probes, permits measurement of amplified product as the reaction proceeds. By adding a DNA-binding dye such as SYBR Green, postreaction melt analysis of amplicons can also be conducted to confirm amplicon identity directly in the reaction tube. At least three real-time amplification methods for the detection of *C. michiganensis* subsp. *sepedonicus* have been used. A nucleic acid sequence based amplification (NASBA) method, designed for epidemiological studies, enabled the detection of viable *C. michiganensis* subsp. *sepedonicus* cells. A second method targeting the intergenic ribosomal DNA region and utilizing conserved primers and variable TaqMan probes was developed for differentiating subspecies of *C. michiganensis*. A third method was formulated as a real-time BIO-PCR assay in which target bacteria are multiplied in a semi-selective medium prior to DNA extraction. An internal reaction control was integrated into a TaqMan polymerase chain reaction (PCR) assay for the detection of *C. michiganensis* subsp. *sepedonicus*. The reaction control, cloned into plasmid pCmsC4, consisted of a sequence unrelated to *C. michiganensis* subsp. *sepedonicus* flanked by the primer sequences used in the TaqMan PCR. Inclusion of the reaction control plasmid in the TaqMan assay had no effect on either the limit of detection or the specificity of the method. Addition of SYBR Green permitted melt analysis of PCR products. The 242-bp reaction control amplicon, with a melt temperature of approximately 94.5°C, could easily be distinguished from the 152-bp primary diagnostic target amplicon, which had a melt temperature of about 85.5°C. Electrophoretic analysis showed that appearance of either melt peak correlated well with the presence of the appropriate amplicon. Two different substances, guanidine-HCl and humic acid, inhibited the amplification of the reaction control at concentrations lower than those that inhibited the primary diagnostic target, demonstrating the reaction control's effectiveness in detecting inhibition or reaction failure. Using the reaction control plasmid, a quantitative threshold for inhibitor detection was established. This permitted the validation of negative results, and thus facilitated the use of TaqMan real-time PCR in the routine testing of diagnostic samples for *C. michiganensis* subsp. *sepedonicus*(Smith *et al.*, 2008).

Table 2: List of semi-selective medium for each specific pathogen

Primary Target	Medium	References
Agrobacterium tumefaciens	MacConkey agar Clark's selective medium (NASA)	Bopp *et al.*, 1999 Serfontein and Staphorst, 1994
*Clavibacter*sp.	D2	Kado and Heskett, 1970
Clavibacter michiganensis	mSCM	Waters and Bolkan,1992
Clavibacter michiganensis subsp. *sepedonicus*	NCP-88	de la Cruz *et al.*, 1992
Pseudomonas spp.	S1 & S2	Gould *et al.*, 1985
P. syringae pathovar	BC*BRVB*	Braun-Kiewnick and Sands, 2001
P. syringae pv. *tomato*	VBTar	Cuppels and Elmhirst 1999; Cuppels *et al.*, 1990
Ralstonia solanacerum	SMSA, TTC	Elphinstone *et al.*,1996, Singh *et al.*, 2014
Xanthomonas spp.	Tween A,B,C	McGuire *et al.*, 1986

Table 3: List of primer sets for detection and identification of phytopathogenic bacteria

Phytopathogenic bacteria	Primer sequences	Product of primer	References
Agrobacterium strains	Primer VCF: 5'- ATC ATT TGT AGC GACT-3'Primer VCR:5'- AGC TCA AAC CTG CTT C-3'	730bp	Sawada *et al.*, 1995
A. vitis, *A. rubi* or *Agrobacteriumtumefaciens biovar 1, 2*	UFf: 5'- GTAAGAAGCGAACGCAGGGAACT-3' B1Rr: 5'-GACAATGACTGTTCTACGCGTAA-3B2Rr: 5'-TCCGATACCTCCAGGGCCCCTCACAA-3'vRr: 5- AACTAACTCAATCGCGCTATTAACA-3'rRr: 5'- AAAACAGCCACTACGACTGTCTT-3'	184 bp (bv-1)1066 bp (bv-2)478 bp (*A. vitis*), 1006 bp *(A. rubi)*	Pulawska and Sobiczewski, 2005
Clavibacter michiganensis sub sp. *michiganensis*	CMM5: 5'- GCG AAT AAG CCC ATA TCA A-3' CMM6:CGT CAG GAG GTC GCT AAT A-3'	614bp	Dreier *et al.*, 1995
Clavibacter michiganensis sub sp. *michiganensis*	PSA-4: 5'-TCA TTG GTC AAT TCT GTCTCC C-3' PSA-R: 5'-TAC TGA GAT GTT TCA CTT CCC C-3'	279 bp	Flores *et al.*, 2009
C. michiganensis subsp. *sepedonicus*	fD2: 5'- AGA GTT TGA TCA TGG CTC AG-3'rD1: 5'- AAG GAG GTG ATC CAG CC-3'	1600bp	*Weisburg et al.*, 1991
C. michiganensis subsp. *sepedonicus*	CMS6: 5'- CGCTCTCCCTCACCAGACTC-3'CMS7: 5'- TCCCGTGCTTGCCTGCGTTG-3'	450 bp	Schneider *et al.*, 1993; Hu *et al.*, 1995
C. michiganensis subsp. *sepedonicus*plant-specific primer	PSA-1: 5'- CTC CTT GTG GGG TGG GAA AA-3' PSA-R: TAC TGA GAT GTT TCA CTT CCC C-3'S-7-F: 5'-GAG GCA ATA ACA GGT CTG TGA TGC-3'NS-8-R: 5'- TCC GCA GGT TCA CCT ACG GA-3'	502 bp377 bp	Pastrik, 2000
C. michiganensis subsp. *sepedonicus*	ivr-fl: 5'- CCGGATCGTCATGCTCTACA-3'ivr-rl : 5'- GTGCCGATCGCGTAGTAGTC-3'	495bp	Smith *et al.*, 2008
Dickeya sp. *(Pectobacterium chrysanthemi)*	5'-GAAGTCGTAACAAGG-3'5'-CAAGGCATCCACCGT-3'	171bp	Peiqian Li *et al.*,2011
E. carotovora sub sp.	Y45: 5'- TCA CCG GAC GCC GAA CTG TGG CGT-3'Y46:	438bp	Frechon *et al.*, 1995

atroseptica	5'- TCG CCA ACG TTC AGC AGA ACA AGT-3'		
E. chrysanthemi	ADE1: 5'- GATCAGAAAGCCCGCAGCCAGAT-3'ADE2:5' -CTGTGGCCGATCAGGATGGTTTTGTCGTGC-3'	420bp	Nassar *et al.*, 1996
Pseudomonas	Ps-for: 5'- GGT CTG AGA GGA TGA TCA GT-3'Ps-rev: TTA GCT CCA CCT CGC GGC-3'	1018bp	Widmer *et al*, 1998
P. syringae pv. *tomato*	MM5F:5'- GAACGAGCTGAAGGAAGACA-3' MM5R: 5'-CAGCCTGGTTAGTCTGGTTA-3'	532 bp	Bereswill *et al.*, 1994
P. corrugataP. mediterranea	PcoFw: 5'-GGTGGTATCGGTTGCGTAGCG-3' PcoRew: 5'-GTGGGAACGTTTGGGCCTGG-3' PmeFor:5'-CTGTCCGAGACGATGGCGAC-3') PmeRew: 5' -CAGACGTGGCCTCAAGCAGAT-3'	149 bp85 bp	Licciardello *et al.*, 2011
P. fluorescens, *P. aureofaciens*	PCA2a: 5'- TTG CCA AGC CTC GCT CCA AC-3'PCA-3b: 5'- CCG CGT TGT TCC TCG TTC AT-3'	1150bp	Raaijmakers *et al.*, 1997
P. syringae	D21: 5'- AGCCGTAGGGGAACCTGCGG-3'D22: 5'-TGACTGCCAAGGCATCCACC-3'	558bp	Manceau and Horvais, 1997
P. syringae	Primer1: 5'- GGCGCTCCCTCGCACTT-3'Primer2: GGTATTGGCGGGGGTGC-3'	650bp	Bereswill *et al.*,1994
P. syringae pv. *syringae*, *atrofaciens, aptata*	B1: 5'- CTTTCCGTGGTCTTGATGAGG-3'B2: TCGATTTTGCCGTGATGAGTC-3'	752bp	Sorensen *et al.*, 1998
Ralstonia solanacearum	Y2: 5'- CCCACTGCTGCCTCCCGTAGGAGT-3'OLII: 5'-GGGGGTAGCTTGCTACCTGCC-3'	288bp	Seal *et al.*, 1993
R. *solanacearum*	759: 5'- GTCGCCGTCAACTCACTTTCC-3'760: 5'-GTCGCCGTCAGCAATGCGGAATCG-3'	281bp	Ito *et al.*, 1998; Opina*et al.*, 1997
R. solanacearum	PS96-H:5'-TCACCGAAGCCGAATCCGCGTCCATCAC-3' PS96-I: AAGGTGTCGTCCAGCTCGAACCCGCC-3'	148bp	Hartung *et al.*, 1998; Seal *et al.*, 1992
R. solanacearum	pehA#3: 5'- CAGCAGAACCCGCGCCTGATCCAG-3'pehA# 6: 5'- ATCGGACTTGATGCGCAGGCCGTT-3'	504bp	Gillings *et al.*, 1993
R. solanacearum	FP: 52 -TGGTAGTCCACGCCTAAAC-32 RP: 52		
R. solanacearum	-CTGGAAAGTTCCGTGGATGT-32	210bp 2012 Singh *et al.*, 2014	Chandrashekar *et al.*,

Streptomyces spp.	NecF1: 5'-ACCTCGCCTGCAGAGAGGAC-3'	462bp	Cullen and Lees, 2007
Conventional PCR	NecR1: 5'-GTTTCGTACTCTCCGAGCGG-3		
Nested PCRReal	NecNF1: 5'-CACTCTTGGAGATCTCATGC-3'		
Time- PCR	NecNR2: 5'-CGGTACAGTTCATGGAGGTC-3'	279 bp	
TaqMan Probe	NecTqF1: 5'-TCGCACTCTTGGAGATCTCATG-3'		
	NecTqR1: 5'-TCGTAAGAACGCGACGCTTT-3'		
	NecTqP1: GTGACGCCAAAGACTCAATCAAGTTCGC	83 bp	

Table 4: Detection plant pathogenic bacteria from seed and plant parts by using different genes in various PCR based techniques.

PCR Genomic assay	Phyopathogenic Bacteria	Host	Part of Detection	Reference(s)
PCR(16S rRNA)	*Ralstonia solanacearum*	Tomato	Plant and soil	Umesha *et al.*,2012
SCAR	*R. solanacearum*	Tobacco	Leaves	Gund *et al.*, 2011
PCR (*rhs* gene)	*X. campestris* pv. *vesicatoria*	Pepper and Tomato Leaves	Park *et al.*, 2009	
PCR (16S–23S) 2002	*R. solanacearum*		Pastrik *et al.*,	ribosomal
PCR (*syr*D gene)	*P. syringae* pv. *syringae*	- Gheysen, 1999	-	Bultreys and
PCR (using competitor DNA template from *E. coli*)	*E. carotovora* subsp. *atroseptica*	Potato	Potato Tubers	Hyman *et al.*, 2000
PCR (*hrp* gene)	*R. solanacearum*	Bacteria	-	Poussier *et al.*, 1999
PCR (*rec* A gene)	*Erwinia* sp.	Bacteria	-	Waleron *et al.*, 2002
PCR (pathogenic locus)	Soft rot Erwinias	-	-	Toth *et al.*, 2001; Toth *et al.*, 1999, Goncalves and Rosato, 2002
qPCR (YD repeat protein gene)	*Pectobacterium wasabiae*	Bacteria	-	Kim *et al.*, 2012
Real time PCR (Cytochrome o ubiquinol oxidase II gene)	*Pseudomonas syringae*	Tomato	leaves	Xu and Tambong, 2011
16S–23S rRNA	*Clavibacter michiganensis* subsp. *sepedonicus*	Potato	Tuber	Pastrik, 2000
16S rDNA gene	*Clavibacter michiganensis*subsp. *sepedonicus*	Potato	Tuber	Weisburg *et al.*, 1991

References

Alfano JR, Collmer A (1997) The type III (Hrp) secretion pathway of plant pathogenic bacteria: trafficking harpins, Avr proteins, and death. *J Bacteriol* 179:5655-5662.

Anonymous (2005) *Clavibacter michiganensis* subsp. *michiganensis*. PM 7/42. Bull. OEPP/ EPPO *Bulletin* 35:275-283.

Araujo ER, Ferreira MA, Quezado-Duval AM (2013) Specific primers for *Xanthomonasvesicatoria*, a tomato bacterial spot causal agent. *Eur J Plant Pathol* 137: 5-9.

Arora RK, Sharma J (2007) Eco-friendly alternatives to pesticides in management of soil and tuberborne diseases of potato in organic farming. In: Sustainable Environmental Management: Dr Jayashree Deshpande Fests chrift Volume (eds. L.V. Gangawane and V.C. Khilare). Daya Publishing House, New Delhi. 1-6.

Arora RK, Sharma J, Singh RK (2006) Soil solarization. In: Technologies in Aid of Healthy Seed Production. Technical Bulletin No.35, *Central Potato Research Institute, Shimla* 1:1-7.

Baharuddin B, Rudolph K, Niepold F (1994) Production of mono specific antiserum against the blood disease bacterium affecting banana and plantain. *Phytopathology* 84:570–5.

Baysal O, Mercati F, Ikten H, Yýldýz RC, Carimi F, Aysan Y, da Silva JAT (2011) *Clavibacter michiganensis* subsp. *michiganensis*: Tracking strains using their genetic differentiations by ISSR markers in Southern Turkey. *Physiol Mol Plant Pathol* 75:113-119.

Beran P, Mraz I (2013) Species-specific PCR primers for detection of *Xanthomonas vesicatoria*. *Crop Prot* 43:213-215.

Bereswill S, Bugert P, Volksch B, Ullrich M, Bender, CL, Geider K (1994) Identification and relatedness of coronatine-producing *Pseudomonas syringae* pathovars by PCR analysis and sequence determination of the amplification products. *Appl Environ Microbiol* 60:2924-2930.

Bopp CA, Brenner FW, Wells JG, Strockbine NA (1999) Manual of Clinical Microbiology. 7th Edn., ASM Press, Washington, D.C., USA.

Braun-Kiewnick A, Sands DC (2001) Gram negative bacteria, In: Schaad, N.W., Jones, J.B., Chun, W. (Eds.), Laboratory guide for identification of plant pathogenic bacteria, 3rd Edition. APS Press, St. Paul, MN 84-120.

Bultreys A, Gheysen II (1999) Biological and molecular detection of toxic lipodepsipeptide producing *Pseudomonas syringae* strains and PCR identification in plants. *Appl Environ Microbiol* 65:1904–1909.

Catara V, Arnold D, Cirvilleri G, Vivian A (2000) Specific oligonucleotide primers for the rapid identification and detection of the agent of tomato pith necrosis, *Pseudomonas corrugata*, by PCR amplification: evidence for two distinct genomic groups. *Eur J Plant Pathol* 106:753-762.

Catara V, Sutra L, Morineau A, Achouak W, Christen R, Gardan L (2002) Phenotypic and genomic evidence for the revision of *Pseudomonas corrugata* and proposal of *Pseudomonas mediterranea* sp. nov. *Int J Syst Evol Microbiol* 52:1749-1758.

Chakravarti SK, Shekhawat GS, Gadewar AV, Gopal J (1993) Selection of bacterial wilt tolerant potato germ plasma. In: seminar on crop protection held at Shimla, India, abstract and souvenir.

Chandrashekar S, Umesha S, Chandan S (2012) Molecular detection of plant pathogenic bacteria using polymerase chain reaction single-strand conformation polymorphism. *Acta Biochim Biophys Sin* 44:217–223.

Cullen DW, Lees AK (2007) Detection of the nec1 virulence gene and its correlation with pathogenicity in *Streptomyces* species on potato tubers and in soil using conventional and real-time PCR. *J Appl Microbiol* 102:1082- 1094.

Cullen DW, Lees AK, Toth IK, Bell KS, Duncan JM (2000) Detection and quantification of fungal and bacterial potato pathogens in plant and soil. In: EPPO Conference on diagnostic techniques for plant pests, Waddington, Netherlands. *Bulletin-OEPP*. 30: 485-488.

Cuppels DA, Elmhirst J (1999) Disease development and changes in the natural *Pseudomonassyringae* pv. *tomato* populations on field tomato plants. *Plant Dis* 83:759-764.

Cuppels DA, Moore RA, Moms VL (1990) Construction and use of a nonradioactive DNA hybridization probe for detection of *Pseudomonas syringae* pv. *tomato* on tomato plants. *Appl Environ Microbiol* 56:1743-1749.

Czajkowski R (2015) Bacteriophages of soft rot Enterobacteriaceae - a minireview. FEMS Microbiol Lett 363: fnv230.

Davis MJ, Gillasie AG Jr., Vidaver AK, Harris RW (1984)*Clavibacter*: a new genus containing some phytopathogenic coryneform bacteria, including *Clavibacter xyli* subsp. *xyli* sp. nov., subsp. nov. and *Clavibacter xyli* subsp. *cynodontis* subsp. nov., pathogens that cause ratoon stunting disease of sugarcane and Bermudagrass stunting disease. *Int J Syst Bacteriol* 34: 107–117.

de la Cruz AR, Wiese MV, Schaad NW (1992) A semi selective agar medium for isolation of *Clavibacter michiganensis* subsp. *sepedonicus* from potato tissues. *Plan Dis* 76:830-834.

Dreier J, Bermpohl A, Eichenlaub R (1995) Southern hybridization and PCR for specific detection of phytopathogenic *Clavibacter michiganensis* subsp. *michignaensis.Phytopathology* 85:464-468.

Dye DW (1978) Genus IX. *Xanthomonas*. Dowson 1939. In: Young JM, Dye DW, Bradbury JF, Panagopoulos CG & Robbs CF. A proposed nomenclature and classification for plant pathogenic bacteria. *New Zeal J Agr Res* 21:153–177.

Elphinstone JG, Hennessy J, Wilson JK, Stead DE (1996) Sensitivity of different methods for the detection of *Ralstoniasolanacearum* in potato tuber extracts. *Bull OEPP/EPPO Bulletin* 26:663-678.

Fackrell HB, Sinha RC (1983) Serological Analysis of *Pseudomonas syringae* pv. *tomato*. *Phytopathology* 73:178-181.

Fiori M, Carta C, Franceschini A (1983) Il saggio immunoenzimatico (ELISA) per la diagnosi precoce e rapida della necrosi del midollo di pomodoro da *Pseudomonas corrugata* Roberts et Scarlett. *Phytopathol Mediterr* 22:22-26.

Flores JB, Puente EOR, Felix EA, Ponce JF, Cruz M, Juarez OG, Ortega AMG (2009) Detection of *Clavibacter michiganensis* subspecies *michiganensis* in tomato of the state of Sonora, Mexico. *Rev Fitotec Mex* 32:319-326.

Frechon D, Exbrayat P, Gallet O, Guillot E, Le Clerc V, Payet N, Bertheau Y (1995) Sequences nuceotidiques pour la detection des *Erwinia carotovora* subsp. *atroseptica*. Institut National de la Recherche Agronomique, Institut National Agronomique Paris-Grignon, Sanofi Diagnostics Pasteur. *Brevet* 95:12-803.

Ftayeh R, Von Tiedemann A, Koopmann B, Rudolph K (2008) First record of *Clavibactermichiganensis* subsp. *michiganensis* causing canker of tomato plants in Syria. Plant Dis 92: 649. https://doi.org/10.1094/PDIS-92-4-0649C

Ftayeh R, Von Tiedemann A, Koopmann B, Rudolph K (2009) Reliability and sensitivity of diagnostic methods for detection of *Clavibacter michiganensis* subsp. *michiganensis*in seeds and plant material. Paper presented in Dossenheim, September 3, 2009.

Gardan L, Gouy C, Christen R, Samson R (2003) Elevation of three subspecies of *Pectobacteriumcarotovorum* to species level: *Pectobacteriumatrosepticum* sp. nov., *Pectobacteriumbetavasculorum* sp. nov. and *Pectobacteriumwasabiae* sp. nov. *Int J Syst Evol Microbiol* 53:381-391.

Garibaldi A, Minuto A, Scortichini M, Gullino ML (2007) First report of syringae leaf spot caused by *Pseudomonas syringae* pv. *syringae* on Tomato in Italy. *Plant Dis* 91:1518.

Gillings M, Fahy P, Davies C (1993) Restriction analysis of an amplified polygalacturonase gene fragment differentiates strains of the phytopathogenic bacterium *Pseudomonas solanacearum*. *Lett Applied Microbiol* 17:44-48.

Goncalves ER, Rosato YB (2002) Phylogenetic analysis of *Xanthomonas* species based upon 16S-23S rDNA intergenic spacer sequences. *Int J Syst Evol Microbiol* 52:355–361.

Gould WD, Hagedorn C, Bardinelli TR, Zablotowicz RM (1985). New selective media for enumeration and recovery of fluorescent pseudomonads from various habitats. *Appl* Environ *Microbiol* 49:28–32.

Gund SV, Moger N, Krishnaraj PU, Bhat R, Kamanna BC (2011) Development of race specific SCAR marker for detection of *Ralstonia solanacearum* (race 2). *J Appl Biosci* 37:91-96.

Hartung F, Werner R, Muhlbach HP, Buttner C (1998) Highly specific PCR-diagnosis to determine *Pseudomonas solanacearum* strains of different geographical origins. *TheorAppl Genet* 96:797-802.

Hauben L, Moore ERB, Vauterin L, Steenackers M, Mergaert J, Verdonck L, Swings J (1998) Phylogenetic position of phytopathogens within the Enterobacteriaceae. *System Appl Microbiol* 21:384-397.

Hu X, Lai FM, Reddy ASN, Ishimaru CA (1995) Quantitative detection of *Clavibactermichiganensis* subsp. *sepedonicus* by competitive polymerase chain reaction. *Phytopathology* 85:1468–1473.

Hyman LJ, Birch PR, Dellagi A, Avrova AO, Toth IK (2000) A competitive PCR based method for the detection and quantification of *Erwinia carotovora* subsp. *atroseptica* on potato tubers. *Lett Appl Microbiol* 30:330–335.

Ito S, Ushijima Y, Fujii T, Tanaka S, Kameya-Iwaki M, Yoshiwara S, Kish F (1998) Detection of visible cells of *Ralstonia solanacearum* in soil using a semi selective medium and a PCR technique. *J Phytopathol* 146:379-384.

Jones JB, Lacy GH, Bouzar H, Stall RE, Schaad NW (2004) Reclassification of the xanthomonads associated with bacterial spot disease of tomato and pepper. *Syst Appl Microbiol*. 27:755-762.

Jones JB, McCarter SM, Gitaitis RD (1981) Association of *Pseudomonas syringae* pv. *syringae* with a leaf spot disease of tomato transplants in Southern Georgia. *Phytopathology* 71: 1281-1285.

Kado CI, Haskett MG (1970) Selective Media for Isolation of *Agrobacterium*, *Corynebacterium*, *Erwinia*, *Pseudomonas*, and *Xanthomonas*. *Phytopathology* 60:969-976.

Kelman A (1954). The relationship of pathogenicity in *Pseudomonas solanacearum* to colony appearance on a tetrazolium medium. *Phytopathology* 44: 693-695.

Khakvar R, Sijan K, Wong MY, Radu S, Thong KL (2008) Improving a PCR-Based Method for Identification of *Ralstonia Solanacearum* in Natural Sources of West Malaysia. *Am J Agric Bio Sci* 4:490-49.

Kim MH, Cho MS, Kim BK, Choi HJ, Hahn JH, Kim CK, Kang MJ, Kim SH, Park DS (2012) Quantitative real-time polymerase chain reaction assay for detection of *Pectobacterium wasabiae* using YD repeat protein gene-based primers. *Plant Dis*. 96:253-257.

Koenraadt H, Van Betteray B, Germain R, Hiddink G, Jones JB, Oosterhof J (2007) Development of specific primers for the molecular detection of bacterial spot of pepper and tomato. *Acta Hortic* 808:99-102.

Lazarovits G, Zutra D, Bar-Joseph M (1987) Enzyme-linked immunosorbent assay on nitrocellulose membranes (dot-ELISA) in the serodiagnosis of plant pathogenic bacteria. *Can J Microbiol* 33:98-103.

Lee IM, Bartoszyk IM, Gundersen DE, Mogen B, Davis RE (1997) Nested PCR for ultrasensitive detection of the potato ring rot bacterium, *Clavibacter michiganensis* subsp. *sepedonicus*. Appl. *Environ Microbiol* 63:2625–2630.

Licciardello G, Bella P, Catara V (2011) Quantitative detection of *Pseudomonas corrugata* and *Pseudomonas mediterranea* in tomato plants by duplex Real-Time PCR. *J Plant Pathol* 93:595-602.

Manceau C, Horvais A (1997) Assessment of genetic diversity among strains of *Pseudomonas syringae* by PCR- restriction fragment length polymorphism analysis of rRNA operons with special emphasis on *P. syringae* pv. *tomato*. *Appl Environ Microbiol* 63:498-505.

McGuire RG, Jones JB, Sasser M (1986) Tween media for semiselective isolation of *Xanthomonascampestris* pv. *vesicatoria* from soil and plant material. *Plant Dis* 70:887-891.

Mitrev S, Gardan L, Samson R (2000) Characterization of bacterial strains of *Pseudomonassyringae* pv. *syringae* isolated from pepper leaf spot in Macedonia. *J Plant Pathol* 82:227-231.

Moretti C, Amatulli MT, Buonaurio R (2009) PCR based assay for the detection of *Xanthomonaseuvesicatoria* causing pepper and tomato bacterial spot. *Lett Appl Microbiol* 49:466-471.

Murugesan S, Manoharan C, Vijayakumar R, Paneerselvam A (2010) Isolation and Characterization of *Agrobacterium rhizogenes* from the root nodules of some leguminous plants. *Int J Microbiol Res* 1:92-96.

Nassar A, Darrasse A, Lemattre M, Kotoujansky A, Dervin C, Vedel R, Bertheau Y (1996) Characterization of *Erwinia chrysanthemi* by pectinolytic isozyme polymorphism and restriction fragment length polymorphism analysis of PCR- amplified fragments of pel genes. *Appl Environ Microbiol* 62:2228-2235.

Naumann, K, Griesbach E, Lattauschke E (1990) Occurrence and importance of bacterial stem pith necrosis of tomato plants in GDR, 473-478. In Proceedings of the 7th International Conference on Plant Pathogenic Bacteria. Akademiai Kiad6, Budapest.

Nemeth J, Vuurde JWL van (2006) Development of immunofluorescence colony staining (IFC) for detection of *Xanthomonas campestris* pv. *vesicatoria* and *Clavibacter michiganensis* subsp.*michiganensis* in tomato seeds. *Seed Sci Technol* 34:85-100.

Notomi T, Okayama H, Masubuchi H, Yonekawa T, Watanabe K, Amino N, Hase T (2000) Loop-mediated isothermal amplification of DNA. *Nucleic Acids Res* 28: E63.

OEPP/EPPO (1992) Quarantine procedures. *Xanthomonas campestris* pv. *vesicatoria*-seed-testing method. Bulletin EPPO/EPPO *Bulletin* 22:247-252.

Opina N, Tavner F, Hollway G, Wang JF, Li TH, Maghirang R, Fagan M, Hayward AC, Krishnapillai V, Hong WF, Holloway BW Timmis JN (1997) A novel method for development of species and strain-specific DNA probes and peR primers for identifying *Burkholderiasolanacearum* (formerly *Pseudomonas solanacearum*). *Asia-Pacific J Molec Biol Biotechnol* 5:19-30.

Ozakman M, Schaad NW (2003) A real-time BIO-PCR assay for detection of *Ralstoniasolanacearum* race 3, biovar 2, in asymptomatic potato tubers. *Can J Plant Patho* 25: 232-239.

Park DS, Shim JK, Kim JS, Lim CK, Shrestha R, Hahn JH, Kim HG (2009) Sensitive and specific detection of *Xanthomonas campestris* pv. *vesicatoria* by PCR using pathovar-specific primers based on rhs family gene sequences. *Microbiol Res* 164:36-42.

Pastrik KH, Elphinstone JG, Pukall R (2002) Sequence analysis and detection of *Ralstoniasolanacearum* by multiplex PCR amplification of 16S–23S ribosomal intergenic spacer region with internal positive control. *Eur J Plant Pathol* 108:831–42.

Pastrik KH (2000) Detection of *Clavibacter michiganensis* subsp. *sepedonicus* in potato tubers by multiplex PCR with coamplification of host DNA. *Eur J Plant Pathol* 106:155–165.

Pastrik KH, Rainey FA (1999) Identification and differentiation of *Clavibacter michiganensis* subspecies by polymerase chain reaction-based techniques. J Phytopathol 147: 687–693.

Peiqian L, Birun L, Huifang S, Xiaoming P (2011) Species-specific detection of *Dickeya* sp. (*Pectobacterium chrysanthemi*) in infected banana tissues, soil and water. *Afr J Biotechnol* 10:16774-16780.

Peng J, Zhan Y, Zeng F, Long H, Pei Y, Guo J (2013) Development of a real-time fluorescence loop-mediated isothermal amplification assay for rapid and quantitative detection of *Fusarium oxysporum* f. sp. *niveum* in soil. *FEMS Microbiol Lett* 349:127–134.

Potrykus M, Golanowska M, Hugouvieux-Cotte-Pattat N, Lojkowska E (2014) Regulators involved in *Dickeya solani*virulence, genetic conservation, and functional variability. *Mol Plant–Microbe Interact* 27: 700–711.

Poussier S, Vandewalle P, Luisetti J (1999) Genetic diversity of African and worldwide strains of *Ralstonia solanacearum* as determined by PCR restriction fragment length polymorphism analysis of the hrp gene region. *Appl Environ Microbiol* 65:2184-2194.

Powell M, Gundersen B, Miles CA, Humann JL, Schroeder BK, Inglis DA (2013) First report of tomato pith necrosis (*Pseudomonas corrugata*) on tomato (*Solanum lycopersicum*) in Washington. *Plant Dis* 97:1381.

Przewodowski W, Przewodowska A (2017) Development of a sensitive and specific polyclonal antibody for serological detection of *Clavibacter michiganensis* subsp. *sepedonicus*. *PLoS One* 12:e0169785.

Pulawska J, Sobiczewski P (2005) Development of a semi nested PCR based method for sensitive detection of tumorigenic *Agrobacterium* in soil. *J Appl Microbiol* 98:710-721.

Raaijmakers JM, Weller DM, Thomasshow LS (1997) Frequency of antibiotic producing *Pseudomonas* spp. in natural environment. *Appl Environ Microbiol* 63:881-887.

Ranjan RK, Singh D, Baranwa VK (2016) Simultaneous detection of brown rot- and soft rot-causing bacterial pathogens from potato tubers through multiplex PCR. *Curr Microbiol* 73:652-659.

Robinson-Smith A, Jones P, Elphinstone JG, Forde SMD, (1995) Production of antibodies to *Ralstonia solanacearum*, the causative agent of bacterial wilt. *Food Agric Immunol* 7:67–79.

Saygili H, Aysan Y, Ustun N, Mirik M, Sahin F (2008) Tomato Pith Necrosis Disease Caused by *Pseudomonas* species in Turkey. In: Fatmi M. et al. (eds.) Pseudomonas syringae Pathovars and Related Pathogens – Identification, Epidemiology and Genomics. Springer, Dordrecht 357-366.

Sawada H, Ieki H, Matsuda J (1995) PCR detection of Ti and Ri plasmids from phytopathogenic *Agrobacterium* strains. *Appl Environ Microbiol* 61:821-831.

Scarlett CM, Fletcher JT, Roberts P, Lelliott RA (1978) Tomato pith necrosis caused by *Pseudomonas corrugata* n. sp. *Ann Appi Biol* 88:105-114.

Schneider BJ, Zhao JL, Orser CS (1993) Detection of *Clavibacter michiganensis* subsp. *sepedonicus* by DNA amplification. *FEMS Microbiol Lett* 109:207-212.

Scortichini M, Marchesi U, Dettori MT, Rossi MP (2003) Genetic diversity, presence of syrB gene, host preference and virulence of *Pseudomonas syringae* pv. *syringae*strains from woody and herbaceous host. *Plant Pathol* 52:277–286.

Seal SE, Jackson LA, Daniels MJ (1992) Isolation of a *Pseudomonas solanacearum*- specific DNA probe by subtraction hybridization and construction of species - specific oligonucleotide primers for sensitive detection by polymerase chain reaction. *Appl Environ Microbiol* 58:3751- 3758.

Seal SE, Jackson LA, Young JPW, Daniels MJ (1993) Differentiation of *Pseudomonas solanacearum*, *Pseudomonas syzigii*, *Pseudomonas pickettii* and the blood disease bacterium by partial 16S rRNA sequencing: construction of oligonucleotide primers for sensitive detection by polymerase chain reaction. *J Gen Microbial* 139:1587-1594.

Sebastien M, Nagy C, Jijakli MH (2014) Development of the simultaneous detection of *Ralstoniasolanacearum* race 3 and *Clavibacter michiganensis* subsp. *sepedonicus* in potato tubers by a multiplex real-time PCR assay. *Eur J Plant Pathol* 138:29-37.

Serfontein S, Staphorst JL (1994) Crown gall of hop caused by *Agrobacteriumtumefaciens* biovar 1 in South Africa. *Plant Pathol* 43:1028-1030.

Shams M, Campillo T, Lavire C, Muller D, Nesme X, Vial L (2012) Rapid and efficient methods to isolate, type strains and determine species of *Agrobacterium* spp. in pure culture and complex environments. Biochemical Testing, InTech.

Shenge KC, Stephan D, Mabagala RB, Mortensen CN, Wydra K (2008) Molecular characterization of *Pseudomonas syringae* pv. *tomato* isolates from Tanzania. *Phytoparasitica* 36:338-351.

Singh D, Sinha S, Yadav DK (2014) Detection of *Ralstonia solanacearum* from asymptomatic tomato, irrigation water and soil through non-selective enrichment medium with hrp Gene-based Bio-PCR. *Curr Microbiol* 69: 127-134.

Singh D, Sinha S, Yadav DK, Sharma JP, Srivastava DK, Lal HC, Mondal KK, Jaiswal RK (2010) Characterization of biovar/races of *Ralstonia solanacearum*, the incitant of bacterial wilt in solanaceous crops. *Indian Phytopath* 63:261-265.

Siverio F, Cambra M, Gorris MT, Corzo J, Lopez MM (1993) Lipopolysaccharides as determinants of serological variability in *Pseudomonas corrugata*. *Appl Environ Microbiol* 59:1805-1812.

Smith DS, De Boer SH, Gourley J (2008) An internal reaction control for routine detection of *Clavibacter michiganensis* subsp. *sepedonicus* using a real-time TaqMan PCR-based assay. *Plant Dis* 92:684-693.

Sorensen KN, Kim KH, Takemoto JK (1998) PCR detection of cyclic lipodepsinonapeptide-producing *Pseudomonas syringae* pv. *syringae* and similarity of strains. *Appl Environ Microbiol* 64:226-230.

Stall RE, Jones JB, Minsavage GV (2009) Durability of resistance in tomato and pepper to Xanthomonads causing bacterial spot. *Annu Rev Phytopathol* 47: 265-284.

Stead DE, Sellwood JE, Wilson J, Viney I (1992) Evaluation of a commercial microbial identification system based on fatty acid profiles for rapid, accurate identification of plant pathogenic bacteria. *J App Bacteriol* 72:315– 21.

Toth IK, Avrova AO, Hyman LJ (2001) Rapid identification and differentiation of the soft rot *Erwinias*by 16S-23S intergenic transcribed spacer-PCR and restriction fragment length polymorphism analyses. *Appl Environ Microbiol* 67:4070-4076.

Toth IK, Bertheau Y, Hyman LJ, Laplaze L, Lopez MM (1999) Evaluation of phenotypic and molecular typing techniques for determining diversity in *Erwinia carotovora* subsp. *atroseptica*. *J Appl Microbiol* 87:770–781.

Umesha S, Chandan S, Swamy LN (2012) Colony PCR-single strand confirmation polymorphism for the detection of *Ralstonia solanacearum* in tomato. *Int J Integr Biol* 13:45-51.

Vauterin L, Hoste B, Kersters K, Swings J (1995) Reclassification of *Xanthomonas*. *Int J Syst Evol Microbiol* 45:472-489.

Waleron M, Waleron K, Podhajska AJ, Lojkowska E (2002) Genotyping of bacteria belonging to the former *Erwinia* genus by PCR-RFLP analysis of a recA gene fragment. *Microbiology* 148:583– 595.

Waters CM, Bolkan HA (1992) An improved semi-selective medium and method of extraction for detecting *Clavibacter michiganensis* subsp. *michiganensis* in tomato seeds. *Phytopathology* 82:1072.

Weisburg WG, Barns SM, Pelletier DA, Lane DJ (1991) 16S ribosomal DNA amplification for phylogenetic study. *J Bacteriol* 173:697-703.

Weller SA, Elphinstone JG, Smith NC, Boonham N, Stead DE (2000). Detection of *Ralstoniasolanacearum* strains with a quantitative, multiplex, real-time, fluorogenic PCR (TaqMan) assay. *Appl Environ Microbiol* 66: 2853–2858.

Weller SA, O'Neill TM (2006) Crown gall in organically grown UK tomato caused by tumorigenic strains of *Agrobacterium radiobacter*. New Dis. Rep. 13:2.

Widmer F, Seidler RJ, Gillevet PM, Watrud LS, Di Giovanni GD (1998). A high elective PCR protocol for detecting 16S RNA genes of the genus *Pseudomonas* (*sensu stricto*) in environmental samples. *Appl Environ Microbiol* 64:2545-2553.

Xu R, Tambong JT (2011) A Taq Man real-time PCR assay targeting the cytochrome o ubiquinol oxidase subunit II gene for detection of several pathovars of *Pseudomonas syringae*. Can *J Plant Pathol* 33:318-331.

Yabbuuchi E, Kosako Y, Yano I, Hotta H, Nishiunchi Y (1995) Transfer of two *Burkholderia* and an *Alcaligenus* species to *Ralstonia* gen. nov. *Ralstonia solnacearum* (Smith, 1986) comb.Nov. and *Ralstonia eutropha* (Davis, 1969) comb. Nov. *Microbiol Immunol* 39: 897- 904.

Zaccardelli M, Spasiano A, Bazzi C, Merighi M (2005) Identification and in planta detection of *Pseudomonas syringae* pv. *tomato* using PCR amplification of hrpZPst. *Eur J Plant Pathol.* 111:85–90.

21

Assessment on Farmers Information Need and Network for Designing ICT Tools for Better Decision Making in Plant Health Management and Agronomic Practices

Chandan Kumar Panda[1], Anil Paswan[1], Chandrashekhar Azad[2] Shashank Tyagi[3] and Shashikant Divakar[1]

[1]*Department of Extension Education, Bihar Agricultural University, Sabour, Bhagalpur, Bihar, India*

[2]*Department of Plant Pathology, Bihar Agricultural University, Sabour, Bhagalpur, Bihar, India*

[3]*Department of Agronomy, Bihar Agricultural University, Sabour, Bhagalpur, Bihar, India*

Abstract

Information and Communication Technology (ICT) played and continue to play pivotal role in better decision making of farmers for plant health management under the climate change scenario. For judicious plant health management by farmers through the use of ICT tools (viz. interactive Kiosk, Mobile Apps, Whatsapp, Webportal), information need and information access network to be assessed. Based on farmers' information need and network, information delivery tree should be designed in ICT tools. Under this backdrop this research work was carried out among the farmers of Bhagalpur district of Bihar. The sample size was 120. From the study it was noted that the major information needs of the farmers were seed availability, crop disease management, insect pest management, weed management and weather information and pesticide application. Farmers were enthusiastic to improve their knowledge on insect pests and disease identification and management. Specifically, farmers need information on insect pest management of wheat (aphid), maize (stem borer), vegetables (fruit borer), pulses (pod borer) and oilseeds (aphid) and also disease management of wheat (leaf blight and spot blotch disease), maize (Turcicum leaf blight), vegetables (wilt and leaf spot) and pulses (wilt disease). Farmers decision making was positively and significantly correlated with crop disease management(0.196), insect pest management of crop(0.208*) and weed management(0.239**). Through the Path Analysis it was noted that farmers decision making on disease management was mediated by the variables - Bihar Agricultural University-Kisan Diary, Mobile Apps(Bihar Krishi Apps) and Kisan Salahkar. So, it can be concluded that these much needed information should be provided to the farmers though different ICT tools and extension personnel should be trained to operate these ICT tools for accelerated use of ICT tools by the farmers.*

***Keywords*:** Plant Disease, Path Analysis, Bihar Krishi Apps, Plant health management

Introduction

Farmers need timely information for management of plant health. With the increase of cropping intensity and changing climatic condition, the extent of disease and insect pest infestation is gradually increasing. Farmers spent about 30% of their input cost for this purpose, however, this expenditure vary from crop to crop. Farmers sprayed more pesticide in vegetable cultivation and some other cash crops. Plant disease epidemiology, overlapping symptom of plant diseases and nutrient deficiency creates confusion among the farmers on taking right decision of disease management. Farmers also face similar problems on selection of insecticide. Due to change in climatic condition, minor disease and insect pests are emerging as major pest and farmers find it difficult to control those pests. The use of pesticide was observed to be high, with over 40 different formulations, probably because farmers assume that the only solution to pest problems is to spray more frequently and using different types of pesticides (Dinham, 2003).However, farmers decision on selection pesticide depends on its performance and effectiveness, awareness and information, technical and operational knowledge, environmental criteria, and financial and accessibility criteria(Sharifzadeh,2018).Farmers decision on selection of pesticide is also influenced by inputs dealers persuasion (NSSO,2005).Although, with the rapid advent of Information and Communication Technology(ICT), there are number of ICT tools viz. interactive Kiosk, Mobile Apps, Whatsapp, Webportal can help the farmers to take right decision on plant health management. Under this backdrop this study was conducted with the objectives to assess farmers information needs and networks on better decision making through the use of ICT tools in judicious plant health management and other agronomic practices.

Materials and Methods

Bhagalpur district of Bihar state is selected purposively for the study. Data was collected from 120 (one hundred twenty) farmers. The data collection schedule was pretested among 15 number non-respondent farmers and pertinent changes were made. Farmers having farming was main occupation and minimum 10 years of farming experiences were within the sampling frame. From the sampling frame, 120 (one hundred twenty) respondents were selected through random sampling method. Although data collection schedule were prepared in English language, but during interview it was translated to local language. The data was collected from the respondents during March 2018 to July 2018. The summative scale and Likert Scale were used. The statistical tools included were Mean, Per cent, Standard Deviation, Rank, Pearson's Correlation Coefficient and Path Analysis. For analysis of data IBM SPSS 21 was employed.

Results and Discussion

A. Socio-economic Profile and crops grown

Farmers' socio economic profile and the crops grown by the respondents are presented in the Table 1 & 2.

Table 1: Socio-economic profile of the farmers

n=120

Characteristics	Categories	*f*	Per cent	Cumulative Per cent	
1. Age Groups (in Years)	Upto 35(Young)	36	30.00	30.00	Mean= 37.07
	> 35 to ≤ 55 (Middle Age)	55	45.83	75.83	SD = 12.13
	> 55 (Older)	29	24.17	100	CV=32.72%
2. Education Level	Illiterate	8	06.67	06.67	
	Functional literacy	12	10.00	16.67	
	Upto primary	8	6.67	23.34	
	Upto secondary	40	33.33	56.67	
	Upto higher Secondary	44	36.66	93.33	
	Graduate and above	8	6.67	100	
3. Farming Experiences (in years)	>10 to ≤ 11	25	20.83	20.83	
	>11 to ≤ 20	29	24.17	45.00	
	>20 to ≤ 30	48	40.00	85.00	
	> 30	18	15.00	100	

From the study, it was noted that 45.83 per cent farmers belonged to middle age group with mean age of 37.07 years and CV of 32.72%. It was also noted that 36.66 per cent farmers education level is upto higher secondary, followed by 33.33 per cent farmers' education level was upto secondary and only 6.67%

were illiterate. In relation to the farmers farming experience, 40.00 per cent farmers had farming experience of 20 to 30 years and only 20.83 per cent farmers farming experience is 10 years(Table 1).

Table 2: Main crops grown and its acreage

Crops grown	Respondents*		Acreage		
	Per cent	Mean	SD	Min.	Max.
Wheat	26.20	4.40	4.19	0.5	6.0
Maize	27.10	3.67	3.11	1.00	7.5
Vegetables	25.11	2.43	0.98	0.05	4.0
Pulses	23.16	2.94	2.73	1.00	6.3
Oilseeds	11.20	1.57	1.97	0.60	4.0
Others	02.32	1.97	1.57	0.40	3.60

*Multiple responses

In the study area, most of the farmers belonged to small and marginal categories. The major crops grown by the farmers were wheat (26.20%), Maize (27.10%),Vegetables (25.11%), Pulses(23.16%), Oilseeds (11.20%) and others (2.32%)(Table 2).

B. Farmers Information Sources and its nature of interaction

Farmers received information on plant health management and other agronomic practices from different sources and their nature of interaction with these sources are also different. The perusal of these is presented in the Table 3 & 4 and Figure 1.

Table 3: Rank position of different sources of information (agriculture related activities)

Sl.No.	Information Sources(Agriculture related Activities)	Weighted Mean	Rank
1.	Progressive Farmer(FIS1)	4.87	I
2.	Neighbour Farmer(FIS2)	4.67	II
3.	Kisan Salahkar(FIS3)	4.25	IV
4.	Assistant Technical Manager(FIS4)	3.21	XII
5.	Block Technological Manager(FIS5)	3.12	XIII
6.	Agriculture Coordinator(FIS6)	3.95	VII
7.	Scientists of Bihar Agricultural University(FIS7)	4.06	VI
8.	Kisan Call Centre(FIS8)	2.89	XIV
9.	BAU,Kisan Help Line(FIS9)	3.86	VIII
10.	Bihar Krishi Apps(Mobile Apps) (FIS10)	4.12	V
11.	Radio(FIS11)	2.17	XV
12.	Television(FIS12)	3.23	XI
13.	Newspaper(FIS13)	3.78	IX
14.	BAU Kisan Diary(FIS14)	3.67	X
15.	Input Dealers(FIS15)	4.45	III

(FIS= Farmers' Information Source. This code is used in Dedrogram)

Farmers received information from different sources. From the study, it was noted that farmers received information related to agriculture activities from fifteen sources. Among the different sources, it was noted that major sources of information were Progressive Farmer(Ranked I), Neighbour Farmer(Ranked II), Input Dealers(Ranked III), Kisan Salahkar (Ranked IV) and Bihar Krishi Apps(Mobile Apps)(Ranked V) and other information sources as shown in Table 3. It was also noted that farmers accessed on an average eight information sources and out of which five sources(average) was tried. The mean frequency of use of sources were 3.4 i.e. the respondents used 'tried information sources' from fortnightly to monthly(Table 4)

Table 4: Summary statistics for variables used in information search

Sl.No.	Variables	Mean	SD	Max.	Min.
1.	Number of sources accessed	8.34	2.34	10.00	3.00
2.	Number of sources from which information tried	5.43	2.12	7.00	2.00
3.	Mean of frequency of use(6=daily,5 =weekly, 4=fortnight, 3=monthly, 2=seasonal, 1=yearly, 0=none)	3.40	1.30	6.00	0

Max.=Maximum, Min.=Minimum

Farmers received agricultural related information from number of sources. Considering types of information disseminated by sources, modus operand of sources and ease to access; it became imperative to group or club or cluster similar type of sources. Hence clustering of the sources was done through the Dendrogram using Single Linkage. It was noted that the information sources- *Agriculture Coordinator(FIS6), Input Dealers(FIS15), Kisan Salahkar (FIS3), BAU Kisan Diary(FIS14) and BAU, Kisan Help Line(FIS9)* have similar type of implication and these were in one cluster. Most interesting thing to note that *Bihar Krishi Apps (Mobile Apps) (FIS10)* is alone stand in Dendrogram, it implied that this mobile apps is enough to support farmers with so many information independently(Figure 1).

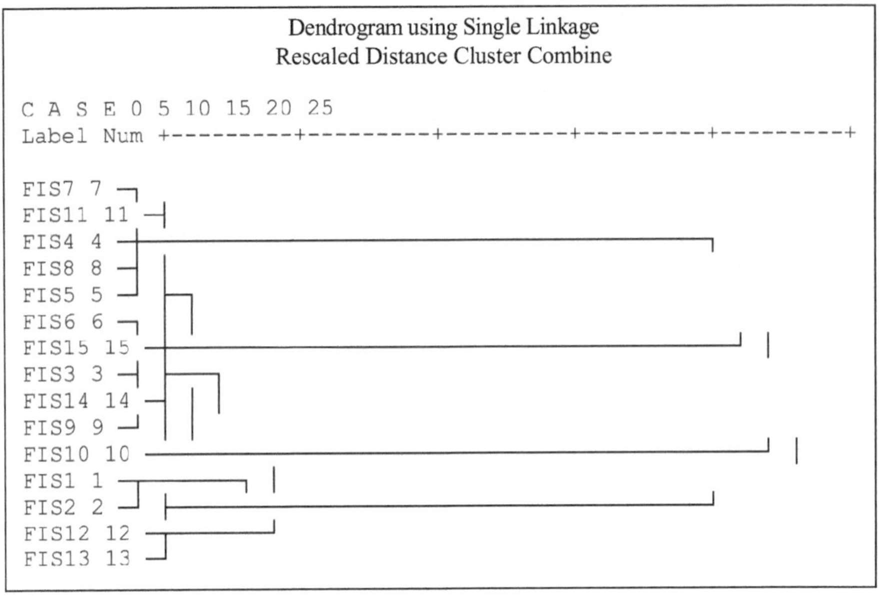

Fig. 1: Dendogram of cluster analysis on information sources used by the farmers

C. Farmers Information Need, Decision Making and Usage of ICT tools

Farmers need different types of information for plant health management and other agronomic practices. The perusal of information need is presented in remaining tables

Table 5: Broad areas of farmers' information need related to crop cultivation

n=120

Sl.No.	Broad Areas of Farmers' Information Need	Weighted Mean	Rank
1.	Seed availability	4.38	I
2.	Crop disease management	4.21	II
3.	Insect pest management	4.13	III
4.	Weed management	3.89	IV
5.	Weather information	3.82	V
6.	Inputs availability and price(i.e. fertilizers, pesticide *etc.*)	3.76	VI
7.	Best agriculture practices(Package of practices)	3.43	VII
8.	Soil health Card and soil health management	3.26	VIII
9.	Agricultural machineries/implements	3.11	IX
10.	Irrigation management	2.86	X
11.	Pesticide application	2.36	XI
12.	Fertilizer application	2.34	XII
13.	Seed treatment	2.11	XIII
14.	Post harvest management	1.98	XIV
15.	Storage and grading	1.86	XV
16.	Time of planting	1.56	XVI

Farmers need different types of information, however, it is necessary to specify the broad areas of information need of the farmers. Accordingly, the respondents information need was assessed. From the study, it was noted that the major information need of the farmers were Seed availability(Rank I),Crop disease management (Rank II),Insect pest management (Rank III),Weed management (Rank IV), Weather information(Rank V) and reaming were as shown in table 5.

Table 6: Correlation coefficient between information need and decision making of the respondents

Sl.No.	Independent Variables	Correlation Co-efficient (r)
1.	Seed availability of different crops(X_1).	0.290**
2.	Crop disease management (X_2).	0.196*
3.	Insect pest management of crop(X_3).	0.208**
4.	Weed management(X_4).	0.239**
5.	Weather information(X_5).	0.103
6.	Inputs availability and price(i.e. fertilizers, pesticide, seed *etc.*) (X_6).	0.248**
7.	Best agriculture practices(Package of practices) (X_7)	-0.078
8.	Soil health Card and soil health management(X_8)	-0.120
9.	Agricultural machineries/implements(X_9).	0.067
10.	Irrigation management(X_{10}).	0.057
11.	Pesticide application techniques and timing(X_{11}).	-0.042
12.	Fertilizer application techniques and timing(X_{12}).	0.095
13.	Seed treatment of different crops(X_{13}).	0.099
14.	Post harvest management(X_{14}).	-0.073
15.	Storage and grading of agricultural produces(X_{15}).	0.062
16.	Time of planting of different crops(X_{16}).	0.060

**Correlation is significant at the 0.01 level.*Correlation is significant at the 0.05 level .

It was noted that farmers decision making was positively and significantly correlated with the variable X_1, this implied that if the farmers were informed on availability of seed of different crops, then they could take good decision for all agricultural practices. Again, it was noted that farmers decision making was positively and significantly correlated with variables X_2 and X_3. From this correlation, it could be concluded that insect pest and disease management decision is immensely influenced by available information and its timeliness(Table 6).

Table 7: Direct and indirect effect of independent variables to dependent variable (decision making)

Independent Var.	Direct Effect	Total Indirect Effect	Substantial Indirect Effect through		
			I	II	III
X_1	0.05197	0.05263	0.00914(X_2)	0.00911(X_5)	0.00823(X_9)
X_2	-0.05703	-0.06432	0.01015(X_4)	0.0085(X_0)	0.00244(X_3)
X_3	0.09969	0.18379	0.03927(X_5)	0.03501(X_5)	0.03501(X_{16})
X_4	0.02637	0.01312	0.00882(X_6)	0.00833(X_2)	0.00464(X_1)
X_5	0.10309	0.03822	0.04061(X_3)	0.02489(X_6)	0.01281(X_9)
X_6	0.12145	0.0625	0.04063(X_{13})	0.0406(X_4)	0.02933(X_5)
X_7	-0.08814	0.15335	0.04032(X_{15})	0.04032(X_{16})	0.03768(X_9)
X_8	0.03583	-0.01376	0.01384(X_{14})	0.01063(X_{11})	0.00862(X_7)
X_9	0.0633	0.05296	0.01973(X_3)	0.01971(X_{10})	0.01704(X_{13})
X_{10}	0.01826	0.00391	0.00676(X_{11})	0.00569(X_9)	0.00183(X_8)
X_{11}	-0.0719	-0.04321	0.01839(X_6)	0.01262(X_{13})	0.00719(X_9)
X_{12}	0.05173	0.10853	0.0223(X_{15})	0.0223(X_{16})	0.0187(X_{13})
X_{13}	0.03295	0.04473	0.01191(X_{12})	0.01102(X_6)	0.00887(X_9)
X_{14}	-0.06813	0.00693	0.0169(X_9)	0.01391(X_5)	0.01346(X_{13})
X_{15}	-0.11562	-0.24213	0.05289(X_7)	0.01467(X_8)	0.00593(X_{10})
X_{16}	-0.0442	-0.11654	0.29823(X_9)	0.2101(X_5)	0.15829(X_6)

Residual = 0.28500

In order to comprehend indirect effect of independent variables to the dependent variable, path analysis was conducted (Table 7). From the study it was noted that information need of farmers on Seed availability of different crops(X_1) was substantiated through the variables crop disease management (X_2), Weather Information (X_5) and Agricultural machineries/implements (X_9). Among the different independent variables, it was noted variables X_9 had maximum times of substantial effects, followed by variables X_6 and $X_{13.}$ The residual is only 0.285, it implied that, the sixteen variables altogether explained around 71 per cent of relationship. As the variables X_9 had maximum times of substantial effects, so, whatever, the information need of farmers were being assessed should considered in relation to the availability of agricultural machineries and implements.

Table 8: Result of stepwise multiple regression on decision making of farmers to three important areas of crop information need

R	R Square	Adjusted R Square
0.573[a]	0.328	0.324
0.594[b]	0.353	0.344
0.609[c]	0.371	0.359 #

a. Predictors: (Constant), X_1(Seed availability of different crops)
b. Predictors: (Constant), X_1, X_2(Crop disease management)
c. Predictors: (Constant), X_1, X_2 and X_5(Weather information)

While in natural science research it is not uncommon to get R square values as high as 0.99, a much lower value (0.10 – 0.20) of R square is acceptable in social science research (Gaur and Gaur, 2006).

Result of the Stepwise Multiple Regression reveals that variables X_1, X_2 and X_5 had explained 35.90 per cent of the variance of the dependent variable decision making. R-value i.e. *multivariate equivalent* indicates the strong relationship between the combination of independent variables (X_1, X_2 and X_5) and the dependent variable (Decision Making). Results also showed that variable X_1 was the best single predictor of job satisfaction.

Table 9: Farmers' perception on value of information

Sl.No.	Information need		Weighted Mean	SD
1.	Seeds Availability		4.45	0.758
2.	Seed treatment		4.16	0.958
3.	Soil testing		3.33	0.958
4.	Fertiliser availability		3.66	0.758
5.	Fertilizer application methods		2.56	0.678
6.	Knowledge about pest(i.e. identifying insect pests, disease symptoms, identifying weeds)		3.26	0.996
7.	Knowledge about pesticide application		4.23	0.935
8.	Pesticide availability	Insecticide	3.78	0.844
		Fungicide	3.56	0.853
		Herbicide/weedicide	2.89	0.634
9.	Application of pesticide	Insecticide	3.60	0.621
		Fungicide	3.80	0.406
		Herbicide/weedicide	2.53	0.776
10.	Farm Machinery	Tillage implements	3.80	0.406
		Sprayer availability	4.13	0.436
		Weed control	3.56	0.319
		Harvesting implements	3.20	0.484
11.	Weather information		4.43	0.859

Farmers need different types of information for their better agricultural activities, however, they do not value all information equally. Keeping this in mind, an assessment was made through this study to know, how the farmers valued each type of information. To assess this, five point Likert Scale was used. It was noted from the study, farmers valued more to the information on Seeds Availability(4.45), Weather information(4.43), Knowledge about pesticide application (4.23), Seed treatment(4.16), Sprayer availability(4.13) and remaining are as shown in table 9.

Table 10: Specific Information needed by farmers for insect pest and plant disease management

n=120

Sl.No.	Specific Information Need of farmers	Weighted Mean	Rank
1.	Need information on insect pest management of		
	a) Wheat (Aphid)	3.76	V
	b) Maize (Stem borer)	3.89	IV
	c) Vegetables (fruit borer)	4.86	I
	d) Pulses (pod borer)	4.12	III
	e) Oilseeds (Aphid)	4.43	II
2.	Need information on Disease management of		
	a) Wheat (leaf blight and spot blotch disease)	3.87	V
	b) Maize (Turcicum leaf blight)	3.79	II
	c) Vegetables (wilt and leaf spot)	4.26	IV
	d) Pulses (Wilt disease)	4.76	I
	e) Oilseeds (Wilt disease)	4.12	III
3.	Need advisory on seed treatment of		
	a) Wheat	4.67	I
	b) Maize	3.89	IV
	c) Vegetables	4.21	III
	d) Pulses	4.53	II
	e) Oilseeds	3.76	V

Farmers specific information need on insect pest and disease management was assessed. It was noted that farmers need information specifically on control measure of fruit borers of vegetables (rank I), followed by Aphids of Oilseeds (Rank II), pod borer of pulses(Rank III). They also need information to control diseases on wilt of pulses(Rank I), Turcicum leaf blight of maize(Rank II) and wilt disease of oilseeds(Rank III). The respondents also need information on seed treatments of different crops(Table 10).

Table 11: ICT tools usage by farmers

n=120

Sl.No.	ICT tools	*f**	Per cent
1.	Whatsapp Group	70	58.33
2.	Mobile SMS	95	79.17
3.	Bihar Krishi Apps(Mobile Apps)	54	45.00
4.	Video Screening through LCD Projectors	110	91.67
5.	Video Screening from Youtube (Social Media)	58	48.33
6.	Attending farmers personal phone call	40	33.33
7.	E-leaflet	55	45.83

*Multiple response

Due to the progress of Information and Communication Technology(ICT) and high penetration of mobile technology and mobile network in rural areas, the farmers are using number of ICT tools. Farmers ICT tool usage was assessed. From the study, it was noted that farmers used number of ICT tools – Mobile SMS(79.17%), WhatsApp(58.33%), Bihar Krishi Apps(45.00%), Youtube (48.33%) and remaining as shown in table 11.

Conclusion

From the study it is concluded that the most of the farmers belonged to middle age group with farming experiences more than ten years. So, these farmers should be continuously strengthen in use of ICT through; as there is a limited chance of leaving the farming by them as they are doing farming more than ten years. Among the different sources of information to the farmers, the major sources of information were Progressive farmers, Input Dealers and Neighbor farmers. Bihar Krishi Apps popularity is increasing among the farmers. Different extension personnel should be trained in use of ICT tools for plant health management. However, to reduce the cost of training extension personnel should be trained in altogether viz. Assistant Technical Manager & Block Technological Manager, Agril. Coordinator, Input Dealers, Kisan Salahkar and, Locatlite extension personnel viz. progressive farmers. Major broad areas of information need of the farmers related to plant health management and other agronomic practices were Seed availability, Insect Pest and disease management, Weed management (wheat) and Weather information. Farmers' decision making is positively and significantly correlated with Seed availability, insect pest and disease pest management. The information need of farmers were being assessed should considered in relation to the availability of agricultural machineries and implements as this variable have maximum times of substantial effect to other variables as indirect effect. Farmers specific information need are control measure of fruit borers of vegetables, Aphids of Oilseeds, Pod borer of pulses, wilt of pulses, Turcicum leaf blight of maize, and wilt disease of oilseeds. It was also noted that farmers use ICT tools of Mobile SMS, WhatsApp, Bihar Krishi Apps and Youtube.

References

Dinham B (2003) Growing Vegetables in Developing Countries for Local Urban Populations and Export Markets: Problems Confronting Small-Scale Producers. *Pest Manag. Sci.*, 59(5): 575–582.

Gaur AS, Gaur, Sanjaya S (2006) Statistical Methods for Practice and Research – A Guide to Data Analysis Using SPSS, New Delhi: Response Books, A Division of Sage Publications India Pvt. Ltd.

National Sample Survey Organisation (2005) Situation Assessment Survey of Farmers: Access to Modern Technology for Farming. Ministry of Statistics and Programme Implementation Government of India, Report No. 499(59/33/2).

Sharifzadeh MS, Abdollahzadeh G, Damalas CA, Rezaei R (2018) Farmers' Criteria for Pesticide Selection and Use in the Pest Control Process. *Agriculture,* 8: 24.

FSC
www.fsc.org
MIX
Papier | Fördert gute Waldnutzung
FSC® C083411

Zeitfracht Medien GmbH
Ferdinand-Jühlke-Straße 7
99095 Erfurt, Deutschland
produktsicherheit@kolibri360.de